Navigating Melanoma Treatment Challenges

This book delves into the complexities of melanoma, offering an in-depth examination of the disease alongside the latest advancements in diagnosis and treatment. The initial chapter provides a comprehensive overview of melanoma, covering its fundamentals and introducing the latest technologies shaping the understanding of the disease. The book introduces advanced molecular diagnostics in identifying targetable mutations and tailoring therapies for personalized and effective melanoma treatment. Additionally, it investigates the role of artificial intelligence in melanoma diagnostics and the advancements in imaging technologies for the monitoring and assessment of melanoma. It also reviews novel, innovative immunotherapeutic approaches designed to enhance the body's immune response against melanoma cells. Further, the book delves into the development and application of targeted therapies and nanomedicine in treating melanoma. A dedicated chapter highlights the advantages of a multi-omics approach, integrating genomic, proteomic, and other omics data to achieve a holistic understanding of melanoma. Toward the end, the book examines the potential of combination therapies to improve treatment outcomes in melanoma. The book is a valuable source for cancer researchers, medical oncologists, and clinicians.

Navigating Melanoma Treatment Challenges

Next-Generation Strategies and Solutions

Edited by

Zodwa Dlamini

CRC Press
Taylor & Francis Group
Boca Raton London New York

CRC Press is an imprint of the
Taylor & Francis Group, an **informa** business

Designed cover image: Zodwa Dlamini

First edition published 2025
by CRC Press
2385 NW Executive Center Drive, Suite 320, Boca Raton, FL 33431

and by CRC Press
4 Park Square, Milton Park, Abingdon, Oxon, OX14 4RN

CRC Press is an imprint of Taylor & Francis Group, LLC

ISBN: 978-1-032-84193-9 (hbk)
ISBN: 978-1-032-84194-6 (pbk)
ISBN: 978-1-003-51162-5 (ebk)

DOI: 10.1201/9781003511625

Typeset in Times
by KnowledgeWorks Global Ltd.

Contents

Editor

Zodwa Dlamini is a Professor of Molecular Oncology and the founding Director and the Executive Head of the Pan African Cancer Research Institute (PACRI) in South Africa. She is the Director of the South African Medical Research Council (SAMRC) Precision Oncology Research Unit (PORU). She is the DSTI/NRF SARChI Chair in Precision Oncology and Cancer Prevention (POCP). She is a member of the American Association for Cancer Research (AACR) Advisory Group on Sub-Saharan Africa. She is a member of the AACR Pathology Resources in Africa Advisory Group. Professor Dlamini is a member of the African Organisation for Research and Training in Cancer (AORTIC) Research Committee Scientific Advisory Board. She is an elected member of the Academy of Science of South Africa. Professor Dlamini is an overseas Fellow of the Royal Society of Medicine (London) and a member of the New York Academy of Sciences.

Contributors

Mohammed Alaouna
SAMRC Precision Oncology Research Unit (PORU)
DSTI/NRF SARChI Chair in Precision Oncology and Cancer Prevention (POCP)
Pan African Cancer Research Institute (PACRI)
University of Pretoria
Pretoria, South Africa

Onyemaechi O. Azu
Department of Medical Biosciences
University of the Western Cape Bellville
Cape Town, South Africa

Jyotsna Batra
Faculty of Health
Centre for Genomics and Personalized Health
Translational Research Institute
School of Biomedical Sciences
Queensland University of Technology
Brisbane, Australia

Cebo Beja
Department of Surgery
Steve Biko Academic Hospital
Faculty of Health Sciences
University of Pretoria
Pretoria, South Africa

Carmen Besliu
Fortrea Inc.
Durham, North Carolina, USA

Meshack Bida
Department of Anatomical Pathology
National Health Laboratory Service
University of Pretoria
Pretoria, South Africa

Nkhensani Chauke-Malinga
SAMRC Precision Oncology Research Unit (PORU)
DSTI/NRF SARChI Chair in Precision Oncology and Cancer Prevention (POCP)
Pan African Cancer Research Institute (PACRI)
University of Pretoria
Pretoria, South Africa

Ian C. Chikanza
International Arthritis & Hypermobility Center
London, UK
and
Faculty of Medicine
Catholic University
and
Department of Pediatrics & Child Health
University of Zimbabwe
Harare, Zimbabwe

Talent Chipiti
SAMRC Precision Oncology Research Unit (PORU)
DSTI/NRF SARChI Chair in Precision Oncology and Cancer Prevention (POCP)
Pan African Cancer Research Institute (PACRI)
University of Pretoria, Faculty of Health Sciences
Pretoria, South Africa

Paulina Czajka-Francuz
Fortrea Inc.
Durham, North Carolina, USA

Botle Precious Damane
Department of Surgery
Faculty of Health Sciences
Steve Biko Academic Hospital
University of Pretoria
Pretoria, South Africa

Ashokkumar Deenabandu
Fortrea Inc.
Durham, North Carolina, USA

Demetra Demetriou
SAMRC Precision Oncology Research Unit (PORU)
DSTI/NRF SARChI Chair in Precision Oncology and Cancer Prevention (POCP)
Pan African Cancer Research Institute (PACRI)
University of Pretoria
Pretoria, South Africa

Dineo Disenyane
Division of Anatomical Pathology
National Health Laboratory Service
University of Pretoria
Pretoria, South Africa

Zodwa Dlamini
SAMRC Precision Oncology Research Unit (PORU)
DSTI/NRF SARChI Chair in Precision Oncology and Cancer Prevention (POCP)
Pan African Cancer Research Institute (PACRI)
University of Pretoria
Pretoria, South Africa

Innocent Edagha
Department of Human Anatomy
School of Medicine
Moi University
Eldoret, Kenya

Jose Espinoza
Fortrea Inc.
Durham, North Carolina, USA

Olalekan Fadebi
SAMRC Precision Oncology Research Unit (PORU)
DSTI/NRF SARChI Chair in Precision Oncology and Cancer Prevention (POCP)
Pan African Cancer Research Institute (PACRI)
Department of Medical Oncology
Faculty of Health Sciences
Steve Biko Academic Hospital
University of Pretoria
Pretoria, South Africa

Rodney Hull
SAMRC Precision Oncology Research Unit (PORU)
DSTI/NRF SARChI Chair in Precision Oncology and Cancer Prevention (POCP)
Pan African Cancer Research Institute (PACRI)
University of Pretoria
Pretoria, South Africa

Mark Jose
Life Fourways Hospital
Sandton, South Africa

Mahlatse Kgokolo
Department of Dermatology
University of Pretoria
Pretoria, South Africa

Richard Khanyile
Department of Medical Oncology
Faculty of Health Sciences
Steve Biko Academic Hospital
University of Pretoria
Pretoria, South Africa

Elisa Marie Ledet
Tulane Cancer Center's Prostate Cancer Biorepository
Tulane Cancer Center
Tulane University
New Orleans, Louisiana, USA

Georgios Lolas
SAMRC Precision Oncology Research Unit (PORU)
DSTI/NRF SARChI Chair in Precision Oncology and Cancer Prevention (POCP)
Pan African Cancer Research Institute (PACRI)
University of Pretoria
Pretoria, South Africa
and
Research Unit of Advanced Composite Nano-Materials and Nanotechnology School of Chemical Engineering
National Technical University of Athens
and
University of Athens
Athens, Greece

Thifhelimbilu Emmanuel Luvhengo
Department of Surgery
University of the Witwatersrand
Johannesburg, South Africa

Lloyd Mabonga
Pan African Cancer Research Institute (PACRI)
Department of Medical Oncology
University of Pretoria, Faculty of Health Sciences
Pretoria, South Africa

Anil Madaree
University of KwaZulu-Natal
Nelson R. Mandela School of Medicine Umbilo
Berea, Durban, South Africa

Stylianos Makrogkikas
Research Unit of Advanced Composite Nano-Materials and Nanotechnology
School of Chemical Engineering
National Technical University of Athens
Zografos, Athens, Greece

Tania Maphoso
Department of Surgery
Steve Biko Academic Hospital
Faculty of Health Sciences
University of Pretoria
Pretoria, South Africa

Rahaba Marima
SAMRC Precision Oncology Research Unit (PORU)
DSTI/NRF SARChI Chair in Precision Oncology and Cancer Prevention (POCP)
Pan African Cancer Research Institute (PACRI)
University of Pretoria
Pretoria, South Africa

Tebogo Marutha
SAMRC Precision Oncology Research Unit (PORU)
DSTI/NRF SARChI Chair in Precision Oncology and Cancer Prevention (POCP)
Pan African Cancer Research Institute (PACRI)
University of Pretoria
Pretoria, South Africa

Sikhumbuzo Z. Mbatha
Department of Surgery
Steve Biko Academic Hospital
University of Pretoria
Pretoria, South Africa

Zukile Mbita
Department of Biochemistry Microbiology and Biochemistry
University of Limpopo
Sovenga, South Africa

Langanani Mbodi
Department of Obstetrics and Gynecology, Gynecologic Oncology Unit
University of the Witwatersrand
Parktown, South Africa

Michelle McCabe
Division of Anatomical Pathology
National Health Laboratory Service
University of Pretoria
Pretoria, South Africa

Sandra McGuigan
Fortrea Inc.
Durham, North Carolina, USA

Ravi Mehrotra
SAMRC Precision Oncology Research Unit (PORU)
DSTI/NRF SARChI Chair in Precision Oncology and Cancer Prevention (POCP)
Pan African Cancer Research Institute (PACRI)
University of Pretoria
Pretoria, South Africa
and
Indian Cancer Genome Atlas Bhageerath
Pune, Maharashtra, India
and
Centre for Health Innovation and Policy (CHIP) Foundation
Noida, Uttar Pradesh, India

Thabiso Victor Miya
SAMRC Precision Oncology Research Unit (PORU)
DSTI/NRF SARChI Chair in Precision Oncology and Cancer Prevention (POCP)
Pan African Cancer Research Institute (PACRI)
University of Pretoria
Pretoria, South Africa

Thulo Molefi
Department of Medical Oncology
Faculty of Health Sciences
Steve Biko Academic Hospital
University of Pretoria
Pretoria, South Africa

Benny Mosoane
Department of Anatomical Pathology
National Health Laboratory Services
Tshwane Academic Division
Faculty of Health Sciences
University of Pretoria
Pretoria, South Africa

Thanyani Mulaudzi
Department of Surgery
Steve Biko Academic Hospital
Faculty of Health Sciences
University of Pretoria
Pretoria, South Africa

Thendo Netshiongolwe
Department of Plastic and Reconstructive Surgery
Faculty of Health Sciences
Steve Biko Academic Hospital
University of Pretoria
Pretoria, South Africa

Lesedi Nevondo
Department of Anatomical Pathology
National Health Laboratory Services
Tshwane Academic Division
Faculty of Health Sciences
University of Pretoria
Pretoria, South Africa

Edward Ngwenya
ARWYP Medical Centre
Kempton Park, South Africa

Paulo Nunes
Fortrea Inc.
Durham, North Carolina, USA

Dakalo Ramali
Department of Surgery
Steve
Biko Academic Hospital
Faculty of Health Sciences
University of Pretoria
Pretoria, South Africa

Kamal S. Saini
Fortrea Inc.
Durham, North Carolina, USA
and
Addenbrooke's Hospital
Cambridge University Hospitals NHS Foundation Trust
Cambridge, UK

Daniel Sambili
Department of Plastic and Reconstructive Surgery
Faculty of Health Sciences
Steve Biko Academic Hospital
University of Pretoria
Pretoria, South Africa

Shobana Sampath
Department of Biotechnology
Vel Tech Rangarajan Dr. Sagunthala R&D Institute of Science and Technology
Avadi, Chennai, India

Philemon Ubanako
Department of Internal Medicine
School of Clinical Medicine
Faculty of Health Sciences
University of the Witwatersrand
Parktown, South Africa

Richard C. Wu
Division of Medical Oncology
The Ohio State University James Comprehensive Cancer Center
Columbus, Ohio, USA

1 Understanding Melanoma
From Basics to Cutting-Edge Insights

Zodwa Dlamini and Rodney Hull
SAMRC Precision Oncology Research Unit (PORU), DSTI/NRF SARChI Chair in Precision Oncology and Cancer Prevention (POCP), Pan African Cancer Research Institute (PACRI), University of Pretoria, Pretoria, South Africa

Thulo Molefi and Richard E. Khanyile
Faculty of Health Sciences, Steve Biko Academic Hospital, University of Pretoria, Pretoria, South Africa

Langanani Mbodi
University of the Witwatersrand, Parktown, South Africa

Thifhelimbilu Emmanuel Luvhengo
University of the Witwatersrand, Johannesburg, South Africa

Ian C. Chikanza
International Arthritis & Hypermobility Center, Harley Street Clinic, London, UK
Faculty of Medicine, Catholic University, Harare, Zimbabwe
University of Zimbabwe, Harare, Zimbabwe

INTRODUCTION

Melanoma develops as the result of several genetic mutations, notably in the *btaf, nras, c=kt, kras,cdkn2a,* and *gnaq/gna11* genes, which affect critical signaling pathways, with ultraviolet (UV) radiation often acting as a mutagenic risk factor (Kim and Kim, 2024). Understanding the molecular signaling pathways of different types of melanomas will allow better characterization and provide tools for the development of targeted therapies.

The most lethal type of skin cancer is malignant melanoma, which accounts for less than 5% of all skin cancers (Erdei and Torres, 2010). This lethality is due to its aggressive nature, which can result in early metastasis. This limits the use of surgical resection as an effective treatment in many cases (Califano and Nance, 2009). Melanoma is characterized by the uncontrolled proliferation of melanocytes, the melanin-producing cells that are located in the bottom layer of the epidermis (Abdel-Malek et al., 1995). Melanocytes are capable of expressing many signaling molecules since they originate from the neural crest. The development and progression of melanoma are promoted

DOI: 10.1201/9781003511625-1

by the increase in migration and metastasis, promoted by the perturbation of these signaling molecules and pathways (Saginala et al., 2021). For instance, the PI3K-AKT signaling cascades are upregulated in melanoma, while dysregulation of the MAPK pathway is associated with sustained ERK activity, which leads to uncontrolled melanocyte proliferation, increased survival, invasion, metastasis, and the promotion of angiogenesis (Juszczak et al., 2022).

The microphthalmia-associated transcription factor (MITF), which regulates the development and survival of melanocytes, also exhibits oncogenic propensity in 20% of melanomas. The altered function of proteins that interact with MITF also plays a role. For instance, MAPK activates MITF and ERK, while BRAF can enhance the expression of MITF (Wellbrock and Arozarena, 2015). About 10–15% of melanomas show *braf* mutation and increased MITF expression (Castellani et al., 2023). The nuclear factor-kappa B (NFκB) regulates several genes involved in immune and inflammatory reactions and the development of neoplastic disorders and their progression. Classically, the NFκB pathway is activated by TNF, IL-1β, and Toll-like receptor (TLR) signaling. It can also be activated by perturbed MAPK and PI3K-AKT signaling in melanoma, leading to enhanced cell proliferation and cell survival by inducing resistance to apoptosis (Ueda and Richmond, 2006).

Melanoma places a large burden on the public health systems of countries worldwide. This is demonstrated by the 288% increase in the cost of treating melanoma in the United States over the ten years between 2010 and 2020. As such, many programs have been instituted in various countries aimed at preventing melanoma. These prevention programs normally consist of trying to encourage responsible sunbathing and outdoor behavior, such as avoiding extended periods of exposure of the bare skin to sunlight or the use of sunscreen. Alongside prevention, new technologies and strategies are being developed to increase the efficiency of melanoma diagnosis and treatment. This chapter serves as an introduction to melanoma, its subtypes, classes, and epidemiology. The chapter then reviews current and future methods for melanoma diagnosis as well as current and new strategies for melanoma treatment.

EPIDEMIOLOGY OF MELANOMA

The incidence of melanoma has increased in the past 50 years at a rate higher than any other type of cancer (Bray et al., 2024; Guy et al., 2015; Rigel and Carucci, 2000). This is especially true in areas or countries where the population is predominantly light-skinned, as this is a major risk factor for most types of melanomas (Sung et al., 2021). As such, there are geographic variations in the incidence of melanoma, which is influenced by the population's genetic background, the clinical phenotype of the population, and the environment, i.e., UV radiation exposure (Jhappan et al., 2003). Fair-skinned people are more prone to developing the disease, especially those with red hair and light eyes. Unlike other cancers, melanoma normally affects younger or middle-aged individuals (Siegel et al., 2020). UV radiation is a major contributor to melanoma genesis as it damages both the skin and the DNA in cutaneous melanocytes (Sample and He, 2018). Apart from exposure to the sun, this damage can result from UV-A rays from artificial sources (D'orazio et al., 2013). Apart from skin color, other risk factors include the presence and number of benign moles present on an individual's skin. Genetic effects play a role, and as such, a family history of melanoma acts as an important risk factor (Bevona et al., 2003).

In 2022, there were a recorded 187,952 new cases of melanoma with 121,388 melanoma-related deaths. Cancer is more common in males than females (Bray et al., 2024). Men of European ancestry with light skin have an incidence (per 100,000) of melanoma of 34.7 compared to 22.1 for females of European ancestry. Among men of African ancestry, the incidence (per 100,000) is 1.0, compared to 0.9 for females of African ancestry (Saginala et al., 2021). Currently, the mortality rate is approximately 1 in 4 or 25% of all cases (Rastrelli et al., 2014), accounting for 80% of deaths related to skin cancer while only accounting for only 1% of skin cancers (Saginala et al., 2021). The number of melanoma-related deaths in 2022 was 58,667, according to GLOBOCAN (Bray et al., 2024).

The regional distribution of melanoma is indicated in **Figures 1.1A and C**, while the mortality distribution is indicated in **Figures 1.1B and C**. Australia and New Zealand have the highest number of cases and the highest number of deaths. Despite the high incidence in specific high-income countries, especially in Europe and North America, having a high incidence rate, the mortality rates in these regions are relatively low compared to those in Africa and Latin America.

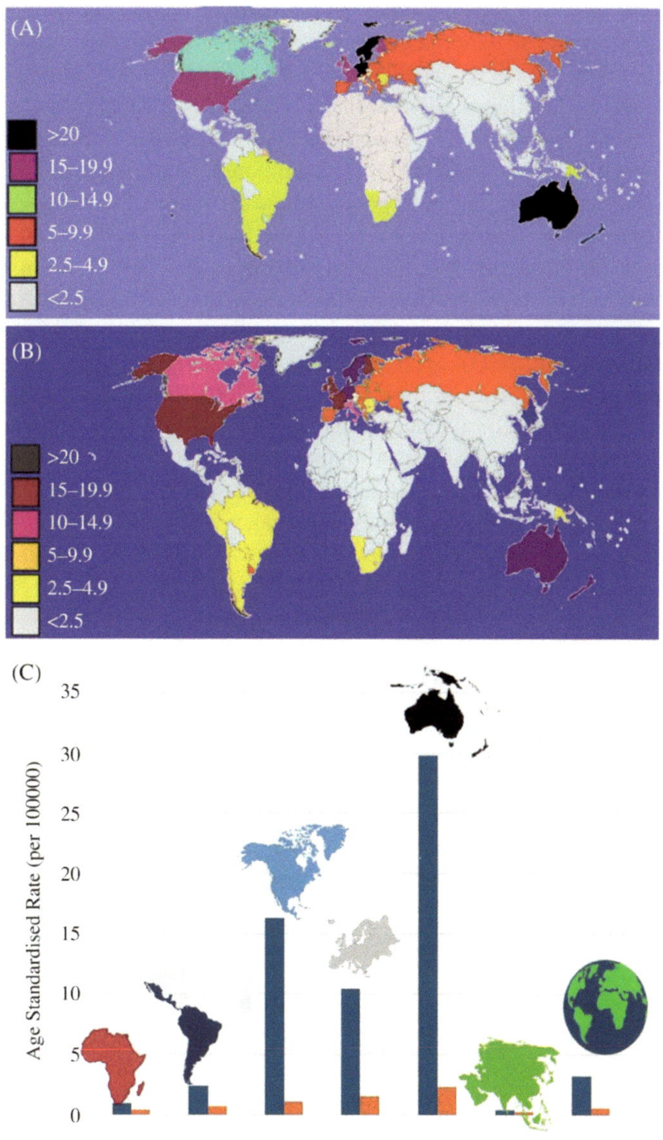

FIGURE 1.1 **Incidence and mortality rates for melanoma in various regions of the world.** (A) The incidence rates (age-standardized incidence rate per 1000,000) across the world. The highest incidence rates are found in Australia and New Zealand as well as in the Scandinavian countries. This is followed by the US and various countries in Western and Central Europe. (B) The mortality rates (age-standardized incidence rate per 1000,000) show that those countries with the highest incidence rate have equivalently high mortality rates. (C) The age-standardized incidence rates by region show once again that Oceania has the highest incidence rates, followed by North America and then Europe. This is due to both Canada and the US having relatively high incidence rates, while many European countries have fairly low incidence rates to offset those high rates in the Scandinavian countries.

CHARACTERISTICS OF MELANOMA

Different clinical types of melanomas differ from each other based on their presentation, causes, and outcomes (**Table 1.1**). The most common type of skin (cutaneous) melanoma is superficial spreading melanoma. It starts on the skin surface in a preexisting mole or as a new lesion. It spreads outward but at later stages invades the lower layers of the skin (Apostu et al., 2023; Greenwald et al., 2012). The next most common type of melanoma is nodular melanoma, which starts as a raised bump or nodule. This type of melanoma grows rapidly, penetrates deeper into the skin layers, and is normally only diagnosed at the later stages with a resulting poorer outcome (Greenwald et al., 2012). This is followed by Lentigo malignant melanoma (LMM), which requires the presence of a precancerous condition of the top skin layer and becomes LMM when this cancer spreads to deeper skin layers. Its slow growth rate means that it is commonly diagnosed timeously and has a more favorable outcome (Kallini et al., 2013). In contrast to other types of melanomas, acral lentiginous melanoma occurs on sections of skin that are not normally exposed to direct sunlight. As such, sun exposure is not a risk factor for this type. It is an aggressive melanoma and quickly penetrates the deeper layers of the skin. This type is relatively rare but is diagnosed more commonly in people with darker skin, being the most common type of melanoma diagnosed in people of African American and Asian descent (Bian et al., 2021).

Desmoplastic melanoma appears as a pink or skin-colored lump that can resemble scar tissue or a skin lesion, normally found on the head or neck. This is a rare type of melanoma that is often unpigmented and, as such, can be difficult to notice or diagnose (Huayllani et al., 2019). Similar to desmoplastic melanoma, amelanotic melanoma does not express melanin and therefore appears skin-colored with slightly defined edges. This also makes it difficult to diagnose and often goes unnoticed (Karmilkar and Norem, 2023). Nevoid melanomas resemble benign moles and as such are difficult to diagnose, and they are also rare (Martín-Alcalde et al., 2021). A benign skin lesion is known as a spitz nevus, and this is the reason that spitzoid melanoma is given its name. This melanoma resembles a round lump that is red or dark in color. It is a rare melanoma that normally appears on the head, arms, or legs. They progress rapidly, and although they commonly spread to the lymph nodes, they do not normally result in distant metastasis (Chacón et al., 2020). Eye or ocular melanoma occurs on the uvea, the middle layer of the eye. In some cases, it can also originate in the conjunctiva, the tissue covering the white of the eye. The melanoma appears as a growing spot on the eye (iris), or it can cause changes to the shape of the pupil. The disease is rare, and the most common symptoms include blurred vision, the development of a blind spot, seeing flashing lights, and increased sensitivity to sunlight (Jager et al., 2017).

Mucosal melanoma affects the mucus membranes, such as the nose, mouth, or vulva. It appears as a sore or discolored area. The symptoms experienced by the patient depend on where the tumor arises. This is a very rare condition. Mucosal melanoma is aggressive and has a poor prognosis. Like LMM, exposure to the sun is not a risk factor (Santeufemia et al., 2023). A specific type of mucosal melanoma is melanoma that originates in the female genital tract, affecting the vulva, vagina, cervix, and urethra. This type of melanoma is known as malignant melanoma of the female genital tract, and it is extremely rare, accounting for only 3% of all melanomas diagnosed in females and making up only 18% of all cases of mucosal melanoma (Mihajlovic et al., 2012). It is most commonly found in the vulva, making up 95% of the cases of this type of melanoma. This is followed by the vagina (3% of all cases) and the rest occurring in the urethra and cervix (Mihajlovic et al., 2012). The outcomes for this mucosal melanoma are poor, with the prognosis having a low overall 5-year survival rate that varies based on the tissue of origin. Overall survival numbers range from between 0% and 25% (Baloglu et al., 2009) to between 8% and 60% for vaginal melanoma (Vaysse et al., 2013). They are also difficult to treat and manage and are associated with distant metastasis (Baloglu et al., 2009). Their rarity means they are understudied and are difficult to diagnose, resulting in late diagnosis, which contributes to their poor outcome. This is exacerbated by the

TABLE 1.1
Clinical Types of Melanomas

Type of Melanoma	Risk Factors	Characteristics	References
Superficial spreading melanoma (SSM)	• Age • UV light • Personal and family history • Light skin tone • Atypical moles	• Torso of males and legs of females • Asymmetrical shape with a smudgy border • Variable color • Changes noticeably over time	Apostu et al. (2023)
Nodular melanoma (NM)	• Age • Males • Exposure to UV light • Light skin tone • Personal and family history	• Black, brown, or red skin color • Head or neck	Greenwald et al. (2012)
Lentigo malignant melanoma (LMM)	• Cumulative sun exposure • Females	• Commonly on the head or neck • Tan or brown spot • Abnormal shape • Slow growing	Kallini et al. (2013)
Acral lentiginous melanoma	• Genetic mutations	• Palms of the hands • Bottoms of the feet • Under fingernails • Light to dark brown • Ulceration occurs as the disease progresses	Bian et al. (2021)
Desmoplastic melanoma	• Lots of sun exposure • High mutation rate	• Head or neck, the torso, arms, and legs	Huayllani et al. (2019)
Amelanotic melanoma	• Advanced age • Exposure to UV light • Many benign moles • Atypical moles • Light skin hair and eyes • Weakened immune system	• Sun-exposed areas • Head, neck, torso, and legs	Karmilkar and Norem (2023)
Spitzoid melanoma	• Specific genetic mutations • Frequent in children and adolescents • More common in individuals older than 20 • Regional lymph node spread	• Round lump • Skin-colored, red, or dark in color • Head, arms, or legs	Chacón et al. (2020)
Eye melanoma	• Exposure to sunlight • Light eye color • Preexisting mole in the eye • Advanced age	• The middle layer of the eye • Growing spot on the eye • Change in the shape of the eye	Jager et al. (2017)
Mucosal melanoma	• Environmental toxins Areas in or near the mouth: dentures that don't fit properly/tobacco use • Area of the vulva or vaginal viral infections • Chronic inflammation • Area of the rectum or anus: HIV	• Sinuses • Mouth and throat • Genitals, urinary tract • Rectum and anus • The sore or discolored area	Santeufemia et al. (2023)
Melanoma of unknown primary	• Fair skin, light hair, and light eye color • Excessive sun exposure • Family history of melanoma • Certain genetic conditions • Weakened immune system • Previous diagnosis of skin cancers	• No or unknown primary site • Lymph nodes • Internal organs	Kamposioras et al. (2011)

lack of uniform protocols concerning their staging and treatment as well as their anatomic location (Mihajlovic et al., 2012).

Little progress has been made in the treatment of these tumors, with the survival rates remaining the same over the last few decades. Treatment often cannot be accomplished through surgical resection due to their late diagnosis and metastatic nature (Mihajlovic et al., 2012). Cytotoxic chemotherapy agents, such as cisplatin and other platinum-based compounds, are the main route of treatment. However, they have been shown to be largely unsuccessful (Yi et al., 2011). Currently, immunotherapy is the only promising treatment for melanoma of the female genital tract for the foreseeable future (Chanal et al., 2016).

A small fraction of melanomas does not have a known site of origin and are only diagnosed when the tumor is detected at a distant site. These are known as melanoma of unknown primary (MUP). The sites where it is identified include the lymph nodes and subcutaneous tissue, such as the internal organs. Depending on where the secondary site is will dictate the symptoms the patient experiences. This melanoma has more favorable outcomes than most other melanomas diagnosed at the same stage (Kamposioras et al., 2011).

Initially, the developing melanoma is known as a melanoma *in situ*. This is because it is confined to the outermost skin layer, or epidermis. At this stage (stage 0), there are no signs of spreading or metastasis. As the cancer progresses, it becomes thicker and increases in diameter. At this stage (stage I), the lesion may be classed as IA or IB based on whether the lesion has become ulcerated or if it has increased past 2 mm in size. However, the tumor is still localized. At stage II, the tumor further increases in diameter and thickness. At this stage, the tumor can be divided into IIA, IIB, or IIC based on thickness and its penetration into the epidermis. At stage III, the tumor has penetrated the dermis and spread to nearby lymph nodes. It has also spread to nearby areas of the skin. By stage IV, the tumor has metastasized to distant parts of the body, including distant areas of the skin, the lungs, and the central nervous system (**Figure 1.2**) (Kauffmann and Chen, 2014).

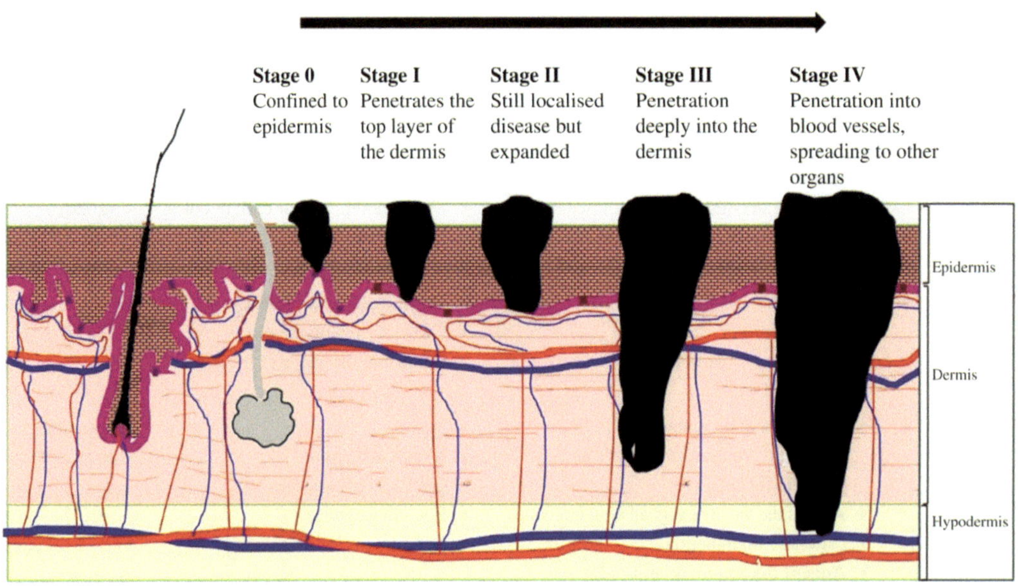

FIGURE 1.2 **Progression of melanoma.** The layers of the skin show that melanoma develops in the epidermis, initiating from the melanocytes in the layer between the epidermis and the dermis. As the disease progresses, it begins to penetrate the top layer of the dermis in stage I. By stage II, the tumor is still confined to the epidermis, but it expands in size. At stage III, the tumor penetrates deeper into the dermis, and by stage IV it reaches the blood vessel, allowing for the cancer to metastasize and spread.

Apart from the contribution of the gut microbiome to the development and progression of various cancers, melanoma, like other skin cancers, has a special relationship with the microbiome of the skin. Under normal conditions, this microbiome is dominated by Gram-positive bacteria, such as *Staphylococcus* and *Veillonella*. These bacteria play an important role in various processes, such as wound healing. Certain pathogenic bacteria on the skin surface, such as *Cutibacterium acnes*, *Staphylococcus vulgaris*, and *Staphylococcus aureus*, play important roles in the development of conditions, such as acne, psoriasis, diabetic foot ulcers, and lupus erythematosus. Non-melanoma skin cancer is characterized by an increase in the number of *S. aureus* species present (Madhusudhan et al., 2020). Skin swabs taken from 27 acral melanoma patients show this form of melanoma is associated with an increase in the number of *Corynebacteriu* species (Mizuhashi et al., 2021). This increase was more noticeable as the disease progressed to later stages. The presence of these bacteria promoted the growth of melanoma by stimulating the immune system to recruit IL-17-producing Th17 cells. IL-17 is known to promote melanoma growth (Chen and Gao, 2019).

MELANOMA IN SOUTH AFRICA

In South Africa, there has only been a slight increase in the number of recorded cases and the age-standardized rate of melanoma. This increase is seen in both males and females (**Figures 1.3A and C**), but it can be seen that the majority of this increase is seen in South Africans of European ancestry (**Figures 1.3B and D**). It has been reported that South Africans of African ancestry only have 10% of the number of cases of melanoma seen in South Africans of European ancestry (Norval and Wright, 2017). In South Africans of European ancestry, the incidence has continued to rise,

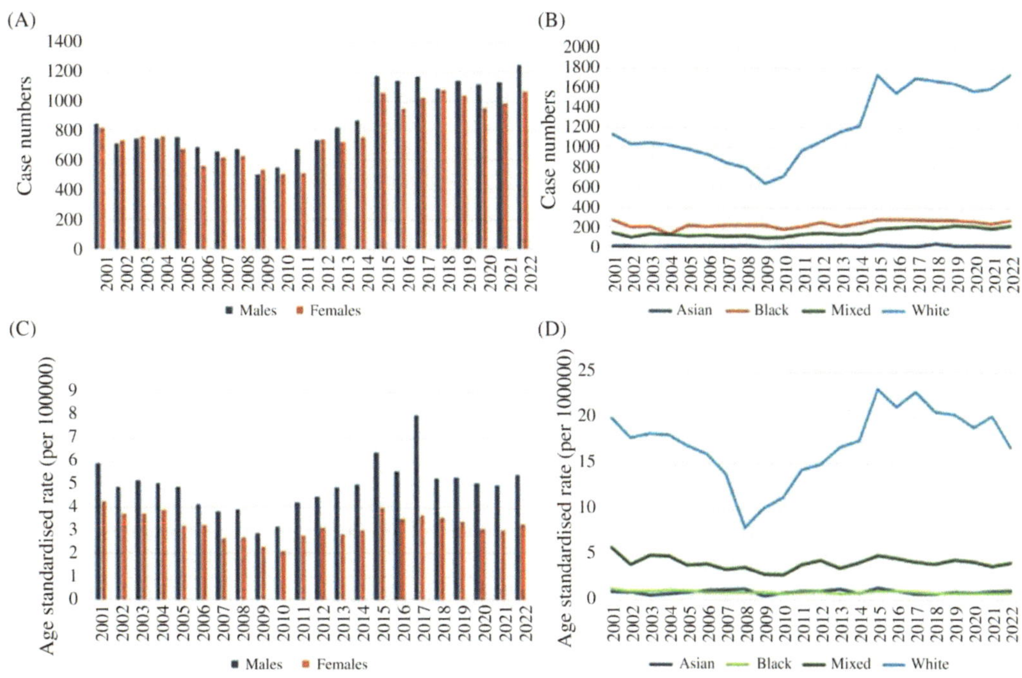

FIGURE 1.3 **Melanoma case number and age-standardized rates in South Africa (2001–2022).** (A) The case numbers for melanoma according to the South African national cancer registry from 2001–2022. (B) Case numbers by race show that the highest number of cases occurs in those of European ancestry, "white." (C) Age-standardized rate for melanoma in South Africa from 2001–2022. (D) Age-standardized rate for melanoma in South Africa from 2001–2022 per population group, once again shows the highest number of cases in South Africans of European ancestry.

while the same is not observed in South Africans of African ancestry (Norval and Wright, 2017). Superficial spreading melanoma is the most common type of melanoma observed in South Africa, where the age-standardized incidence and mortality rates are 4.1 and 1.3, respectively (Bray et al., 2024). However, people of African ancestry are normally diagnosed at later stages compared to individuals of European ancestry, and as such, the survival rates in patients of African ancestry are lower (Norval and Wright, 2017).

DIAGNOSIS OF MELANOMA

Proper treatment of melanoma requires accurate diagnosis as well as precise staging and classification of the disease. Early diagnosis is also important since it greatly increases the chance of a positive outcome, especially if the melanoma is diagnosed and treated when the tumor is less than a millimeter thick (Braun et al., 2004). Usually, a clinician will conduct a visual inspection of the skin or use a dermoscopy to capture images of a lesion. If the clinician judges these lesions to be cancerous, a biopsy can be taken for further examination (Argenziano and Soyer, 2001). Visual inspection to diagnose melanoma uses the ABCD rule. Visual inspection examines characteristics of the visual appearance of the skin lesion. These characteristics include asymmetric appearance, border irregularity, color variegation, and the size of the tumor judged by its diameter (Balch et al., 2001). The most basic diagnostic tool following visual inspection by a medical professional is the use of total-body photography (TBP). This can be used to monitor changes in the appearance and number of moles or skin lesions (Tiersten et al., 1991). It has been estimated that 20 years ago, up to 35% of melanomas that were diagnosed prospectively were done so using changes in the appearance of skin lesions (Kelly et al., 1997). Recently, there has been interest in shifting from a two-dimensional TBP protocol to a three-dimensional one involving the use of a three-dimensional representation of the entire cutaneous surface of the patient's body and are especially useful for areas of the body where the body contours decrease skin surface resolution (Rayner et al., 2018).

Dermoscopy

Dermoscopy is an *in vivo* method for the early diagnosis of melanoma and the differential diagnosis of pigmented lesions of the skin. It has been shown to increase diagnostic accuracy over clinical visual inspection in the hands of experienced physicians(Pehamberger et al., 1993). Dermoscopy is also known as epiluminescence microscopy or amplified surface microscopy (Braun et al., 2005). The device itself is a binocular microscope with a built-in light source (Soyer et al., 2001). The differences between the appearance of the skin and the lesion change the reflection, dispersal, or absorption of the light. This is due to changes in the stratum corneum (Anderson and Parrish, 1981). Various immersion liquids can render the skin translucent, allowing for the partial visualization of underlying structures. As such, dermoscopy uses the same visual diagnostic criteria (ABCD) (Anderson and Parrish, 1981; Soyer et al., 2001). Handheld dermoscopy results can be further tracked and confirmed through the use of a record of images using digital dermoscopy to image analyses and store images of the skin lesions (Stanganelli et al., 2015). Ultrasound can also be used to identify and analyze melanocytic lesions, where they appear as echolucent regions. However, it does not give enough information to be used as a diagnostic tool that can be used to monitor disease progression (Blum et al., 2006).

Reflectance Confocal Microscopy

Over the last few decades, the imaging of melanoma for diagnosis and management has advanced dramatically. One of these advancements includes reflectance confocal microscopy (RCM), which uses confocal microscopy to highlight a single point in the skin and magnify it to a single-cell resolution. Visual information obtained from RCM is able to differentiate between benign skin lesions, keratinocyte carcinoma, and melanoma due to differences in chemical and molecular structures in these skin lesions (Witkowski et al., 2017). This procedure is performed *in vivo*, can be performed rapidly, is painless, and has been reported to have a high degree of accuracy (Guitera et al., 2010). Fluorescence confocal microscopy can be used in a similar way to RCM; however, the contrast can be improved through the use of various fluorescent dyes. These include dyes, such as fluorescein, toluidine blue, methylene blue, or Yaroslavsky stains (Busam et al., 2001; Yaroslavsky et al., 2007).

Another advanced imaging procedure is known as multispectral imaging. This procedure involves taking sequential images at different wavelengths. These different wavelengths have different abilities when it comes to penetrating the skin, with some penetrating to a greater depth than others. Depending on this penetration, the different images taken at different wavelengths can give information concerning collagen distribution, melanin levels, and blood vessel density and distribution. These characteristics can be used to diagnose and stratify skin lesions (Marghoob et al., 2007). Artificial intelligence (AI) has also been developed to analyze spectral images, and the resulting artificial neural network has been shown to be capable of coming to the same conclusion as clinicians, with higher sensitivity and specificity (Carrara et al., 2007; Yaroslavsky et al., 2007). Technologies combining spectral imaging and confocal microscopy have also been developed. Spectrally encoded confocal microscopy (SECM) uses white light to scan various points in a line. The resulting scans are analyzed using a spectral filter, and the data generated through this method is converted to separate points with both spatial and resolution data. SECM has the advantage over other line scanning imaging procedures due to the improved contrast it provides (Boudoux et al., 2005).

Positron emission tomography with computed tomography (PET/CT) can be used in melanoma diagnosis, assessment, and monitoring. Using ^{18}F-Fluorodeoxyglucose, skin lesions with altered glucose metabolism can be identified while still providing an indication of anatomic changes like CT and magnetic resonance imaging (MRI) scans (Sachpekidis et al., 2018; Vensby et al., 2017). FDG PET/CT is also useful in identifying all sites of metastasis in order to properly design a treatment plan (Wong et al., 2017).

Histology and Molecular Diagnostics Aspects in Melanoma

Biopsy and histologic examination are the final steps in the diagnosis of melanoma. Following the identification of a skin lesion as a potential malignant tumor, tissue sampling can be performed followed by histopathological examination. Advances have been made in the collection of the biopsy. The main advancement has been the development of micro-punch technique, or fine needle aspiration biopsy (FNAB). This allows for the sampling of a precise area of the tumor that can correspond to a section defined by a dermoscopy image. These biopsies can be guided by CT imaging (Mágori, 2003). Histopathology relies on the recognition of patterns to classify a lesion as melanocytic or not. It can also assess the color of the lesion, especially the presence of steel-blue areas, which defines it as a blue nevus or melanocytic nevus. The lesion can further be judged by border shape, the presence of red patches, and the presence of arborizing telangiectasias or spoke-like structures. The presence of these changes identifies the lesion as not being a melanoma (Gheoca Mutu et al., 2022). The lesion is benign or malignant and can be judged using other criteria known as Color, Architectural order, Symmetry of pattern, and Homogeneity (CASH). Malignant lesions contain multiple colors, are asymmetric, and appear disordered and heterogeneous (Gheoca Mutu et al., 2022).

Ultimately, the histopathological criteria are integrated with the clinical features. These criteria may be subject to interobserver variability, especially in nonconventional lesions. The World Health Organization (WHO) has therefore added the assessment of known aberrations in molecular pathways in melanoma cells from different types of melanomas to the diagnostic pathways and also introduced the concept of "intermediate" lesions. The WHO 2018 criteria now has nine categories/pathways that lead to the diagnosis of melanoma, each with specific genetic markers (**Table 1.2**) (Elder et al., 2020).

TABLE 1.2
Melanoma Classification

UV Exposure	Category	Melanoma Subtype	Key Molecular Genes	
Low UV/CSD	I	Superficial Spreading Melanoma	BRAFV600 mut CDKN2A mut NRAS mut	TERT mut PTEN mut TP53 mut
High UV/CSD	II	Lentigo maligna melanoma	NRAS mut BRAFnon-V600E mut KIT mut TERT mut	CDKN2A mut PTEN mut TP53 mut
	III	Desmoplastic melanoma	NF1 mut NFKBIE mut	NRAS mut PIK3CA mut
Low or no UV/CSD	IV	Spitz melanoma	ALK rearr NTRK1 rearr NRTK3 rearr	CDKN2A mut HRAS mut
	V	Acral melanoma	KIT mut NRAS or BRAF mut ALK rearr NRTK3 rearr	CDKN2A mut CCND1 amp TERT mut
	VI	Mucosal melanoma	KIT mut NRAS or BRAF mut CDKN2A mut SF3B1 mut	CCND1 amp CDK4 mut MDM2 amp
	VII	Melanoma in congenital nevus	NRAS mut	BRAFV600E mut
	VIII	Melanoma in blue nevus	GNA11 mut GNAQ mut CYSLTR2 mut	BAP1 mut EIFAX mut SF3B1 mut
	IX	Uveal melanoma	GNA11 mut GNAQ mut CYSLTR2 mut PLCB4 mut	BAP1 mut EIFAX mut SF3B1 mut

Source: Modified from 2018 World Health Organization Classification (Elder et al., 2020).
Abbreviations: amp, amplification; CSD, cumulative sun damage; mut, mutation; rearr, rearrangement.

Artificial Intelligence in Diagnosis

Diagnosis of skin cancers has been advanced through the use of AI. Machine learning algorithms learn to recognize patterns in large datasets and can use these patterns to classify the cancer. In many cases, the diagnosis of various skin cancers depends on visual interpretation of clinical and dermoscopic images (Brancaccio et al., 2024). AI can provide advantages over traditional diagnosis in multiple ways. Firstly, there is a shortage of qualified dermatologists worldwide, with this shortage being far more extreme in certain regions. AI can alleviate this problem by providing easy access to specialist-level expertise. This can allow for more timeous diagnosis and treatment. Secondly, AI diagnosis may offer more consistent and accurate diagnosis (Esteva et al., 2017). Convolutional neural networks (CNNs) have been shown to be extremely efficient in image-based classification of skin cancers. These neural networks are generally trained using supervised learning techniques. CNNs have been shown to be particularly useful for image analysis. Supervised learning requires that the images used to train the neural network must have been previously analyzed and given a diagnosis or label, and the algorithm will learn based on these previous diagnoses

(Esteva et al., 2017; Tschandl et al., 2020). CNNs can be trained using images of various skin lesions and the diagnoses given by board-certified dermatologists as to whether the lesion is a benign or malignant neoplasm (Haenssle et al., 2018).

AI has also been used to design home diagnosis software for use with smartphones to track suspicious moles on their bodies. While some of these apps merely transmit images for expert analysis, others use AI algorithms to identify high-risk lesions and recommend that the patient seek further medical advice. However, the assessment of these apps carried out in 2018 showed that they performed poorly with different skin colors and showed bias. Additionally, these rely on taking good photos of the lesion using the smartphone camera, and poor photos can result in poor analysis (Chuchu et al., 2018). However, this assessment was carried out in 2018, and these technologies have advanced greatly in recent years. One of these specific apps named MoleMapper™ can be used to photograph and track changes to skin lesions (moles). This app was released in October 2015 and does not act as a diagnostic tool; rather, it allows individuals to track changes in the appearance of moles and advise when a visit to a doctor is necessary. It also collects image data for use in research projects (Petrie et al., 2019).

TREATMENT OF MELANOMA

Advances in the studies on the molecular pathways of melanoma cells have facilitated the development of targeted immunotherapy for stages III and IV melanoma. These therapeutic advances can be divided into either targeted therapies or immunotherapies. Targeted therapies are generally kinase inhibitors that inhibit proteins that are the most commonly mutated in melanoma. Immune therapies consist of antibodies that target molecules that downregulate the immune response (Mcarthur and Ribas, 2013) and others that enhance cell apoptosis.

IMMUNOTHERAPY

Advanced metastatic melanoma is traditionally associated with poor patient outcomes and a low survival rate. The only practical option to effectively treat the disease at this advanced stage was through the use of cytotoxic chemotherapeutic agents. However, this changed with the development of immunotherapy (Knight et al., 2023). Immunotherapy agents are such as interleukin-2 (IL-2), interferon alpha, and immune checkpoint inhibitors. The development and use of immune system activators to treat melanoma resulted in the first of these, the use of the cytokine IL-2. The use of this treatment was limited since it is toxic (Davar et al., 2017). In addition to these, immune checkpoint inhibitors such as antibodies that block CTLA4 and PD1 (Wolchok et al., 2021) were developed. These include ipilimumab which targets and blocks CTLA4 (Robert et al., 2011), while pembrolizumab and nivolumab block programmed cell death protein 1 (PD-1) (Ribas et al., 2015; Topalian et al., 2012). Recently, a combination treatment has been developed consisting of the two antibodies relatlimab and nivolumab. Relatlimab blocks the activity of the LAG-3 surface receptor (Ascierto et al., 2017). Unfortunately, some patients may develop inflammatory rheumatic disorders, such as polymyalgia rheumatica/giant cell arteritis, aortitis, myocarditis, and ovarian and uterine lymphocytic vasculitis (Ralli et al., 2020).

TLRs are a family of immune receptors that recognize pathogen-associated molecular patterns (PAMPS), molecules commonly found on the surface of various diverse pathogens (Bianchi, 2007). Once activated by binding one of these PAMPS, TLRs activate the innate immune system, and this leads to an adaptive immune response. Different members of the family bind different PAMPS and are expressed on different cells or under different circumstances. TLR9 is expressed intracellularly on the surfaces of endoplasmic reticulum and intracellular vesicles. From here they can be exported to the cell membrane via the endocytic transport pathway (Leifer et al., 2004). TLR9 recognizes nucleic acid sequences that contain unmethylated CpG oligonucleotides (Agrawal and Kandimalla, 2007; Kandimalla et al., 2003). This results in the activated TLR9 signaling pathway recruiting T cells to the tumor microenvironment (Moynihan and Irvine, 2017). Efforts have led to the development of TLR9 agonists. The activities of these agonists against melanoma have been examined in clinical trials involving subcutaneous injection (Hofmann et al., 2008). It has been observed that these agonists elicit an inflammatory response and increase the recruitment of tumor-infiltrating lymphocytes (TILs) (Karapetyan et al., 2020). Some of these agonists include Tilsotolimod (IMO-2125), Vittorio (CMP-001), and SD-101 (Davar et al., 2020; Milhem et al., 2019). The use of oncolytic viruses, such as Talimogene and laherparepvec (T-VEC), is well suited for melanoma treatment since it is located on the skin surface and spread across the skin. T-VEC lacks the ability to replicate in neurons but is still able to replicate in tumor cells (Russell and Peng, 2007). The lysis of tumor cells as a result of this virus recruits APC to the tumor, stimulating the immune response (Liu et al., 2003).

Combination therapy can be used to increase treatment efficiency when immune-related therapies and chemotherapy show decreased efficiency with the development of resistance (Mattia et al., 2018; Mishra et al., 2018). The first-line treatment for melanoma is to remove the tumor using surgical procedures. This is the first treatment option at all stages of melanoma. The tumor and an amount of surrounding normal healthy tissue are removed from the area of the tumor. This is generally followed by a skin graft to replace the removed and damaged skin.

TILs migrate toward tumors and attempt to kill the cancer. Adoptive cell therapy (ACT) isolates lymphocytes from tumor tissue, grows them to increase their number, and then inserts them back into the patient via infusion (Lee and Margolin, 2012). Positive responses to this treatment are observed in 72% of patients, with 10–20% of patients achieving melanoma remission following treatment (Rohaan et al., 2018; Wu et al., 2012). Future advances in ACT center around optimizing the process or using ACT in conjunction with other immunotherapies (Mullinax et al., 2018).

Like in most cancers, the role of the immune system in the development and progression of melanoma is vital. As such, factors that can influence the immune system play an important role in melanoma. This includes the host microbiota, which plays an important role in both promoting or suppressing the immune response and, as such, plays an important role in immunotherapy (Beura et al., 2016).

Precision Medicine and Targeted Therapies

Targeted therapies and immunotherapies have both demonstrated the ability to increase the survival times of patients compared to those individuals treated with chemotherapy (Michielin et al., 2019). Precision-oriented medicine relies on specifically targeting the characteristics of the melanoma in the individual patient. Most commonly, this relies on identifying mutations that promote the growth and survival of the melanoma and then using molecular therapies to target these mutations. One of the results of this has been the development of small molecules that bind to or interact with specific targets in melanoma treatment.

One of the most common mutations identified in melanoma is mutations in the serine-threonine protein kinase rapidly accelerated fibrosarcoma isoform B (BRAF). Mutations in the *braf* gene are found in approximately 60% of melanoma. These melanomas show increased activation of the MAPK pathway leading to increased proliferation and decreased apoptosis (Davies et al., 2002). Vemurafenib is a selective BRAF inhibitor, which demonstrated an effective treatment response in around 47% of patients with metastatic melanoma (Sosman et al., 2012). In clinical studies, vemurafenib use led to a 63% decrease in mortality compared to patients treated with dacarbazine (Chapman et al., 2011). As such, vemurafenib has been adopted as the first-line treatment for metastatic melanoma containing *braf* mutation (Davies et al., 2002).

The *c-kit* gene is another gene that is commonly mutated in melanoma. This gene encodes the proto-oncogene KIT, a tyrosine protein kinase also known as CD117 or mast/stem cell growth factor receptor (SCFR). Mutations in this gene or copy number variations in this gene are found in 39% of mucosal melanomas and 36% of acral melanomas. Mutations in this gene are also found in 28% of melanomas that are caused by sun-induced damage (Kushnir and Merimsky, 2013). Imatinib mesylate is a drug that was developed to target KIT mutations in gastrointestinal stromal tumors (GIST) and is being investigated for treating melanomas (Bello et al., 2014; Hodi et al., 2008).

Transmitted genetic mutation contributing to the development is less common in the development of cutaneous melanoma despite a family history of melanoma being present in 5–15% of melanoma patients. True hereditary melanoma occurs in familial atypical multiple mole-melanoma (*FAMMM*) syndrome and melanoma-astrocytoma syndrome. In those families affected by these conditions, the most common mutations occur in cyclin-dependent kinase inhibitor 2A (*CDKN2A*) and cyclin-dependent kinase 4 (*CDK4*) (Rossi et al., 2019). Apart from these, other inherited conditions are linked with the increased risk of developing melanoma. These include xeroderma pigmentosum, familial retinoblastoma, Lynch syndrome type II, and Li–Fraumeni cancer syndrome (Goldstein and Tucker, 2001).

Combination Therapy

Using these new therapies in combination with each other as well as in combination with other treatments, such as chemotherapy and radiotherapy, has proved advantageous. Using separate targeted therapies, such as targeting both BRAF and MEK inhibitors. For instance, combinations of dabrafenib and trametinib (Robert et al., 2015) or combinations of vemurafenib plus cobimetinib (Larkin et al., 2014) showed that inhibiting both BRAF and MEK together was a more effective treatment leading to increased progression-free survival (Larkin et al., 2014; Robert et al., 2015). Resistance to the combination of these treatments has still been observed; however, this resistance develops at a slower rate compared to single-agent therapy (Wagle et al., 2014). This combination also had different side effects compared to those observed with single agents (Gibney and Sondak, 2013).

Nivolumab-ipilimumab used in combination was shown to be far more effective compared to ipilimumab monotherapy, with the combination treatment having a response rate of 61% compared to only 16% for the monotherapy (Postow et al., 2015). These combination immunotherapy treatments do have the disadvantage of showing increased toxicity and more adverse effects. These adverse effects were observed in 55% of patients receiving the combination therapy, compared to 27% in patients receiving ipilimumab monotherapy (Larkin et al., 2015).

Nanotechnology

A strategy to improve treatment efficiency involves the use of nanomedicine to actively target and deliver the drugs to a specific target and to reduce systemic side effects. These include nanoparticles containing these specific drugs. These nanoparticles can target tumors using antibodies, peptides, nucleic acids, or small molecules that can target tumor cell surface receptors. In the case of melanoma, these surface receptors include receptors like transferrin, melanocortin-1, fibroblast growth factor, laminin, somatostatin, and sigma. These intracytoplasmic receptor proteins show increased expression in melanoma (Rigon et al., 2015). Nanomedicine can be used to improve drug delivery as well as increase the concentration of the drug in the tumor tissue due to the nanoparticles increasing the length of time the drug remains stable and circulating in the drug (Rigon et al., 2015). Nanomedicine and nanoparticles can also be used to target melanoma for imaging and diagnostic purposes, especially for diagnostic capabilities (Madamsetty et al., 2020). Various chemical approaches can be used to create these nanoparticles. These include amid and thiol coupling, PEGylation, and biofunctionalization (Madamsetty et al., 2020). Various types of nanoparticles have been used to target melanoma. These need to function as transdermal carriers and include liposomes, niosomes, transferosomes, and particular systems (Song et al., 2021).

The oldest of these are liposomes, which are spherical, microscopic nanoparticles that consist of one or more phospholipid bilayers that surround an aqueous core (Tran et al., 2009). Liposomes are not highly effective in targeting melanoma because they are rigid due to them containing cholesterol. This also limits their ability to penetrate the epidermis and reach deeper layers and release the drug (Sudhakar et al., 2021). Liposome function can be improved through the creation of synthetic versions of the nanoparticle. These are known as niosomes and consist of layers of nonionic surfactant surrounding an aqueous core. These nanoparticles are biodegradable and nonimmunogenic. Their size can be dictated by the surfactant used and can therefore contain a large amount of drug. They are stable and can deliver sensitive drugs through various routes of administration (Gharbavi et al., 2018).

Another lipid-based vesicle, named transferosomes, are flexible elastic structures that consist of phospholipids, surfactants, and an ethanol and water vehicle (Zylberberg and Matosevic, 2016). Yet another lipid-based nanoparticle, ethosomes, also consists of a phospholipid bilayer containing a high percentage of ethanol, which gives the lipid particle its name. The inner core is aqueous and is also flexible due to the high concentration of ethanol. Another characteristic of these particles allows for them to efficiently permeate the skin. This is the ethosome effect, which describes the ability of the ethosome to fuse with skin lipids (Zylberberg and Matosevic, 2016). These two can be combined to create transethosomes, consisting of lipid, ethanol, and surfactant. Transethosomes are better than either ethosomes or transferosomes in transdermal drug delivery (Salem et al., 2019). Cubosomes are not circular in shape; rather, they are honeycomb-shaped and contain internal aqueous channels with a resulting large area of contact between these structures. They consist of amphiphilic lipids and self-assemble in water. They characteristically form a thin surface film of liquid crystal. As such, these particles are useful for topical drug administration by forming a film on the skin surface and can be used to protect the skin (Dhadwal et al., 2020). Other important nanoparticles that can be used to target melanoma include dendrimers, cyclodextrins (Michel et al., 2012), solid lipid nanoparticles (Geszke-Moritz and Moritz, 2016), and inorganic nanocarriers (Kumari et al., 2022).

OMICS TECHNOLOGIES AND THEIR APPLICATION TO MELANOMA MANAGEMENT

Advances in the characterization of the molecular basis of melanoma have been advanced through developments in the "omics" technologies. These include genomics (the genetic characterization of the DNA sequences), epigenomics (epigenetic modifications of the DNA), transcriptomics (mRNA sequences), proteomics (protein expression and activity), metabolomics (metabolites present in the patient), and microbiomics (the populations of microbes present in the patient) (Yang et al., 2020). The interplay between these different omics allows for greater identification of molecular patterns since they provide more information on the molecular characterization of the individual. In other words, the genomic and epigenomic profiles provide information on the transcriptomic profile, which, in turn, provides information on the proteomic profile (Lim et al., 2024). The proteomic profile can be considered to be the observable patient's observable phenotype. As such, the genomics and proteomic profile represent either end of the molecular basis for melanoma. Metabolomics and microbiomics represent the effect of the interplay between the environment and the phenotype of the patient (You et al., 2023).

These technologies allow for the discovery and application of patterns of biomarkers for the diagnosis, prognosis, and treatment response prediction in melanoma. Biomarkers have been identified for screening, diagnosis, staging, and predictions. They also provide insight into targets for the development of new therapies (Das et al., 2023). Biomarkers can be detected through various means with various starting materials. These sources of starting material range from tissue biopsies and liquid or circulating biopsies (Calapre et al., 2017).

Genomics is the best studied of the omics, supplying data concerning mutations, amplifications, gene fusions, and deletions. The rapid expansion of genomics databases has occurred thanks to technologies, such as next-generation sequencing and array-based comparative genomic hybridization (Array-CGH) (Manzoni et al., 2018). Next-generation sequencing is two of the most-used techniques, and the latter is an accessible, reliable, and economical tool. One of the first uses of Array-CGH was reported in mouse melanoma to study the chromosomal aberrations in melanomas with the same phenotype (Guhan et al., 2021).

The most common genomic changes are associated with genes involved in MAP-kinase pathway activation. These included mutations and chromosomal aberrations in *braf, nras, hras, gnaq, gna11, nap1, ctnnb1, map2k1, prkar1a,* and *nf1*. Additionally, fusions were found in *alk, ros1, ntrk1, ret, met, braf. Ntrk3,* and *prkca* (Urso, 2019). An important part of the definition of the proteome is that it is time- and state-dependent (Graves and Haystead, 2002). Mass spectrometry (MS) is the technique responsible for advancing proteomics, allowing for the identification and quantification of proteins in a complex mixture of proteins. MS allows for the protein biomarkers to be used to evaluate the progression of the disease and treatment effectiveness due to the dynamic nature of the proteome (Tully et al., 2019). Expression of the mutated forms of proteins has been shown to be related to survival in melanoma patients. These include proteins such as BRAF and V600E (Hugdahl et al., 2016).

The vast amount of data generated through omics technologies means that the analysis and interpretation of the data become difficult and, in many cases, impractical. The use of AI alongside machine learning and deep learning has revolutionized the use of omics data. The MM500 study is a joint Swedish-Hungarian study that aims to "identify and define the overall melanoma proteome." This data concerning the localization and expression of proteins can be combined with genome and transcriptome sequencing information as well as digital pathology (DP) and clinical information to discover new prognostic and predictive markers for melanoma (Betancourt et al., 2021).

The discovery of genetic mutations in melanoma also raises the possibility that gene therapy can be used in melanoma management. Here specific genetic mutations are repaired or silenced in order to reverse the pro-melanoma effects of these mutated genes and gene products (Menezes et al., 2018).

PATIENT-CENTRIC TECHNOLOGIES: EMPOWERING INDIVIDUALS IN MELANOMA CARE

Patient-centered care is defined as care that respects a patient's wishes while also responding to and changing to suit the preferences of the patient. The implication is that all treatment decisions will respect the patient's wishes, and the patient plays a proactive role in their treatment (Institute of Medicine Committee on Quality of Health Care in America, 2001). Many of these new strategies used to achieve this are the use of digital technologies, such as telehealth, electronic health (eHealth), and digital technologies. At the same time, it also includes mobile health (mHealth) (Njoroge et al., 2017).

mHealth interventions are defined as the use of mobile devices to support personal and public healthcare. This includes the use of technologies, such as mobile phones, patient monitoring devices, personal digital assistance, and wireless devices (Bradway et al., 2017). The effectiveness of these mobile devices remains to be established (Michie et al., 2017). Alternatively, although eHealth or digital technologies include similar technologies to mHealth, these also include devices or technologies that do not rely on mobile devices. These can include software that can be used to monitor patient admission and records of care in a hospital setting or methods to educate patients at clinics or hospitals, such as Smart Boards and Smart TVs (Lee et al., 2017). A subset of eHealth is known as digital behavior change interventions (DBCIs), where computers are used to change the behavior of patients. These interventions can be accomplished through the use of educational websites, smartphone apps, or text messages. It can also include monitoring technologies through the use of wearable devices (Michie et al., 2017).

Social media is also being used to generate data around a patient's actual lived experience (Humphrey et al., 2017). These include patients sharing their experiences with others through social media as well as using the Internet and asking others with the same diagnosis various health-related questions (Chauhan et al., 2022). These can provide insights into a patient's psychological well-being and any specific needs they may require (Taylor and Pagliari, 2019). A study performed in a European setting used social media to gather information regarding the experiences of patients living with melanoma. Peaks in costs concerning melanoma occurred following public education campaigns and World Melanoma Day. These posts were found to discuss the side effects of various treatments, with surgery being discussed positively most often. Chemotherapy, on the other hand, was most commonly discussed with negative associations. These negative discussions are related to side effects and ineffective treatment. Patients also asked questions around diagnosis and treatment, information that should be provided by healthcare professionals (Chauhan et al., 2022).

CONCLUSION

This book aims to provide a comprehensive overview of melanoma, covering its fundamentals and introducing the latest technologies shaping our understanding of the disease. From molecular insights to AI applications, readers will gain a holistic understanding of melanoma's landscape (**Figure 1.4**).

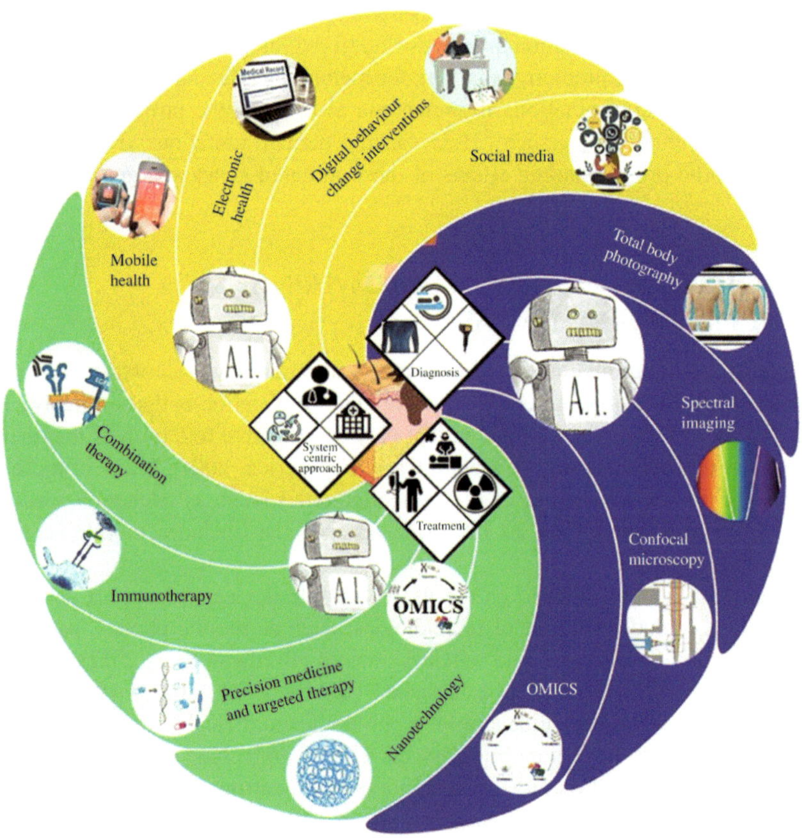

FIGURE 1.4 **Advances in the treatment and diagnosis of melanoma.** This figure summarizes the content and topics covered by this book. This book covers advances in the diagnosis and treatment of melanoma, as well as the shift to patient-centered treatments. The squares in the center of the diagram display the current and well-established techniques to manage melanoma, and the diagram shows how these techniques are being replaced or improved through new advanced technologies. Surgery, radiotherapy, and chemotherapy are all traditional treatments for melanoma. These are being used in combination with new, more specific treatments such as targeted therapy and immunotherapy alongside new drug delivery systems based on nanotechnology. These treatments can be improved by monitoring their effectiveness using AI to monitor changes in the proteome or transcriptome. AI and Omics technologies are also being used to improve diagnosis using various biomarkers. Traditional diagnosis relied on visual inspection of the skin through whole-body photography, dermoscopy, and PET/CT scans. New imaging techniques are being developed based on confocal imaging and spectral refraction. Finally, system centers that provide healthcare where the patient is a passive participant are being replaced with patient-centric models using digital health to allow patients to participate more actively in their own treatment.

Chapter 2 discusses the use of precision medicine in transforming melanoma treatment and will describe the latest molecular profiling technologies. It explores the power of advanced molecular diagnostics in identifying targetable mutations and tailoring therapies for personalized and effective treatment. Chapter 3 describes the integration of AI in melanoma diagnostics. From AI-driven imaging analysis to predictive modeling. It provides insights into how cutting-edge technologies are revolutionizing the early detection and accurate diagnosis of melanoma. In Chapter 4, the authors focus on the latest immunotherapeutic advancements and explore how technology is enhancing our ability to harness the immune system against melanoma. It covers diverse topics ranging from the use of immune checkpoint inhibitors or adoptive cell therapies to the technological frontiers driving breakthroughs in melanoma immunotherapy. Chapter 5 investigates the latest advancements in targeted therapies and nanomedicine, showcasing how these technologies offer precise interventions at the molecular level. These include topics ranging from the use of small molecule inhibitors to nanocarriers. The chapter also discusses innovative strategies for combating melanoma with minimal collateral damage. Chapter 6 focuses on treatment resistance, and it delves into the latest molecular insights surrounding treatment resistance. The chapter describes how cutting-edge technologies are unraveling the complexities of resistance mechanisms and guiding the development of innovative solutions. Chapter 7 explores the synergy of genomics and proteomics in a comprehensive multi-omics approach to melanoma treatment. The chapter provides insights into how the latest technologies in genomics and proteomics are providing a holistic view of melanoma, paving the way for integrated therapeutic solutions. In Chapter 8, next-generation approaches to imaging technologies are being discussed. It examines how these approaches are revolutionizing melanoma monitoring and assessment. These advanced imaging modalities include AI-driven analyses and the latest tools enhancing our ability to track and evaluate melanoma progression. Chapter 9 shifts the focus from general treatment and management strategies to patient-centric technologies. This chapter explores how digital health, wearables, and patient-centric apps are empowering individuals in their melanoma care journey. The chapter describes the latest technologies being developed to promote active patient involvement in the treatment and management of melanoma. Chapter 10 expands on the burgeoning landscape of combination therapies for melanoma, uncovering synergistic possibilities and future prospects to revolutionize treatment efficacy and patient outcomes while mitigating adverse effects. The penultimate chapter, Chapter 11, highlights the unique challenges faced by melanoma research and management in Low to middle income countries around the world, with a special focus on Africa. It examines attempts to address cancer disparities. These include the limited access these countries have to advanced retirements and diagnostics as well as the emergence of drug resistance in these countries. Finally, the chapter will make a case for the need of low cost solutions for the control and treatment of melanoma in these countries. The final chapter (Chapter 12) maps out a technological roadmap for collaborative solutions to future melanoma challenges. These include interdisciplinary collaborations and data sharing.

REFERENCES

Abdel-Malek, Z., Swope, V. B., Suzuki, I., Akcali, C., Harriger, M. D., Boyce, S. T., Urabe, K. and Hearing, V. J. 1995. Mitogenic and melanogenic stimulation of normal human melanocytes by melanotropic peptides, *Proceedings of the National Academy of Sciences of the United States of America*, 92, pp. 1789–1793.

Agrawal, S. and Kandimalla, E. R. 2007. Synthetic agonists of Toll-like receptors 7, 8 and 9, *Biochemical Society Transactions*, 35, pp. 1461–1467.

Anderson, R. R. and Parrish, J. A. 1981. The optics of human skin, *Journal of Investigative Dermatology*, 77, pp. 13–19.

Apostu, A. P., Ungureanu, L., Halmagyi, S. R., Trufin, I. I. and Şenilă, S. C. 2023. Multiple primary melanomas: A literature review, *Medicine (Baltimore)*, 102, p. e34378.

Argenziano, G. and Soyer, H. P. 2001. Dermoscopy of pigmented skin lesions—a valuable tool for early diagnosis of melanoma, *Lancet Oncology*, 2, pp. 443–449.

Ascierto, P. A., Del Vecchio, M., Robert, C., Mackiewicz, A., Chiarion-Sileni, V., Arance, A., Lebbé, C., Bastholt, L., Hamid, O., Rutkowski, P., Mcneil, C., Garbe, C., Loquai, C., Dreno, B., Thomas, L., Grob,

J. J., Liszkay, G., Nyakas, M., Gutzmer, R., Pikiel, J., Grange, F., Hoeller, C., Ferraresi, V., Smylie, M., Schadendorf, D., Mortier, L., Svane, I. M., Hennicken, D., Qureshi, A. and Maio, M. 2017. Ipilimumab 10 mg/kg versus ipilimumab 3 mg/kg in patients with unresectable or metastatic melanoma: A randomised, double-blind, multicentre, phase 3 trial, *Lancet Oncology*, 18, pp. 611–622.

Balch, C. M., Buzaid, A. C., Soong, S. J., Atkins, M. B., Cascinelli, N., Coit, D. G., Fleming, I. D., Gershenwald, J. E., Houghton, A. Jr., Kirkwood, J. M., Mcmasters, K. M., Mihm, M. F., Morton, D. L., Reintgen, D. S., Ross, M. I., Sober, A., Thompson, J. A. and Thompson, J. F. 2001. Final version of the American Joint Committee on Cancer staging system for cutaneous melanoma, *Journal of Clinical Oncology*, 19, pp. 3635–3648.

Baloglu, A., Bezircioglu, I., Cetinkaya, B. and Yavuzcan, A. 2009. Primary malignant melanoma of the vagina, *Archives of Gynecology and Obstetrics*, 280, pp. 819–822.

Bello, D. M., Dematteo, R. P. and Ariyan, C. E. 2014. The GIST of targeted therapy for malignant melanoma, *Annals of Surgical Oncology*, 21, pp. 2059–2067.

Betancourt, L. H., Gil, J., Kim, Y., Doma, V., Çakir, U., Sanchez, A., Murillo, J. R., Kuras, M., Parada, I. P., Sugihara, Y., Appelqvist, R., Wieslander, E., Welinder, C., Velasquez, E., De Almeida, N. P., Woldmar, N., Marko-Varga, M., Pawłowski, K., Eriksson, J., Szeitz, B., Baldetorp, B., Ingvar, C., Olsson, H., Lundgren, L., Lindberg, H., Oskolas, H., Lee, B., Berge, E., Sjögren, M., Eriksson, C., Kim, D., Kwon, H. J., Knudsen, B., Rezeli, M., Hong, R., Horvatovich, P., Miliotis, T., Nishimura, T., Kato, H., Steinfelder, E., Oppermann, M., Miller, K., Florindi, F., Zhou, Q., Domont, G. B., Pizzatti, L., Nogueira, F. C. S., Horvath, P., Szadai, L., Tímár, J., Kárpáti, S., Szász, A. M., Malm, J., Fenyö, D., Ekedahl, H., Németh, I. B. and Marko-Varga, G. 2021. The human melanoma proteome atlas-defining the molecular pathology, *Clinical and Translational Medicine*, 11, p. e473.

Beura, L. K., Hamilton, S. E., Bi, K., Schenkel, J. M., Odumade, O. A., Casey, K. A., Thompson, E. A., Fraser, K. A., Rosato, P. C., Filali-Mouhim, A., Sekaly, R. P., Jenkins, M. K., Vezys, V., Haining, W. N., Jameson, S. C. and Masopust, D. 2016. Normalizing the environment recapitulates adult human immune traits in laboratory mice, *Nature*, 532, pp. 512–516.

Bevona, C., Goggins, W., Quinn, T., Fullerton, J. and Tsao, H. 2003. Cutaneous melanomas associated with nevi, *Archives of Dermatology*, 139, pp. 1620–1624; discussion 1624.

Bian, S. X., Hwang, L., Hwang, J., Ragab, O., In, G. K., Peng, D. and Lin, E. 2021. Acral lentiginous melanoma-population, treatment, and survival using the NCDB from 2004 to 2015, *Pigment Cell & Melanoma Research*, 34, pp. 1049–1061.

Bianchi, M. E. 2007. DAMPs, PAMPs and alarmins: All we need to know about danger, *Journal of Leukocyte Biology*, 81, pp. 1–5.

Blum, A., Schmid-Wendtner, M. H., Mauss-Kiefer, V., Eberle, J. Y., Kuchelmeister, C. and Dill-Müller, D. 2006. Ultrasound mapping of lymph node and subcutaneous metastases in patients with cutaneous melanoma: Results of a prospective multicenter study, *Dermatology*, 212, pp. 47–52.

Boudoux, C., Yun, S., Oh, W., White, W., Iftimia, N., Shishkov, M., Bouma, B. and Tearney, G. 2005. Rapid wavelength-swept spectrally encoded confocal microscopy, *Optic Express*, 13, pp. 8214–8221.

Bradway, M., Carrion, C., Vallespin, B., Saadatfard, O., Puigdomènech, E., Espallargues, M. and Kotzeva, A. 2017. mHealth assessment: Conceptualization of a global framework, *JMIR Mhealth and Uhealth*, 5, p. e60.

Brancaccio, G., Balato, A., Malvehy, J., Puig, S., Argenziano, G. and Kittler, H. 2024. Artificial intelligence in skin cancer diagnosis: A reality check, *Journal of Investigative Dermatology*, 144, pp. 492–499.

Braun, R. P., Rabinovitz, H. S., Oliviero, M., Kopf, A. W. and Saurat, J.-H. 2005. Dermoscopy of pigmented skin lesions, *Journal of the American Academy of Dermatology*, 52, pp. 109–121.

Braun, R. P., Saurat, J. H. and French, L. E. 2004. Dermoscopy of pigmented lesions: A valuable tool in the diagnosis of melanoma, *Swiss Medical Weekly*, 134, pp. 83–90.

Bray, F., Laversanne, M., Sung, H., Ferlay, J., Siegel, R. L., Soerjomataram, I. and Jemal, A. 2024. Global cancer statistics 2022: GLOBOCAN estimates of incidence and mortality worldwide for 36 cancers in 185 countries, *CA: A Cancer Journal for Clinicians*, 74, pp. 229–263.

Busam, K. J., Charles, C., Lee, G. and Halpern, A. C. 2001. Morphologic features of melanocytes, pigmented keratinocytes, and melanophages by in vivo confocal scanning laser microscopy, *Modern Pathology*, 14, pp. 862–868.

Calapre, L., Warburton, L., Millward, M., Ziman, M. and Gray, E. S. 2017. Circulating tumour DNA (ctDNA) as a liquid biopsy for melanoma, *Cancer Letters*, 404, pp. 62–69.

Califano, J. and Nance, M. 2009. Malignant melanoma, *Facial Plastic Surgery Clinics of North America*, 17, pp. 337–348.

Carrara, M., Bono, A., Bartoli, C., Colombo, A., Lualdi, M., Moglia, D., Santoro, N., Tolomio, E., Tomatis, S., Tragni, G., Santinami, M. and Marchesini, R. 2007. Multispectral imaging and artificial neural network: Mimicking the management decision of the clinician facing pigmented skin lesions, *Physics in Medicine and Biology*, 52, pp. 2599–2613.

Castellani, G., Buccarelli, M., Arasi, M. B., Rossi, S., Pisanu, M. E., Bellenghi, M., Lintas, C. and Tabolacci, C. 2023. BRAF mutations in melanoma: Biological aspects, therapeutic implications, and circulating biomarkers. *Cancers (Basel)*, 15, p. 4026.
Chacón, M., Pfluger, Y., Angel, M., Waisberg, F. and Enrico, D. 2020. Uncommon subtypes of malignant melanomas: A review based on clinical and molecular perspectives. *Cancers (Basel)*, 12, p. 2362.
Chanal, J., Kramkimel, N., Guegan, S., Moguelet, P., Fourchotte, V. and Avril, M. F. 2016. Locally advanced unresectable vaginal melanoma: Response with anti-programmed death receptor 1, *J Low Genit Tract Dis*, 20, pp. e4–e5.
Chapman, P. B., Hauschild, A., Robert, C., Haanen, J. B., Ascierto, P., Larkin, J., Dummer, R., Garbe, C., Testori, A., Maio, M., Hogg, D., Lorigan, P., Lebbe, C., Jouary, T., Schadendorf, D., Ribas, A., O'day, S. J., Sosman, J. A., Kirkwood, J. M., Eggermont, A. M., Dreno, B., Nolop, K., Li, J., Nelson, B., Hou, J., Lee, R. J., Flaherty, K. T. and Mcarthur, G. A. 2011. Improved survival with vemurafenib in melanoma with BRAF V600E mutation, *New England Journal of Medicine*, 364, pp. 2507–2516.
Chauhan, J., Aasaithambi, S., Márquez-Rodas, I., Formisano, L., Papa, S., Meyer, N., Forschner, A., Faust, G., Lau, M. and Sagkriotis, A. 2022. Understanding the lived experiences of patients with melanoma: Real-world evidence generated through a European social media listening analysis, *JMIR Cancer*, 8, p. e35930.
Chen, C. and Gao, F. H. 2019. Th17 cells paradoxical roles in melanoma and potential application in immunotherapy, *Frontiers in Immunology*, 10, p. 187.
Chuchu, N., Takwoingi, Y., Dinnes, J., Matin, R. N., Bassett, O., Moreau, J. F., Bayliss, S. E., Davenport, C., Godfrey, K., O'connell, S., Jain, A., Walter, F. M., Deeks, J. J. and Williams, H. C. 2018. Smartphone applications for triaging adults with skin lesions that are suspicious for melanoma, *The Cochrane Database of Systemaic Reviews*, 12, p. Cd013192.
D'orazio, J., Jarrett, S., Amaro-Ortiz, A. and Scott, T. 2013. UV radiation and the skin, *International Journal of Molecular Sciences*, 14, pp. 12222–12248.
Das, S., Dey, M. K., Devireddy, R. and Gartia, M. R. 2023. Biomarkers in cancer detection, diagnosis, and prognosis. *Sensors (Basel)*, 24, p. 37.
Davar, D., Ding, F., Saul, M., Sander, C., Tarhini, A. A., Kirkwood, J. M. and Tawbi, H. A. 2017. High-dose interleukin-2 (HD IL-2) for advanced melanoma: A single center experience from the University of Pittsburgh Cancer Institute, *Journal for Immunotherapy of Cancer*, 5, p. 74.
Davar, D., Karunamurthy, A., Hartman, D., Deblasio, R., Chauvin, J.-M., Ding, Q., Pagliano, O., Rose, A., Kirkwood, J. and Zarour, H. 2020. 303 Phase II trial of neoadjuvant nivolumab (Nivo) and intratumoral (IT) CMP-001 in high-risk resectable melanoma (Neo-C-Nivo): Final results, *Journal for Immunotherapy of Cancer*, 8(3).
Davies, H., Bignell, G. R., Cox, C., Stephens, P., Edkins, S., Clegg, S., Teague, J., Woffendin, H., Garnett, M. J., Bottomley, W., Davis, N., Dicks, E., Ewing, R., Floyd, Y., Gray, K., Hall, S., Hawes, R., Hughes, J., Kosmidou, V., Menzies, A., Mould, C., Parker, A., Stevens, C., Watt, S., Hooper, S., Wilson, R., Jayatilake, H., Gusterson, B. A., Cooper, C., Shipley, J., Hargrave, D., Pritchard-Jones, K., Maitland, N., Chenevix-Trench, G., Riggins, G. J., Bigner, D. D., Palmieri, G., Cossu, A., Flanagan, A., Nicholson, A., Ho, J. W., Leung, S. Y., Yuen, S. T., Weber, B. L., Seigler, H. F., Darrow, T. L., Paterson, H., Marais, R., Marshall, C. J., Wooster, R., Stratton, M. R. and Futreal, P. A. 2002. Mutations of the BRAF gene in human cancer, *Nature*, 417, pp. 949–954.
Dhadwal, A., Sharma, D. R., Pandit, V., Ashawat, M. S. and Kumar, P. 2020. Cubosomes: A novel carrier for transdermal drug delivery, *Journal of Drug Delivery and Therapeutics*, 10, pp. 123–130.
Elder, D. E., Bastian, B. C., Cree, I. A., Massi, D. and Scolyer, R. A. 2020. The 2018 World Health Organization classification of cutaneous, mucosal, and uveal melanoma: Detailed analysis of 9 distinct subtypes defined by their evolutionary pathway, *Archives of Pathology Laboratory Medicine*, 144, pp. 500–522.
Erdei, E. and Torres, S. M. 2010. A new understanding in the epidemiology of melanoma, *Expert Rev Anticancer Ther*, 10, pp. 1811–1823.
Esteva, A., Kuprel, B., Novoa, R. A., Ko, J., Swetter, S. M., Blau, H. M. and Thrun, S. 2017. Dermatologist-level classification of skin cancer with deep neural networks, *Nature*, 542, pp. 115–118.
Geszke-Moritz, M. and Moritz, M. 2016. Solid lipid nanoparticles as attractive drug vehicles: Composition, properties and therapeutic strategies, *Material Science & Engineering: C*, 68, pp. 982–994.
Gharbavi, M., Amani, J., Kheiri-Manjili, H., Danafar, H. and Sharafi, A. 2018. Niosome: A promising nanocarrier for natural drug delivery through blood-brain barrier, *Advances in Pharmacological Sciences*, 2018, p. 6847971.
Gheoca Mutu, D. E., Avino, A., Balcangiu-Stroescu, A. E., Mehedințu, M., Bălan, D. G., Brîndușe, L. A., Popescu, A. M., Ionescu, D., Cristea, B. M., Tomescu, L. F., Jecan, C. R. and Răducu, L. 2022. Histopathological evaluation of cutaneous malignant melanoma: A retrospective study, *Experimental and Therapeutic Medicine*, 23, p. 402.

Gibney, G. T. and Sondak, V. K. 2013. Has targeted therapy for melanoma made chemotherapy obsolete? *Lancet. Oncology*, 14, pp. 676–677.

Goldstein, A. M. and Tucker, M. A. 2001. Genetic epidemiology of cutaneous melanoma: A global perspective, *Archives of Dermatology*, 137, pp. 1493–1496.

Graves, P. R. and Haystead, T. A. 2002. Molecular biologist's guide to proteomics, *Microbiology and Molecular Biology Reviews*, 66, pp. 39–63.

Greenwald, H. S., Friedman, E. B. and Osman, I. 2012. Superficial spreading and nodular melanoma are distinct biological entities: A challenge to the linear progression model, *Melanoma Research*, 22, pp. 1–8.

Guhan, S., Klebanov, N. and Tsao, H. 2021. Melanoma genomics: A state-of-the-art review of practical clinical applications, *British Journal of Dermatology*, 185, pp. 272–281.

Guitera, P., Pellacani, G., Crotty, K. A., Scolyer, R. A., Li, L. X., Bassoli, S., Vinceti, M., Rabinovitz, H., Longo, C. and Menzies, S. W. 2010. The impact of in vivo reflectance confocal microscopy on the diagnostic accuracy of lentigo maligna and equivocal pigmented and nonpigmented macules of the face, *Journal of Investigative Dermatology*, 130, pp. 2080–2091.

Guy, G. P. Jr., Thomas, C. C., Thompson, T., Watson, M., Massetti, G. M. and Richardson, L. C. 2015. Vital signs: Melanoma incidence and mortality trends and projections—United States, 1982–2030, *MMWR. Morbidity and Mortality Weekly Report*, 64, pp. 591–596.

Haenssle, H. A., Fink, C., Schneiderbauer, R., Toberer, F., Buhl, T., Blum, A., Kalloo, A., Hassen, A. B. H., Thomas, L., Enk, A., Uhlmann, L., Alt, C., Arenbergerova, M., Bakos, R., Baltzer, A., Bertlich, I., Blum, A., Bokor-Billmann, T., Bowling, J., Braghiroli, N., Braun, R., Buder-Bakhaya, K., Buhl, T., Cabo, H., Cabrijan, L., Cevic, N., Classen, A., Deltgen, D., Fink, C., Georgieva, I., Hakim-Meibodi, L. E., Hanner, S., Hartmann, F., Hartmann, J., Haus, G., Hoxha, E., Karls, R., Koga, H., Kreusch, J., Lallas, A., Majenka, P., Marghoob, A., Massone, C., Mekokishvili, L., Mestel, D., Meyer, V., Neuberger, A., Nielsen, K., Oliviero, M., Pampena, R., Paoli, J., Pawlik, E., Rao, B., Rendon, A., Russo, T., Sadek, A., Samhaber, K., Schneiderbauer, R., Schweizer, A., Toberer, F., Trennheuser, L., Vlahova, L., Wald, A., Winkler, J., Wölbing, P. and Zalaudek, I. 2018. Man against machine: Diagnostic performance of a deep learning convolutional neural network for dermoscopic melanoma recognition in comparison to 58 dermatologists, *Annals of Oncology*, 29, pp. 1836–1842.

Hodi, F. S., Friedlander, P., Corless, C. L., Heinrich, M. C., Mac Rae, S., Kruse, A., Jagannathan, J., Van Den Abbeele, A. D., Velazquez, E. F., Demetri, G. D. and Fisher, D. E. 2008. Major response to imatinib mesylate in KIT-mutated melanoma, *Journal of Clinical Oncology*, 26, pp. 2046–2051.

Hofmann, M. A., Kors, C., Audring, H., Walden, P., Sterry, W. and Trefzer, U. 2008. Phase 1 evaluation of intralesionally injected TLR9-agonist PF-3512676 in patients with basal cell carcinoma or metastatic melanoma, *Journal of Immunotherapy*, 31, pp. 520–527.

Huayllani, M. T., Sisti, A., Restrepo, D. J., Boczar, D., Cochuyt, J. J., Spaulding, A. C., Bagaria, S. P., Rinker, B. D. and Forte, A. J. 2019. Desmoplastic melanoma: Clinical characteristics and survival in the US population, *Cureus*, 11, p. e4931.

Hugdahl, E., Kalvenes, M. B., Puntervoll, H. E., Ladstein, R. G. and Akslen, L. A. 2016. BRAF-V600E expression in primary nodular melanoma is associated with aggressive tumour features and reduced survival, *British Journal of Cancer*, 114, pp. 801–808.

Humphrey, L., Willgoss, T., Trigg, A., Meysner, S., Kane, M., Dickinson, S. and Kitchen, H. 2017. A comparison of three methods to generate a conceptual understanding of a disease based on the patients' perspective, *Journal of Patient-Reported Outcomes*, 1, p. 9.

Institute of Medicine Committee on Quality of Health Care in America. 2001. *Crossing the Quality Chasm: A New Health System for the 21st Century*. Washington (DC): National Academies Press.

Jager, M. J., Dogrusöz, M. and Woodman, S. E. 2017. Uveal melanoma: Identifying immunological and chemotherapeutic targets to treat metastases, *Asia-Pacific Journal of Ophthalmology (Philadelphia)*, 6, pp. 179–185.

Jhappan, C., Noonan, F. P. and Merlino, G. 2003. Ultraviolet radiation and cutaneous malignant melanoma, *Oncogene*, 22, pp. 3099–3112.

Juszczak, A. M., Wöelfle, U., Končić, M. Z. and Tomczyk, M. 2022. Skin cancer, including related pathways and therapy and the role of luteolin derivatives as potential therapeutics, *Medicinal Research Reviews*, 42, pp. 1423–1462.

Kallini, J. R., Jain, S. K. and Khachemoune, A. 2013. Lentigo maligna: Review of salient characteristics and management, *American Journal of Clinical Dermatology*, 14, pp. 473–480.

Kamposioras, K., Pentheroudakis, G., Pectasides, D. and Pavlidis, N. 2011. Malignant melanoma of unknown primary site. To make the long story short. A systematic review of the literature, *Critical Reviews in Oncology/Hematology*, 78, pp. 112–126.

Kandimalla, E. R., Bhagat, L., Cong, Y. P., Pandey, R. K., Yu, D., Zhao, Q. and Agrawal, S. 2003. Secondary structures in CpG oligonucleotides affect immunostimulatory activity, *Biochemical and Biophysical Research Communications*, 306, pp. 948–953.

Karapetyan, L., Luke, J. J. and Davar, D. 2020. Toll-like receptor 9 agonists in cancer, *OncoTargets and Therapy*, 13, pp. 10039–10060.

Karmilkar, K. and Norem, R. F. 2nd. 2023. Amelanotic malignant melanoma: A case report, *Cureus*, 15, p. e41665.

Kauffmann, R. M. and Chen, S. L. 2014. Workup and staging of malignant melanoma, *The Surgical Clinics of North America*, 94, pp. 963–972.

Kelly, J. W., Yeatman, J. M., Regalia, C., Mason, G. and Henham, A. P. 1997. A high incidence of melanoma found in patients with multiple dysplastic naevi by photographic surveillance, *The Medical Journal of Australia*, 167, pp. 191–194.

Kim, H. J. and Kim, Y. H. 2024. Molecular frontiers in melanoma: Pathogenesis, diagnosis, and therapeutic advances. *International Journal of Molecular Sciences*, 25, p. 2984.

Knight, A., Karapetyan, L. and Kirkwood, J. M. 2023. Immunotherapy in melanoma: Recent advances and future directions. *Cancers (Basel)*, 15, p. 1106.

Kumari, S., Choudhary, P. K., Shukla, R., Sahebkar, A. and Kesharwani, P. 2022. Recent advances in nanotechnology based combination drug therapy for skin cancer, *Journal of Biomaterials Science. Polymer Edition*, 33, pp. 1435–1468.

Kushnir, I. and Merimsky, O. 2013. The evolution in melanoma treatment as a reflection of precision-oriented medicine, *Oncology Letters*, 5(2), pp. 424–426. doi: 10.3892/ol.2012.1065.

Larkin, J., Ascierto, P. A., Dréno, B., Atkinson, V., Liszkay, G., Maio, M., Mandalà, M., Demidov, L., Stroyakovskiy, D., Thomas, L., De La Cruz-Merino, L., Dutriaux, C., Garbe, C., Sovak, M. A., Chang, I., Choong, N., Hack, S. P., Mcarthur, G. A. and Ribas, A. 2014. Combined vemurafenib and cobimetinib in BRAF-mutated melanoma, *New England Journal of Medicine*, 371, pp. 1867–1876.

Larkin, J., Hatswell, A. J., Nathan, P., Lebmeier, M. and Lee, D. 2015. The predicted impact of ipilimumab usage on survival in previously treated advanced or metastatic melanoma in the UK, *PLOS ONE*, 10, p. e0145524.

Lee, S. and Margolin, K. 2012. Tumor-infiltrating lymphocytes in melanoma, *Current Oncology Reports*, 14, pp. 468–474.

Lee, S., Cho, Y. M. and Kim, S. Y. 2017. Mapping mHealth (mobile health) and mobile penetrations in sub-Saharan Africa for strategic regional collaboration in mHealth scale-up: An application of exploratory spatial data analysis, *Global Health*, 13, p. 63.

Leifer, C. A., Kennedy, M. N., Mazzoni, A., Lee, C., Kruhlak, M. J. and Segal, D. M. 2004. TLR9 is localized in the endoplasmic reticulum prior to stimulation, *Journal of Immunology*, 173, pp. 1179–1183.

Lim, J., Park, C., Kim, M., Kim, H., Kim, J. and Lee, D. S. 2024. Advances in single-cell omics and multiomics for high-resolution molecular profiling, *Experimental & Molecular Medicine*, 56, pp. 515–526.

Liu, B. L., Robinson, M., Han, Z. Q., Branston, R. H., English, C., Reay, P., Mcgrath, Y., Thomas, S. K., Thornton, M., Bullock, P., Love, C. A. and Coffin, R. S. 2003. ICP34.5 deleted herpes simplex virus with enhanced oncolytic, immune stimulating, and anti-tumour properties, *Gene Therapy*, 10, pp. 292–303.

Madamsetty, V. S., Paul, M. K., Mukherjee, A. and Mukherjee, S. 2020. Functionalization of nanomaterials and their application in melanoma cancer theranostics, *ACS Biomaterials Science & Engineering*, 6, pp. 167–181.

Madhusudhan, N., Pausan, M. R., Halwachs, B., Durdević, M., Windisch, M., Kehrmann, J., Patra, V., Wolf, P., Boukamp, P., Moissl-Eichinger, C., Cerroni, L., Becker, J. C. and Gorkiewicz, G. 2020. Molecular profiling of keratinocyte skin tumors links *Staphylococcus aureus* overabundance and increased human β-defensin-2 expression to growth promotion of squamous cell carcinoma. *Cancers (Basel)*, 12, p. 541.

Mágori, A. 2003. The role of fine needle aspiration biopsy in the diagnosis of melanoma, *Magyar Onkologia*, 47, pp. 41–43.

Manzoni, C., Kia, D. A., Vandrovcova, J., Hardy, J., Wood, N. W., Lewis, P. A. and Ferrari, R. 2018. Genome, transcriptome and proteome: The rise of omics data and their integration in biomedical sciences, *Briefings in Bioinformatics*, 19, pp. 286–302.

Marghoob, A. A., Korzenko, A. J., Changchien, L., Scope, A., Braun, R. P. and Rabinovitz, H. 2007. The beauty and the beast sign in dermoscopy, *Dermatologic Surgery*, 33, pp. 1388–1391.

Martín-Alcalde, J., Gamo-Villegas, R., Floristán-Muruzábal, M. U., Pampín-Franco, A., Pinedo-Moraleda, F. and López-Estebaranz, J. L. 2021. Nevoid melanoma: Dermoscopic and in vivo reflectance confocal microscopic aspects in 4 cases, *JAAD Case Reports*, 11, pp. 132–136.

Mattia, G., Puglisi, R., Ascione, B., Malorni, W., Carè, A. and Matarrese, P. 2018. Cell death-based treatments of melanoma: Conventional treatments and new therapeutic strategies, *Cell Death & Disease*, 9, p. 112.
Mcarthur, G. A. and Ribas, A. 2013. Targeting oncogenic drivers and the immune system in melanoma, *Journal of Clinical Oncology*, 31, pp. 499–506.
Menezes, M. E., Talukdar, S., Wechman, S. L., Das, S. K., Emdad, L., Sarkar, D. and Fisher, P. B. 2018. Prospects of Gene therapy to treat melanoma, *Advances in Cancer Research*, 138, pp. 213–237.
Michel, D., Chitanda, J. M., Balogh, R., Yang, P., Singh, J., Das, U., El-Aneed, A., Dimmock, J., Verrall, R. and Badea, I. 2012. Design and evaluation of cyclodextrin-based delivery systems to incorporate poorly soluble curcumin analogs for the treatment of melanoma, *European Journal of Pharmaceutics and Biopharmaceutics*, 81, pp. 548–556.
Michie, S., Yardley, L., West, R., Patrick, K. and Greaves, F. 2017. Developing and evaluating digital interventions to promote behavior change in health and health care: Recommendations resulting from an international workshop, *Journal of Medical Internet Research*, 19, p. e232.
Michielin, O., Van Akkooi, A. C. J., Ascierto, P. A., Dummer, R. and Keilholz, U. 2019. Cutaneous melanoma: ESMO Clinical Practice Guidelines for diagnosis, treatment and follow-up, *Annals of Oncology*, 30, pp. 1884–1901.
Mihajlovic, M., Vlajkovic, S., Jovanovic, P. and Stefanovic, V. 2012. Primary mucosal melanomas: A comprehensive review, *International Journal of Clinical and Experimental Pathology*, 5, pp. 739–753.
Milhem, M. M., Long, G. V., Hoimes, C. J., Amin, A., Lao, C. D., Conry, R. M., Hunt, J., Daniels, G. A., Almubarak, M. and Shaheen, M. F. 2019. Phase 1b/2, open label, multicenter, study of the combination of SD-101 and pembrolizumab in patients with advanced melanoma who are naïve to anti-PD-1 therapy. American Society of Clinical Oncology.
Mishra, H., Mishra, P. K., Ekielski, A., Jaggi, M., Iqbal, Z. and Talegaonkar, S. 2018. Melanoma treatment: From conventional to nanotechnology, *Journal of Cancer Research and Clinical Oncology*, 144, pp. 2283–2302.
Mizuhashi, S., Kajihara, I., Sawamura, S., Kanemaru, H., Makino, K., Aoi, J., Makino, T., Masuguchi, S., Fukushima, S. and Ihn, H. 2021. Skin microbiome in acral melanoma: Corynebacterium is associated with advanced melanoma, *Journal of Dermatology*, 48, pp. e15–e16.
Moynihan, K. D. and Irvine, D. J. 2017. Roles for innate immunity in combination immunotherapies, *Cancer Research*, 77, pp. 5215–5221.
Mullinax, J. E., Hall, M., Prabhakaran, S., Weber, J., Khushalani, N., Eroglu, Z., Brohl, A. S., Markowitz, J., Royster, E., Richards, A., Stark, V., Zager, J. S., Kelley, L., Cox, C., Sondak, V. K., Mulé, J. J., Pilon-Thomas, S. and Sarnaik, A. A. 2018. Combination of ipilimumab and adoptive cell therapy with tumor-infiltrating lymphocytes for patients with metastatic melanoma, *Frontiers in Oncology*, 8, p. 44.
Njoroge, M., Zurovac, D., Ogara, E. A., Chuma, J. and Kirigia, D. 2017. Assessing the feasibility of eHealth and mHealth: A systematic review and analysis of initiatives implemented in Kenya, *BMC Research Notes*, 10, p. 90.
Norval, M. and Wright, C. Y. 2017. The Epidemiology of Cutaneous Melanoma in the White and Black African Population Groups in South Africa. In: Ward, W. H. and Farma, J. M. (eds.) *Cutaneous Melanoma: Etiology and Therapy*. Brisbane (AU): Codon Publications.
Pehamberger, H., Binder, M., Steiner, A. and Wolff, K. 1993. In vivo epiluminescence microscopy: Improvement of early diagnosis of melanoma, *Journal of Investigative Dermatology*, 100, pp. 356s–362s.
Petrie, T., Samatham, R., Witkowski, A. M., Esteva, A. and Leachman, S. A. 2019. Melanoma early detection: Big data, bigger picture, *Journal of Investigative Dermatology*, 139, pp. 25–30.
Postow, M. A., Manuel, M., Wong, P., Yuan, J., Dong, Z., Liu, C., Perez, S., Tanneau, I., Noel, M., Courtier, A., Pasqual, N. and Wolchok, J. D. 2015. Peripheral T cell receptor diversity is associated with clinical outcomes following ipilimumab treatment in metastatic melanoma, *Journal for Immunotherapy of Cancer*, 3, p. 23.
Ralli, M., Botticelli, A., Visconti, I. C., Angeletti, D., Fiore, M., Marchetti, P., Lambiase, A., De Vincentiis, M. and Greco, A. 2020. Immunotherapy in the treatment of metastatic melanoma: Current knowledge and future directions, *Journal of Immunology Research*, 2020, p. 9235638.
Rastrelli, M., Tropea, S., Rossi, C. R. and Alaibac, M. 2014. Melanoma: Epidemiology, risk factors, pathogenesis, diagnosis and classification, *In Vivo*, 28, pp. 1005–1011.
Rayner, J. E., Laino, A. M., Nufer, K. L., Adams, L., Raphael, A. P., Menzies, S. W. and Soyer, H. P. 2018. Clinical perspective of 3D total body photography for early detection and screening of melanoma, *Frontiers in Medicine (Lausanne)*, 5, p. 152.
Ribas, A., Puzanov, I., Dummer, R., Schadendorf, D., Hamid, O., Robert, C., Hodi, F. S., Schachter, J., Pavlick, A. C., Lewis, K. D., Cranmer, L. D., Blank, C. U., O'day, S. J., Ascierto, P. A., Salama, A. K., Margolin, K. A., Loquai, C., Eigentler, T. K., Gangadhar, T. C., Carlino, M. S., Agarwala, S. S., Moschos, S. J., Sosman, J. A., Goldinger, S. M., Shapira-Frommer, R., Gonzalez, R., Kirkwood, J. M., Wolchok, J. D., Eggermont, A., Li, X. N., Zhou, W., Zernhelt, A. M., Lis, J., Ebbinghaus, S., Kang, S. P. and Daud, A.

2015. Pembrolizumab versus investigator-choice chemotherapy for ipilimumab-refractory melanoma (KEYNOTE-002): A randomised, controlled, phase 2 trial, *Lancet Oncology*, 16, pp. 908–918.

Rigel, D. S. and Carucci, J. A. 2000. Malignant melanoma: Prevention, early detection, and treatment in the 21st century, *CA: A Cancer Journal for Clinicians*, 50, pp. 215–36; quiz 237–240.

Rigon, R. B., Oyafuso, M. H., Fujimura, A. T., Gonçalez, M. L., Do Prado, A. H., Gremião, M. P. and Chorilli, M. 2015. Nanotechnology-based drug delivery systems for melanoma antitumoral therapy: A review, *BioMed Research International*, 2015, p. 841817.

Robert, C., Karaszewska, B., Schachter, J., Rutkowski, P., Mackiewicz, A., Stroiakovski, D., Lichinitser, M., Dummer, R., Grange, F. and Mortier, L. 2015. Improved overall survival in melanoma with combined dabrafenib and trametinib, *New England Journal of Medicine*, 372, pp. 30–39.

Robert, C., Thomas, L., Bondarenko, I., O'day, S., Weber, J., Garbe, C., Lebbe, C., Baurain, J. F., Testori, A., Grob, J. J., Davidson, N., Richards, J., Maio, M., Hauschild, A., Miller, W. H. Jr., Gascon, P., Lotem, M., Harmankaya, K., Ibrahim, R., Francis, S., Chen, T. T., Humphrey, R., Hoos, A. and Wolchok, J. D. 2011. Ipilimumab plus dacarbazine for previously untreated metastatic melanoma, *New England Journal of Medicine*, 364, pp. 2517–2526.

Rohaan, M. W., Van Den Berg, J. H., Kvistborg, P. and Haanen, J. 2018. Adoptive transfer of tumor-infiltrating lymphocytes in melanoma: A viable treatment option, *Journal for Immunotherapy of Cancer*, 6, p. 102.

Rossi, M., Pellegrini, C., Cardelli, L., Ciciarelli, V., Di Nardo, L. and Fargnoli, M. C. 2019. Familial melanoma: Diagnostic and management implications, *Dermatology Practical & Conceptual*, 9, pp. 10–16.

Russell, S. J. and Peng, K. W. 2007. Viruses as anticancer drugs, *Trends in Pharmacological Sciences*, 28, pp. 326–333.

Sachpekidis, C., Anwar, H., Winkler, J. K., Kopp-Schneider, A., Larribere, L., Haberkorn, U., Hassel, J. C. and Dimitrakopoulou-Strauss, A. 2018. Longitudinal studies of the (18)F-FDG kinetics after ipilimumab treatment in metastatic melanoma patients based on dynamic FDG PET/CT, *Cancer Immunology Immunotherapy*, 67, pp. 1261–1270.

Saginala, K., Barsouk, A., Aluru, J. S., Rawla, P. and Barsouk, A. 2021. Epidemiology of melanoma. *Medical Sciences (Basel)*, 9, p. 63.

Salem, H. F., Kharshoum, R. M., Abou-Taleb, H. A., Aboutaleb, H. A. and Abouelhassan, K. M. 2019. Progesterone-loaded nanosized transethosomes for vaginal permeation enhancement: Formulation, statistical optimization, and clinical evaluation in anovulatory polycystic ovary syndrome, *Journal of Liposome Research*, 29, pp. 183–194.

Sample, A. and He, Y. Y. 2018. Mechanisms and prevention of UV-induced melanoma, *Photodermatology, Photoimmunology & Photomedicine*, 34, pp. 13–24.

Santeufemia, D. A., Palmieri, G., Miolo, G., Colombino, M., Doro, M. G., Frogheri, L., Paliogiannis, P., Capobianco, G., Madonia, M., Cossu, A., Lo Re, G. and Corona, G. 2023. Current trends in mucosal melanomas: An overview. *Cancers (Basel)*, 15, p. 1356.

Siegel, R. L., Miller, K. D. and Jemal, A. 2020. Cancer statistics, 2020, *CA: A Cancer Journal for Clinicians*, 70, pp. 7–30.

Song, M., Liu, C., Chen, S. and Zhang, W. 2021. Nanocarrier-based drug delivery for melanoma therapeutics. *International Journal of Molecular Sciences*, 22, p. 1873.

Sosman, J. A., Kim, K. B., Schuchter, L., Gonzalez, R., Pavlick, A. C., Weber, J. S., Mcarthur, G. A., Hutson, T. E., Moschos, S. J., Flaherty, K. T., Hersey, P., Kefford, R., Lawrence, D., Puzanov, I., Lewis, K. D., Amaravadi, R. K., Chmielowski, B., Lawrence, H. J., Shyr, Y., Ye, F., Li, J., Nolop, K. B., Lee, R. J., Joe, A. K. and Ribas, A. 2012. Survival in BRAF V600-mutant advanced melanoma treated with vemurafenib, *New England Journal of Medicine*, 366, pp. 707–714.

Soyer, H. P., Argenziano, G., Chimenti, S. and Ruocco, V. 2001. Dermoscopy of pigmented skin lesions, *European Journal of Dermatology*, 11, pp. 270–276; quiz 277.

Stanganelli, I., Longo, C., Mazzoni, L., Magi, S., Medri, M., Lanzanova, G., Farnetani, F. and Pellacani, G. 2015. Integration of reflectance confocal microscopy in sequential dermoscopy follow-up improves melanoma detection accuracy, *British Journal of Dermatology*, 172, 365–371.

Sudhakar, K., Fuloria, S., Subramaniyan, V., Sathasivam, K. V., Azad, A. K., Swain, S. S., Sekar, M., Karupiah, S., Porwal, O., Sahoo, A., Meenakshi, D. U., Sharma, V. K., Jain, S., Charyulu, R. N. and Fuloria, N. K. 2021. Ultraflexible liposome nanocargo as a dermal and transdermal drug delivery system. *Nanomaterials (Basel)*, 11, p. 2557.

Sung, H., Ferlay, J., Siegel, R. L., Laversanne, M., Soerjomataram, I., Jemal, A. and Bray, F. 2021. Global cancer statistics 2020: GLOBOCAN estimates of incidence and mortality worldwide for 36 cancers in 185 countries, *CA: A Cancer Journal for Clinicians*, 71, pp. 209–249.

Taylor, J. and Pagliari, C. 2019. The social dynamics of lung cancer talk on Twitter, Facebook and Macmillan.org.uk, *NPJ Digital Medicine*, 2, p. 51.

Tiersten, A. D., Grin, C. M., Kopf, A. W., Gottlieb, G. J., Bart, R. S., Rigel, D. S., Friedman, R. J. and Levenstein, M. J. 1991. Prospective follow-up for malignant melanoma in patients with atypical-mole (dysplastic-nevus) syndrome, *Journal of Dermatologic Surgery and Oncology*, 17, pp. 44–48.

Topalian, S. L., Hodi, F. S., Brahmer, J. R., Gettinger, S. N., Smith, D. C., Mcdermott, D. F., Powderly, J. D., Carvajal, R. D., Sosman, J. A., Atkins, M. B., Leming, P. D., Spigel, D. R., Antonia, S. J., Horn, L., Drake, C. G., Pardoll, D. M., Chen, L., Sharfman, W. H., Anders, R. A., Taube, J. M., Mcmiller, T. L., Xu, H., Korman, A. J., Jure-Kunkel, M., Agrawal, S., Mcdonald, D., Kollia, G. D., Gupta, A., Wigginton, J. M. and Sznol, M. 2012. Safety, activity, and immune correlates of anti-PD-1 antibody in cancer, *New England Journal of Medicine*, 366, pp. 2443–2454.

Tran, M. A., Watts, R. J. and Robertson, G. P. 2009. Use of liposomes as drug delivery vehicles for treatment of melanoma, *Pigment Cell & Melanoma Research*, 22, pp. 388–399.

Tschandl, P., Rinner, C., Apalla, Z., Argenziano, G., Codella, N., Halpern, A., Janda, M., Lallas, A., Longo, C., Malvehy, J., Paoli, J., Puig, S., Rosendahl, C., Soyer, H. P., Zalaudek, I. and Kittler, H. 2020. Human-computer collaboration for skin cancer recognition, *Nature Medicine*, 26, pp. 1229–1234.

Tully, B., Balleine, R. L., Hains, P. G., Zhong, Q., Reddel, R. R. and Robinson, P. J. 2019. Addressing the challenges of high-throughput cancer tissue proteomics for clinical application: ProCan, *Proteomics*, 19, p. e1900109.

Ueda, Y. and Richmond, A. 2006. NF-kappaB activation in melanoma, *Pigment Cell Research*, 19, pp. 112–124.

Urso, C. 2019. Melanocytic skin neoplasms: What lesson from genomic aberrations? *American Journal of Dermatopathology*, 41, pp. 623–629.

Vaysse, C., Pautier, P., Filleron, T., Maisongrosse, V., Rodier, J. F., Lavoue, V., Reyal, F., Thomas, L., De La Fouchardière, A. and Delannes, M. 2013. A large retrospective multicenter study of vaginal melanomas: Implications for new management, *Melanoma Research*, 23, pp. 138–146.

Vensby, P. H., Schmidt, G., Kjær, A. and Fischer, B. M. 2017. The value of FDG PET/CT for follow-up of patients with melanoma: A retrospective analysis, *American Journal of Nuclear Medicine and Molecular Imaging*, 7, pp. 255–262.

Wagle, N., Van Allen, E. M., Treacy, D. J., Frederick, D. T., Cooper, Z. A., Taylor-Weiner, A., Rosenberg, M., Goetz, E. M., Sullivan, R. J. and Farlow, D. N. 2014. MAP kinase pathway alterations in BRAF-mutant melanoma patients with acquired resistance to combined RAF/MEK inhibition, *Cancer Discovery*, 4, pp. 61–68.

Wellbrock, C. and Arozarena, I. 2015. Microphthalmia-associated transcription factor in melanoma development and MAP-kinase pathway targeted therapy, *Pigment Cell & Melanoma Research*, 28, pp. 390–406.

Witkowski, A. M., Łudzik, J., Arginelli, F., Bassoli, S., Benati, E., Casari, A., De Carvalho, N., De Pace, B., Farnetani, F., Losi, A., Manfredini, M., Reggiani, C., Malvehy, J. and Pellacani, G. 2017. Improving diagnostic sensitivity of combined dermoscopy and reflectance confocal microscopy imaging through double reader concordance evaluation in telemedicine settings: A retrospective study of 1000 equivocal cases, *PLOS ONE*, 12, p. e0187748.

Wolchok, J. D., Chiarion-Sileni, V., Gonzalez, R., Grob, J.-J., Rutkowski, P., Lao, C. D., Cowey, C. L., Schadendorf, D., Wagstaff, J. and Dummer, R. 2021. *CheckMate 067: 6.5-Year Outcomes in Patients (pts) with Advanced Melanoma*. Wolters Kluwer Health.

Wong, A. N. M., Mcarthur, G. A., Hofman, M. S. and Hicks, R. J. 2017. The advantages and challenges of using FDG PET/CT for response assessment in melanoma in the era of targeted agents and immunotherapy, *European Journal of Nuclear Medicine and Molecular Imaging*, 44, pp. 67–77.

Wu, R., Forget, M. A., Chacon, J., Bernatchez, C., Haymaker, C., Chen, J. Q., Hwu, P. and Radvanyi, L. G. 2012. Adoptive T-cell therapy using autologous tumor-infiltrating lymphocytes for metastatic melanoma: Current status and future outlook, *Cancer Journal*, 18, pp. 160–175.

Yang, K., Oak, A. S. W., Slominski, R. M., Brożyna, A. A. and Slominski, A. T. 2020. Current molecular markers of melanoma and treatment targets. *International Journal of Molecular Sciences*, 21, p. 3535.

Yaroslavsky, A. N., Salomatina, E. V., Neel, V., Anderson, R. and Flotte, T. 2007. Fluorescence polarization of tetracycline derivatives as a technique for mapping nonmelanoma skin cancers, *Journal of Biomedical Optics*, 12, p. 014005.

Yi, J. H., Yi, S. Y., Lee, H. R., Lee, S. I., Lim, D. H., Kim, J. H., Park, K. W. and Lee, J. 2011. Dacarbazine-based chemotherapy as first-line treatment in noncutaneous metastatic melanoma: Multicenter, retrospective analysis in Asia, *Melanoma Research*, 21, pp. 223–227.

You, J., Guo, Y., Zhang, Y., Kang, J. J., Wang, L. B., Feng, J. F., Cheng, W. and Yu, J. T. 2023. Plasma proteomic profiles predict individual future health risk, *Nature Communications*, 14, p. 7817.

Zylberberg, C. and Matosevic, S. 2016. Pharmaceutical liposomal drug delivery: A review of new delivery systems and a look at the regulatory landscape, *Drug Delivery*, 23, pp. 3319–3329.

2 Molecular Profiling in Melanoma

Precision Strategies for Targeted Therapies

Meshack Bida, Dineo Disenyane, and Michelle McCabe
National Health Laboratory Service, University of Pretoria, Pretoria, South Africa

Thabiso Victor Miya and Zodwa Dlamini
SAMRC Precision Oncology Research Unit (PORU), DSTI/NRF SARChI Chair in Precision Oncology and Cancer Prevention (POCP), Pan African Cancer Research Institute (PACRI), University of Pretoria, Pretoria, South Africa

Stylianos Makrogkikas
Research Unit of Advanced Composite Nano-Materials and Nanotechnology, School of Chemical Engineering, National Technical University of Athens, Zografos, Athens, Greece

Georgios Lolas
SAMRC Precision Oncology Research Unit (PORU), DSTI/NRF SARChI Chair in Precision Oncology and Cancer Prevention (POCP), Pan African Cancer Research Institute (PACRI), University of Pretoria, Pretoria, South Africa
and
Research Unit of Advanced Composite Nano-Materials and Nanotechnology, School of Chemical Engineering, National Technical University of Athens, Zografos University of Athens, Athens, Greece

INTRODUCTION

Melanoma is one of the several skin malignancies that are linked with excessive sun exposure arising from melanocytes and occurs after DNA mutation (Handolias et al., 2010). The cumulative pathogenic changes in the genome lead to genomic instability and permanent genomic alterations that disrupt cellular homeostasis (Yeh and Bastian, 2021). Melanomas are more commonly seen in fair-skinned and light-haired individuals and are associated with high sun-exposure environments. Until recently, effective treatment relied on early detection and surgical excision. In the past 20 years or so, progress

DOI: 10.1201/9781003511625-2

in the development of treatment options, which includes the implementation of personalized precision medicine targeting specific molecular biomarkers to eradicate the disease, has been the subject of several clinical trials (Beuret et al. 2011). Ultraviolet radiation is linked with DNA mutations and melanoma carcinogenesis. Several genetic markers have been described in melanomas, including the *BRAF* oncogene, which results from the p.V600E protein substitution, particularly in the low-CSD (cumulative sun damage) cohort. Others include NRAS, NF1, BRAF (non-V600E mutations), and KIT, which are frequently altered in the high-CSD cohort, whereas TERT is also frequently altered in the promoter region and is linked to both cohorts. CDKN2A is the gene that encodes the p16 protein and is commonly mutated in melanomas. p16 is an oncosuppressor that is suppressed during melanoma oncogenesis, either directly or indirectly (Puckett et al., 2022).

Given that melanomas often elicit host immune responses and are regarded as being immunogenic in this regard, this offers an opportunity to explore ICIs as additional treatment targets. The immunological checkpoint is a key regulatory mechanism that limits T-cell responses and prevents detrimental inflammation. The two most thoroughly studied immunological checkpoint receptors are programmed cell death protein-1 (PD-1) and cytotoxic T-lymphocyte-associated protein-4 (CTLA-4). Immune checkpoint inhibition has altered the course of treatment for individuals with metastatic melanoma. Inhibitory receptors block several targets, including PD-1 and CTLA-4, to promote T-cell-mediated antitumor immune responses. In some cases, this improves patient survival. These immune checkpoint inhibitors (ICIs) should be closely watched, though, as they may also cause immunological-related side effects. Common immune-related adverse effects (irAEs) include endocrine, gastrointestinal, and dermatologic toxicity. Cardiotoxicity, neurotoxicity, and pulmonary toxicity are examples of fatal adverse effects from IR. The rate of irAEs is greater in ICI combination therapy than in ICI monotherapy. As amazing as it may sound, immune checkpoint blockage only produces therapeutic improvements in a small percentage of individuals. Thus, more clinically effective predictive biomarkers may determine patients who are most likely to respond to therapy as a result of an enhanced understanding of the mechanisms of action acquired by using basic scientific approaches and clinical experience. Drug options are further restricted in certain patients due to numerous mechanisms of drug resistance that have been reported. Combination treatments are being developed to increase immune checkpoint blockade's therapeutic impact. These combination therapies are useful when drug resistance has emerged and will often bypass the treatment failure due to drug resistance (Rausch and Hastings, 2017).

MOLECULAR PATHWAYS IN MELANOMA ONCOGENESIS

Mutations in Driver Genes and Subsequent Signal Transduction Pathways

Numerous driving gene mutations encoding proteins involved in several signal pathways in melanoma have been identified.

MCR1 Melanocortin Receptor 1 of the Pigmentation Pathway

The tumor suppressor p53 within the ATM/ATR pathway, along with proto-oncogenes such as *MAPK* of the MAPK pathway and *AKT* of the PI3K/AKT pathway, are notable examples. Additionally, the melanocortin receptor 1 (MC1R) mutation is significant in the pigmentation-associated pathway, which, together with cell cycle regulation, is among the pathways implicated in melanoma-driving mutations (Guo et al., 2021). The MAPK mediators, such as ERK, MEK, Ras, and Raf, are activated in response to growth factors (GFs), notably epidermal growth factor (EGF), that bind to tyrosine kinase receptors (RTKs).

In melanoma, hyperactivation of the MAPK pathway is triggered by mutations in crucial signal components like *NF1, BRAFKIT,* and *NRAS* (**Figure 2.1**). BRAF is a Raf family serine/threonine kinase implicated in the signal transduction of the MAPK pathway (Guo et al., 2021). In 2002, a point mutation in *BRAF* was observed to be more frequent in melanoma in contrast to other solid tumor types (Davies et al., 2002). About 50% of melanomas have the BRAF substitution of glutamic acid for valine at codon 600 (V600E), which induces the constitutive BRAF activation (Davies et al., 2002). BRAF ^{V600R}, BRAF ^{V600D}, and BRAF ^{V600K} are among other single-nucleotide polymorphisms (SNPs) that account for approximately 1%, 5%, and 12% of *BRAF* mutations, respectively (Lovly et al., 2012; Rubinstein et al., 2010). *BRAF* mutations indicate a poor outcome for melanoma patients (Long et al., 2011; Mann et al., 2013). The frequency of *BRAF* mutation in mucosal and acral melanoma is approximately 6% and 20%, respectively; significantly lower in comparison to that of cutaneous melanoma (Nassar and Tan, 2020; Yeh et al., 2019). A tiny GTP-binding protein from the RAS family, NRAS t activates RAF. *NRAS* mutations are typically identified at the NRAS ^{Q61}, NRAS ^{G13}, and NRAS ^{G12} locations and account for approximately 25% of melanoma cases (Randic et al., 2021).

Therapeutics against *NRAS* mutations are less developed compared to *BRAF* ^{V600E} mutants. Serine threonine kinase 19 (STK19) has been found to phosphorylate NRAS, enhancing its activity and contributing to melanoma oncogenic signaling. Researchers have been developing small-molecule inhibitors targeting STK19, called STK19 inhibitors, to reduce the phosphorylation and activation of NRAS. STK19 inhibitors specifically target the mutant NRAS signaling pathway, potentially reducing melanoma cell survival and proliferation (Yin et al., 2019). Furthermore, *NF1*, which encodes for a negative modulator of RAS, is the third most often mutated gene in melanoma, after *NRAS* and *BRAF* (Krauthammer et al., 2015; Nissan et al., 2014). In 46% of melanoma cases expressing non-mutated *RAS* and *BRAF*, *NF1* has a null mutation resulting in MAPK pathway over-activation (Andersen et al., 1993).

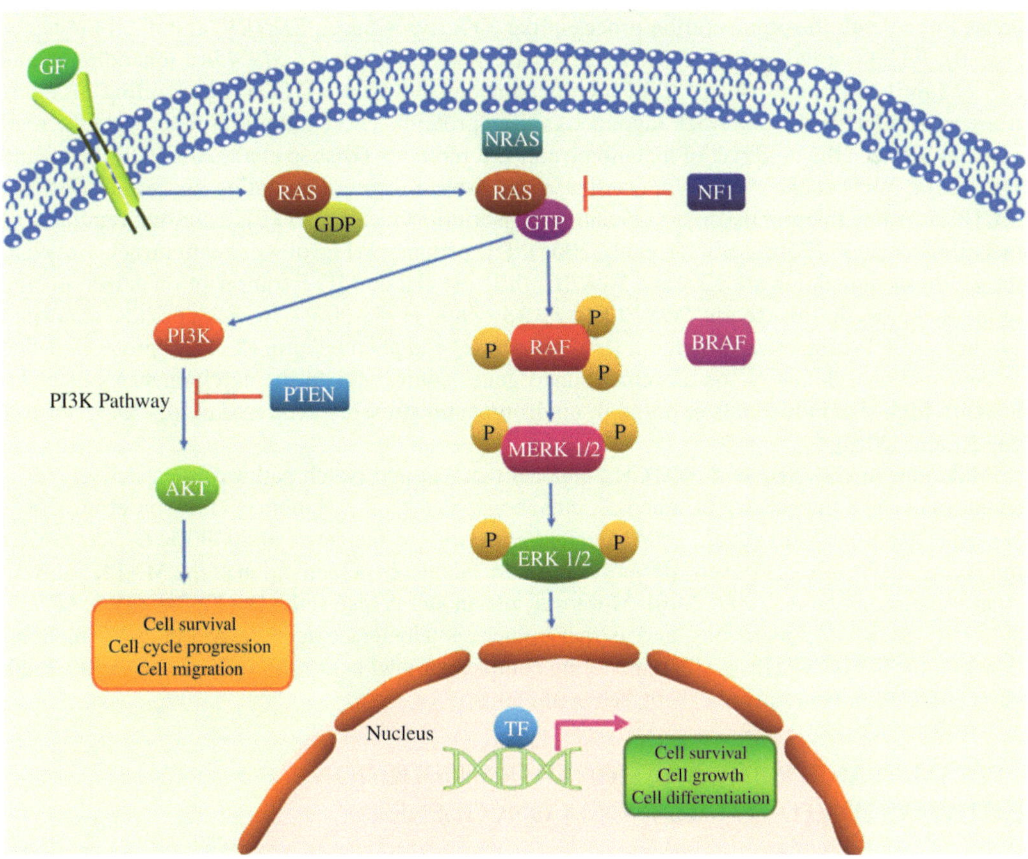

FIGURE 2.1 An illustration of the MAPK pathway. RTKs initiate MAPK signaling, leading to the activation of transcription factors inside the nucleus through the RAS, RAF, MEK, and ERK cascade. Additionally, RAS-GDP facilitates PI3K signaling via AKT activation.

Cyclin-dependent kinase inhibitor 2A (CDKN2A), Cyclin D1, retinoblastoma-associated protein (RB), P 3-kinase, and cyclin-dependent kinase 4/6 (CDK4/6) were reported to be mutated in melanoma. More specifically, over 40% of family melanomas have *CDKN2A* risk loci identified. Two proteins—p16^{Ink4a} and p14^{Arf}—are encoded by *CDKN2A*. By blocking CDK6- or CDK4-mediated phosphorylation, wild-type p16^{Ink4a} inhibits the advancement of the cell cycle. Furthermore, wild-type p14^{Arf} stops the E3 ubiquitin ligase MDM2-modulated p53 degradation. Acral melanoma frequently exhibits abnormalities in the CCND1 and CDK4/6 pathways, with incidences of approximately 40% and 80%, respectively (Kong et al., 2017; Sauter et al., 2002). Mucosal melanoma also frequently exhibits the amplification rates of *CCND1* and *CDK4*, with incidences of 27.7% and 47.0%, respectively (Xu et al., 2019). Treatment for mucosal and acral melanoma is thus anticipated to benefit from targeting the CDK4/6 pathway with a unique inhibitor (Guo et al., 2021).

PTEN loss together with AKT3 overexpression accounts for around 70% of all melanomas' dysregulated activation of the AKT pathway (Stahl et al., 2004). When exogenous GFs stimulate the AKT pathway, activated PI3K upregulates phosphatidylinositol-3,4,5-trisphosphate (PIP3) synthesis (**Figure 2.1**). Since the phosphatase PTEN negatively regulates intracellular levels of PIP3, a functional deficit in PTEN might cause the elevation of PIP3 levels and encourage AKT activation (Robertson, 2005). AKT3 is the major AKT isoform in melanoma (Sharma et al., 2009). PTEN overexpression and siRNA-mediated knockdown of *AKT3* mRNA suppresses AKT3 activity against melanoma (Stahl et al., 2004).

Approximately 90% of melanomas are sporadic cases, which are mainly active by mutations in genes linked with the pigmentation process, like *TYR* (tyrosinase), *EDNRB* (endothelin receptor type B), *PAX3* (paired box 3), *TYRP1* (tyrosinase-related protein-1), *SLC45A2* (encoding solute carrier family 45 members 2), *OCA2* (oculocutaneous albinism II), *SOX10* (encoding SRY-box transcription factor 10), and *ASIP* (agouti signaling protein). These mutations determine the relationship between the high risk of melanoma and UV radiation (Bishop et al., 2009; Hawryluk and Tsao, 2014; Ward et al., 2012). When activated by α-melanocyte-stimulating hormone (α-MSH), MC1R activates microphthalmia-associated transcription factor (MITF), a master regulator of melanin formation (García-Borrón et al., 2005). The primary MITF downstream targets linked to the synthesis of melanin are *TYR* and *TYRP1*, while the classic MITF transcription genes specific to the melanocytic lineage are *SOX10* and *PAX3* (Zhou et al., 2021). In melanocytes, abnormal synthesis of UV-protective eumelanin (UV-protective) and pheomelanin (less UV-protective) due to the functional deficit of the aforementioned genes contributes to the carcinogenesis of melanoma in high-risk individuals exposed to environmental stressors (Maresca et al., 2015; Scherer and Kumar, 2010).

Mutations in *CTNNB1 and* NOTCH2 activate the Wnt and Notch pathways, respectively, contributing to the pathogenesis of mucosal, cutaneous, and acral melanomas (Jönsson et al., 2007; Newell et al., 2020; Worm et al., 2004). Furthermore, with an incidence of 80–90%, *GNA11/GNAQ* mutations are the primary genetic drivers of uveal melanoma hyperactivation of the MAPK pathway (Van Raamsdonk et al., 2009, 2010). Moreover, melanoma is also linked to *TERT, TP53, ARID2, ARID1B*, and MDM2 mutations, and as that influences telomerase activity, p53 pathway modulation, and the SWI/SNF chromatin remodeling complex (Alaiwi et al., 2020; Forschner et al., 2020; Horn et al., 2013; Newell et al., 2019; Yeh et al., 2019).

CRUCIAL TRANSCRIPTIONAL SIGNAL TRANSDUCTION PATHWAYS LINKED TO MELANOMA ONCOGENESIS

Melanoma is derived from epidermal melanocytes. Furthermore, it shares several molecular characteristics with precursors of melanocytes, such as neural crest cells and melanoblasts (Wessely et al., 2021). Several transcriptional factors and signal transduction proteins, like

MITF, SOX10, Notch, and Wnt-β-catenin, play a critical role in melanoma. SOX10 transcription factor (TF) is active in neural crest cells and differentiates into Schwann cells and melanocytes. SOX10 mutations and the expression of the SOX10 protein are valuable tools in the diagnostic process for Schwannian and melanocytic cancers (Antonellis et al., 2008). The use of SOX10 as a specific and highly sensitive marker helps in the accurate identification of these cancers, particularly metastatic melanoma in sentinel lymph nodes (the first lymph nodes to which cancer cells have the highest probability to spread from a primary tumor), thereby aiding in effective clinical decision-making and patient management (Blochin and Nonaka, 2009; Nonaka et al., 2008; Szumera-Ciećkiewicz et al., 2020). SOX10 haploinsufficiency prevents the congenital nevus and melanoma induced by mutant *NRAS*. Knocking down SOX10 expression in melanoma cells reduces their migratory and proliferative capacity *in vitro* and growth *in vivo*. This highlights the significant role of SOX10 in cell survival (Cronin et al., 2013; Graf et al., 2014; Shakhova et al., 2012). SOX10 activates transcription of *MITF*, *SAMMSON*, *RAB7*, and *FOXD3* to modulate mitochondrial function, cell proliferation, and endolysosomal pathways. (Alonso-Curbelo et al., 2014; Han et al., 2018; Harris et al., 2010; Leucci et al., 2016).

SOX10 protein stability modulation and transcriptional activity involve several post-translational modifications like sumoylation, ubiquitination, and phosphorylation (Girard and Goossens, 2006; Han et al., 2018; Lv et al., 2015; Taylor and LaBonne, 2005). Utilizing an shRNA library, Sun et al. determined SOX10 downregulation was a major factor in vemurafenib therapy resistance. SOX10 downregulation activated transforming growth factor-β (TGF-β) signaling, increasing (EGFR) platelet-derived growth factor receptor β (PDGFRβ), and providing resistance against BRAF and MEK inhibitors (Sun et al., 2014).

SOX10 downregulation results in SAMMSON long-non-coding RNA (lncRNA) downregulation, which alerts melanoma cells to MEK and BRAF inhibitors (Han et al., 2018, 2021). On the contrary, upregulating SAMMSON and FOXD3 in the early phases of inhibitor therapy results in adaptive resistance. However, during a prolonged inhibitor treatment, mutationally acquired resistance will take hold, with the RTK overexpression(s). Rather than reducing tumor cell survival, the SOX10 downregulation enhances senescence and activates RTKs (Han et al., 2021; Smith et al., 2016; Zhang and Herlyn, 2014). MITF regulates a variety of melanoma biology signal pathways, such as those related to cell proliferation, phenotypic plasticity, metastasis, metabolism, survival, antitumor immunity, and treatment resistance (Goding and Arnheiter, 2019). Early research on the function of MITF in cell proliferation of melanoma produced conflicting results (Garraway et al., 2005; Loercher et al., 2005), which were subsequently mainly resolved through the "rheostat model" implemented by Carreira et al. (2006). More specifically, a slow-cycling condition marked by the overexpression of cell cycle inhibitors and the activation of invasion and metastasis is linked to low expression of MITF. Moderate MITF expression, on the other hand, induces a phenotypic shift from an invasive to a proliferative phenotype, giving melanoma cells a greater advantage for growth. On the other hand, a differentiation-linked G1 arrest would be restored by further upregulation of MITF expression (Carreira et al., 2006). According to the "rheostat model," there is a strong correlation between the biological function and activity level of MITF. The MITF-modulated cellular phenotype may be related to a combination of aberrant molecules participating in various biological aspects. This is because MITF regulates the expressions of numerous target genes linked with cell cycle propagation (CDK2, CCN1, p16, p21, and p27), cell differentiation (MYO5a, RAB27, TYPR1, TYR, and DCT), and invasive capacity (DIAPH1 and GMPR) (Goding and Arnheiter, 2019). Genes implicated in cell cycle arrest and invasion are mostly activated by low levels of MITF expression. Conversely, MITF expression levels ranging from low to high mainly upregulate downstream targets that promote cell division and proliferation (Guo et al., 2021).

MITF's "rheostat" function in cell proliferation, numerous investigations have offered strong proof of MITF's critical role in melanoma cell survival. MIF1α, c-MET, Bcl2, BRAC1, Bcl2a1, ML-IAP, APE1, HIF1α, and p21 are just a few of the transcriptional targets that MITF regulates to play a pro-survival function in both normal and stressful situations by controlling cell senescence, oxidative stress, DNA damage repair, and carcinogenic pathways (**Figure 2.2**) (Beuret et al., 2011; Carreira et al., 2005; Haq et al., 2013; Hartman and Czyz, 2015; Lazar et al., 2012; McGill et al., 2002). Although there has long been evidence of a link between poor MITF expression and high melanoma cell invasiveness, Bianchi-Smiraglia and colleagues have later explained the underlying mechanism (Bianchi-Smiraglia et al., 2017). According to their research, MITF primarily reduces the invasive capacity through the transcriptional modulation of guanosine monophosphate reductase (GMPR), which lowers intracellular GTP pools and subsequently levels of RHO-A, RHO-C, and active (GTP-bound) RAC1 (Bianchi-Smiraglia et al., 2017). Additionally, during the metastatic phase of melanoma, MITF decrease controls the mediating function of signal transducer and activator of transcription 3 (STAT3) through the transcriptional mediation of cAMP-response element-binding protein (CREB) (Swoboda et al., 2021). This further validates the upregulated invasive attribute in MITF-low melanomas. The MITF is a molecular rheostat that permits reversible switching between multiple cellular states based on activity levels. It does this by directly suppressing the expression of genes linked to the focal adhesion pathways, the extracellular matrix (ECM), and regulators of the epithelial-to-mesenchymal transition (EMT), like CDH2, in human melanoma cells. This has an impact on tumorigenicity and tumor progression. A characteristic of drug-resistant melanomas is an increase in focal adhesion sites upon MITF knockdown. Thus, MITF plays an active role in sculpting the melanoma TME as a repressor of gene expression (Dilshat et al., 2021).

Cell metabolism modification is also linked to MITF control of plasticity observed in melanoma cells. MITF was reported to be a transcriptional activator of stearoyl-CoA desaturase (SCD), which is a crucial lipogenic enzyme modulated by lineage. The widely expressed MITF-mediated proliferation of melanoma cells requires the conversion of saturated fatty acids into mono-unsaturated ones, which is made possible by SCD overexpression. Conversely, the de-differentiation state and enhanced invasive and metastatic potential are brought about by the inhibition of SCD in MITF-low melanoma cells, which also activates inflammation-related signaling (Vivas-García et al., 2020). Apart from the biological impacts, as previously discussed, MITF expression can also determine how sensitive BRAF-mutant melanoma is to targeted therapy that inhibits MAPK, but this function is counterintuitive when considering the stage at which drug resistance is established. Although reduced MITF expression is particularly linked to enhanced resistance in the aging microenvironment and acquired/intrinsic resistance to targeted therapy (Kaur et al., 2016; Müller et al., 2014), MITF overexpression is thought to mediate adaptive resistance within a comparatively brief period following treatment. Furthermore, it is protective against BRAF inhibitor-induced cell death (Goding and Arnheiter, 2019; Smith et al., 2016). In light of this, a drug-repositioning screening revealed that nelfinavir, an HIV-1 protease inhibitor, is a potentially effective medication to triumph over the adaptive resistance to the MAPK pathway inhibitors through the downregulation of the MITF expression (Kim and Ronai, 2016). As such, establishing the phase of drug resistance should be considered when modifying the outcome of targeted therapy through MITF expression modulation (Guo et al., 2021).

The Notch signal pathway is a basic signal channel that influences stem cell differentiation, self-renewal, and cell fate decisions in a range of organs (Asnaghi et al., 2012). Even 20 weeks after stopping therapy in mice, exposure to γ-secretase inhibitor (GSI) blocking the Notch signal affects hair pigmentation. This suggested that Notch is necessary for preserving melanocyte homeostasis (Asnaghi et al., 2012). Melanoma cells have upregulated the Notch expression levels and activity in contrast to healthy melanocytes. Melanocytes that were transfected with the constitutively active intracellular domain of Notch (NICD) exhibit malignant traits akin to melanoma and increased cell proliferation. TME elements like hypoxia and intracellular AKT pathway activation are both involved in the overexpression of Notch in melanoma (Bedogni et al., 2008). Notch can activate the MAPK pathway, upregulate N-cadherin expression, and intensify β-catenin signaling in melanoma.

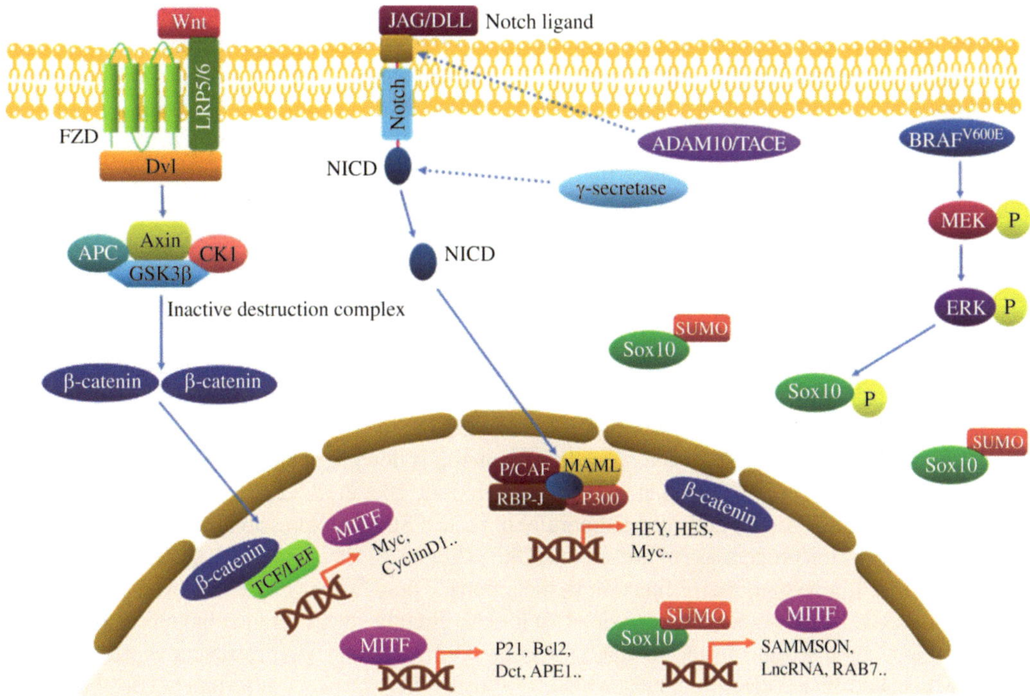

FIGURE 2.2 **Crucial signaling pathways and TFs in melanoma.** MIF1 regulates several transcriptional targets, including MIF1α, Bcl2, HIF1α, APE1, BRAC1, and p21, to perform a pro-survival role in both normal and stressed circumstances by modulating carcinogenic pathways, DNA damage repair, oxidative stress, and cell senescence. *Abbreviations*: ADAM10, ADAM metallopeptidase domain 10; APC, adenomatosis polyposis coli; DVL, disheveled segment polarity protein; FZD, frizzled class receptor; GSK3β, glycogen synthase kinase 3β; JAG, jagged canonical Notch ligand; LEF-1, lymphoid enhancer binding factor 1; LRP5/6, low-density lipoprotein receptor-related protein 5/6; MAML, mastermind-like transcriptional coactivator; NICD, Notch intracellular domain; P/CAF, P300/CBP-associated factor; RBPJ, recombination signal binding protein for immunoglobulin κ J region; TACE, TNFα-converting enzyme.

These mechanisms demonstrate that Notch functions as a nexus node, mediating several carcinogenic signals (Balint et al., 2005; Liu et al., 2006). Notch activation has a significant role in angiogenesis, and it is implicated in the communication between endothelial and tumor cells that mediates tumor migration. (Howard et al., 2013; Murtas et al., 2015).

Specifically, prolonged Notch1 activation triggers endothelial cell senescence and facilitates upregulated expression of vascular cell adhesion molecule 1 (VCAM1). In turn, this promotes neutrophil infiltration, lung colonization, tumor cell attachment to endothelium, invasion, and postsurgical metastasis (Wieland et al., 2017). Moreover, Porcelli et al. (2021) have demonstrated that Notch activation makes *BRAF*-mutant melanoma cells resistant to MEK inhibitors such as cobimetinib (Porcelli et al., 2021). A mechanism that has been conserved throughout evolution, the Wnt signal is involved in cell homeostasis, tissue regeneration, and embryonic development. In the past, the discovery that Wnt is crucial for the development of melanocytes was made based on the finding that animals lacking Wnt had no melanoblasts (Makoto et al., 1997). β-catenin's activation considerably influences the decision of cell fate, from the expansion of melanocytes to the glial derivatives loss.

In melanoma, the Wnt signaling, β-catenin-independent (noncanonical), and β-catenin-dependent (canonical) pathways focus on various elements of cell proliferation and polarity/migration (Grumolato et al., 2010). For the first time, Takeda and colleagues have reported that canonical Wnt-β-catenin signaling activates MITF through LEF-1 (Takeda et al., 2000). This is subsequently shown to be necessary for Wnt's pro-proliferative action in melanoma (Widlund et al., 2002). Suppressing p16 modulates the carcinogenic activity of the Wnt-β-catenin pathway. Consequently, melanoma development in mice with great penetration and short latency can result from the cooperation of Wnt-β-catenin activation and *NRAS* mutation (Delmas et al., 2007). Damsky and colleagues used a melanoma transgenic mouse model with a PTEN deficiency and a *BRAF* oncogenic mutation to show that β-catenin is the principal inducer of tumor propagation to the lung and lymph nodes. (Damsky et al., 2011). Furthermore, β-catenin activation in melanoma cells, resulting from Wnt3a produced from tumor-infiltrating fibroblast, reduces tumor cell adhesion and promotes motility to formulate liver metastases (Sinnberg et al., 2018). Alternative Wnt ligands involved in melanoma metastasis include Wnt11 and Wnt5a, which are generated by myeloid-derived suppressor cells (MDSC) (Douglass et al., 2021; Rodriguez-Hernandez et al., 2020).

Despite thorough research, the precise function of the Wnt-β-catenin signal during the formation of melanoma is still up for debate. Specifically, the data suggest that β-catenin cannot be entirely classified as an oncogene (Chien et al., 2009; Gallagher et al., 2013; Webster and Weeraratna, 2013). It was previously revealed that the expression of nuclear β-catenin is downregulated as melanoma progresses (Kageshita et al., 2001; Mælandsmo et al., 2003). Moreover, Uka et al. (2020) demonstrated that the Wnt/β-catenin signal must be activated temporally to reduce SOX10 expression by proteasome degradation, which halts the progression of melanoma (Uka et al., 2020). These research studies demonstrate Wnt/β-catenin's tumor-suppressive function in melanoma. Thus, further research is warranted to elucidate the precise function of Wnt in various biological circumstances, unique biological processes, and variable genetic settings in melanoma (Guo et al., 2021). Melanocyte precursors express SOX10, Notch, MITF, and Wnt-β-catenin signals, which collectively drive critical transcriptional programs that significantly add to the cancerous transition (melanocyte to melanoma). Interestingly, these same variables, such as ultraviolet-induced DNA damage, mutational burden, and immune microenvironment, that control melanoma cell development and adaptability also determine how well-targeted therapies work. Overcoming the tumor cell's de-differentiation trait could be a helpful tactic to enhance the prognosis of patients receiving MAPK inhibition-targeted therapy (Tsoi et al., 2018).

THE CURRENT STATE OF MOLECULAR BIOMARKERS FOR MELANOMA SCREENING, PROGNOSIS, AND DIAGNOSIS

Melanoma is an aggressive skin cancer that metastasizes even at early stages, with a lifetime risk of 1 in 50 (Kyrgidis, 2017). Melanoma has significant morbidity and mortality rates, with an incidence of nearly 332,000 cases and 60,000 deaths recorded globally (Ferrara and Argenziano, 2021). Despite recent breakthroughs in the treatment of advanced-stage melanoma (e.g., ICIs), there remains a large gap in the surveillance, diagnosis, staging, and monitoring of the disease (Knight et al., 2023). In its early stages, melanoma is highly treatable with high survival rates shown solely with surgery (Davis et al., 2019). After metastasis, however, survival rates are significantly low, and therefore accurate diagnosis is crucial for patients to have a good prognosis. Melanoma misdiagnosis is common in pathology and dermatology practice after breast cancer, and significant improvement in current melanoma biomarker testing and treatment strategies is required in the management of the disease (Davis et al., 2019). Melanoma has been divided into four major subtypes, according to the originator tissue cells from which the tumor develops. These include cutaneous melanoma, arising from non-glabrous (hairy) sites; acral melanoma appearing in glabrous (smooth) skin such as soles of feet and palms of hands; mucosal melanoma develops in melanocytes in the mucosa lining of tissue; and uveal melanoma from uveal tract melanocytes in the eye (Rabbie et al., 2019).

Diagnosis

To clinically diagnose melanoma requires the assessment of a pigmented skin lesion by a clinician to ascertain if benign or abnormal features exist (Deacon et al., 2021). Current methods include the

ABCDE method, which assists clinicians in detecting potential melanomas based on appearances (Duarte et al., 2021). This method includes the asymmetry of the lesion, border irregularity, color inconsistency, diameter or size increase, and evolving or progressive features. If further testing is justified, a biopsy of the lesion is taken for further evaluation by a pathologist to determine if it is malignant or benign. Histopathology remains the gold standard in diagnosing melanomas; however, intra- and inter-observer inconsistencies among pathologists remain a challenge in accurate detection and subtyping (Deacon et al., 2021; Waseh and Lee, 2023). There is therefore a greater need for molecular biomarker development to assist pathologists with ambiguous diagnostic evaluations, staging, and prognosis and to predict more targeted treatment strategies (Deacon et al., 2021).

Melanomas are described by Breslow thickness, with thin (defined as <1 mm), intermediate (1–4 mm), and thick (>4 mm) melanomas. The thickness confers the stage, prognosis, and therapy strategy (Ertekin et al., 2021; Pavlidis and Pavlidis, 2022). When malignant melanoma has been diagnosed, a sentinel lymph node biopsy (SLNB) process is performed to assess for early metastasis in the patient. Approximately 25% of melanomas with a Breslow thickness <4 mm have lymph node involvement at initial diagnosis, and approximately 60% with a thickness >4 mm (Ertekin et al., 2021). Existing pathological and clinical staging is based on the American Joint Committee on Cancer (AJCC) classification of melanocytic lesions and is grouped into 5 classes (Table 2.1): (i) benign, (ii) moderately dysplastic atypical nevus and Spitz nevus, (iii) severely dysplastic nevus, atypical Spitz nevi, (iv) AJCC T1a and T1b invasive melanomas, and (v) AJCC T1b-T4a invasive melanomas. In the absence of metastasis identified during SLNB, these primary melanomas are classified as Stage I-II (Deacon et al., 2021; Elmore et al., 2017).

TABLE 2.1
AJCC Simplified Pathological Diagnostic Classification

I	Benign nevus with or without mild atypia
II	Dysplastic moderately atypical nevi, Spitz nevi
III	Dysplastic severely atypical nevi
IV	Invasive melanomas ≤1.0 mm thick without ulceration
V	Invasive melanomas >1.0 mm thick or ≤1.0 mm thick with ulceration

Prognosis

The AJCC staging criteria is used to direct investigations and manage early disease stages; however, it cannot predict prognosis and survival rates (Rabbie et al., 2019). The clinical diversity of patient melanoma diagnosis and prognosis indicates that the standard approach to the management of the disease does not exist (Deacon et al., 2021). Metastatic melanoma generally is linked with a poor prognosis, and the five-year survival rates of melanoma (**Table 2.2**) show the highest with localized melanoma (stage 0–stage II: 90%–95%) compared to regional melanoma (stage III: up to 66%) and metastatic melanoma (stage IV: ~11%) (Knispel et al., 2021). With the administration of targeted drugs and ICIs, survival rates have improved significantly in patients with melanoma.

An additional prognostic biomarker included in the AJCC staging system is lactate dehydrogenase (LDH) assessment for staging malignant melanoma, and *BRAF* V600E mutation status is utilized as a predictive biomarker of treatment response (Balch et al., 2009). LDH is elevated in metastatic melanoma, due to the hypoxic environment of melanoma cells incapable of producing adenosine triphosphate (ATP) through oxidative phosphorylation, and so LDH converts pyruvate to lactate when oxygen supply is low (Balch et al., 2009).

ICIs (e.g., ipilimumab, nivolumab, and pembrolizumab) target CTLA-4 and PD-1 (Back et al., 2023). Treatment approved for *BRAF* ^{V600}-mutated melanoma includes inhibitors targeting MEK (e.g., trametinib) molecules and BRAF (e.g., vemurafenib) (Waninger et al., 2021).

TABLE 2.2
Prognosis According to the Simplified AJCC Staging System

Stage	Approximate Frequency of 5-Year Survival Rate (%)	Disease
0		*In situ*
1	~90–95	T1a/b, T2a
II	~45–75	T2b, T3a/b, T4a/b
III	~25–65	Involved lymph nodes
IV	~7.5–11	Distant metastases

Current Diagnostic Tests

Currently, immunohistochemistry (IHC) is used in histopathological evaluations to target preferentially expressed antigen in melanoma (PRAME), a cancer test antigen expressed in malignant neoplasms like melanoma (Harvey et al., 2021). PRAME is mostly expressed in cutaneous melanomas, whereas melanocytic nevi do not express PRAME or are limited to a small subpopulation of tumor cells. PRAME differential expression therefore serves as an important marker to differentiate between ambiguous melanocytic neoplasms. Cytogenetic tests, such as fluorescence *in situ* hybridization (FISH) for PRAME and genome-wide array-comparative genomic hybridization (CGH) for melanoma, are usually only supplementary tests requested when additional evidence is required to confirm a diagnosis. Cytogenetic tests, including PRAME FISH and CGH to detect amplifications and deletions, have been reported to be useful in confirming the diagnosis of perplexing melanocytic tumors. However, it does incur higher costs and longer turnaround times (Bastian et al., 2003; Ebbelaar et al., 2021; Harvey et al., 2021). Intermediate neoplasms with ambiguous histopathological characteristics have been found difficult to diagnose. Copy number variations (CNVs) are a reliable classification of benign (nevus) but not malignant (melanoma) tumors diagnosis; however, intermediate lesions versus melanoma CNV thresholds have not been demarcated thus far, and more defined borderlines or cut-off CNVs are required for these classification groups (Gerami et al., 2012).

Future Biomarker Tests

In the recent revision of AJCC guidelines, certain biomarkers have enhanced conventional staging guideline systems (e.g., BRAF and PRAME); however, more relevant molecular biomarker studies and clinical validations are required to effectively manage the disease. The 2018 World Health Organization (WHO) classification of melanomas has been modified according to key molecular genes and nine molecular pathways associated with melanoma subtypes (**Table 2.3**) (Ferrara and Argenziano, 2021). These include mutations in genes like *BRAF, ALK, TP53, NRAS, CDKN2A, PTEN, TERT, BAP1, GNA11*, etc. The most common mutations present in most melanomas include *BRAF* ^{V600} mutations, *TERT* promoter, *CDKN2A*, *TP53*, and *PTEN*. Biomarkers for resistance and response to ICIs are also of interest, as most advanced-stage *BRAF*-mutated melanoma patients with MEK and BRAF inhibitors show relapse within several months (Teixido et al., 2021). Key molecular pathways identified in advanced-stage melanoma progression and drug resistance mechanisms include the PI3K-AKT pathways and MAPK (Teixido et al., 2021). The β-catenin and the interferon-gamma (IFN-γ) signaling pathways were also presented as mechanisms of resistance and responses to ICIs in melanoma, and therefore targets in these pathways are worth further pursuits for biomarker research (Spranger et al., 2015). A study by Ayers and colleagues also showed a 10-gene panel targeting IFN-γ pathways in differentiating RNA expression profiles of ICI-responding versus non-responding patients (Ayers et al., 2017).

TABLE 2.3
Classification of Melanomas Modified According to the 2018 WHO Classification

UV Exposure	Subtype	Category	Altered Genes
Low	Superficial spreading melanoma	I	*BRAFV600*^{mut}, *CDKN2A NRAS, PTEN, TERT, TP53*
High	Lentigo maligna melanoma	II	*BRAF, CDKN2A, KIT, NRAS, PTEN, TERT, TP53*
	Desmoplastic melanoma	III	*NF1, NFKBIE, NRAS, PIK3CA*
Low/No	Spitz melanoma	IV	*ALK, CDKN2A, HRAS, NRTK3, NTRK1*
	Acral melanoma	V	*ALK, BRAF, CDKN2A, CCND1, KIT, NRAS, NRTK3, TERT*
	Mucosal melanoma	VI	*BRAF, CCND1, CDK4, CDKN2A, KIT, MDM2, NRAS, SF3B1*
	Melanoma in congenital nevus	VII	*BRAF* ^{V600E}, *NRAS*
	Melanoma in blue nevus	VIII	*BAP1, CYSLTR2, EIFAX, GNA11, GNAQ, SF3B1*
	Uveal melanoma	IX	*BAP1, CYSLTR2, EIFAX, GNA11, GNAQ, PLCB4, SF3B1*

With more research and larger cohort validation studies, more key biomarkers associated with melanoma subtypes, prognosis, treatment, and resistance predictions are expected to be incorporated in AJCC guidelines shortly to assist clinicians and pathologists in the accurate diagnosis and efficient management of patients with melanoma. Limitations in melanoma research studies include small amounts of available clinical specimens and the huge costs involved in validation-type laboratory experiments to confirm biomarkers and clinically relevant associations (Deacon et al., 2021). It is therefore important to conduct proper assessments to determine the most worthwhile biomarkers to be evaluated, particularly one of an associated clinical decision-making impact, before initiating biomarker validation studies. Varied clinical cohorts representing various subgroups and populations need to be taken into consideration before incorporating them into current clinical practice guidelines. Preceding any biomarker test development, important features required for a test to be considered valuable need to be determined; this way limited funds available will be utilized more cost-effectively for serviceable biomarker screening and validations.

TWO PUTATIVE PROMISING TIL AND TIL-B MARKERS CONFER BETTER SURVIVAL IN MELANOMA PATIENTS

Two promising novel, yet uncharacterized genes, increasing the survival of melanoma patients, are the *PKHD1L1* and *LAX1* genes (Martín-Lluesma et al., 2024). The *PKHD1L1* gene encodes polycystic kidney and hepatic disease 1-like protein 1 and is hypothesized to be a tumor-interfering lymphocyte (TIL) and TIL-B marker (Kang et al., 2024). *PKHD1L1* mRNA expression is markedly lower in skin cutaneous melanoma (SKCM) compared to normal tissues (Kang et al., 2024), and decreased *PKHD1L1* expression is linked with unfavorable overall survival (OS) in patients with melanoma. High PKHD1L1 expression correlates with higher OS rates in melanoma patients, indicating that it could serve as a prognostic biomarker. *PKHD1L1* expression is highly co-expressed with genes involved in immune cell functions, such as LAX1 in melanoma, which is linked with B-cell receptor (BCR) signaling and immune cell activation (Kang et al., 2024).

LAX1 is one of the genes most highly co-expressed with PKHD1L1 in SKCM, suggesting a potential role of LAX1 in melanoma biology, particularly in immune cell functions. LAX1 is an adaptor protein involved in immune cell signaling and it is primarily involved in the signaling pathways of lymphocytes. Similarly to PKHD1L1, LAX1 is also associated with BCR signaling, suggesting LAX1 is also a TIL-B marker. The expression of LAX1, alongside PKHD1L1, is indicative of a favorable prognosis in melanoma; the correlation between LAX1 and PKHD1L1 suggests that higher expression levels are associated with better patient outcomes, likely due to enhanced immune cell activity and infiltration.

The *LAX1* ENSG00000122188 gene, encoded, is a transmembrane adaptor protein primarily mediating the signaling pathways of lymphocytes, particularly T cells, B cells, NK cells, and plasma cells (Willsmore et al., 2020). Besides its expression in B cells, LAX1 shows enhanced expression in tonsils, small intestine, spleen, and appendix. At the protein level, LAX1 is predominantly localized to the plasma membrane, cytosol, and Golgi apparatus in immune cells within the lymphoid tissues and bone marrow. The co-expression of PKHD1L1 and LAX1 suggests that they may work in tandem to facilitate a robust immune response against melanoma, though the exact mechanisms of their potential interaction remain to be further elucidated (Kang et al., 2023).

MOLECULAR TARGETS OF TREATMENT IN MELANOMA

Several genetic alterations as a result of mutagenic risk factors, such as UV radiation, are potential biomarkers and targets of treatment. Through our understanding of the different molecular signaling pathways of melanoma, we can identify and characterize the potential targets for the development of therapies (Stark and Hayward, 2007). The development of immunotherapies is also made possible by these melanoma molecular pathways, particularly in cases with advanced and incurable stages III and IV melanoma. A few of these are in clinical trials or preclinical research, or they have previously received approval for usage in clinical settings (**Figure 2.3**) (**Table 2.4**).

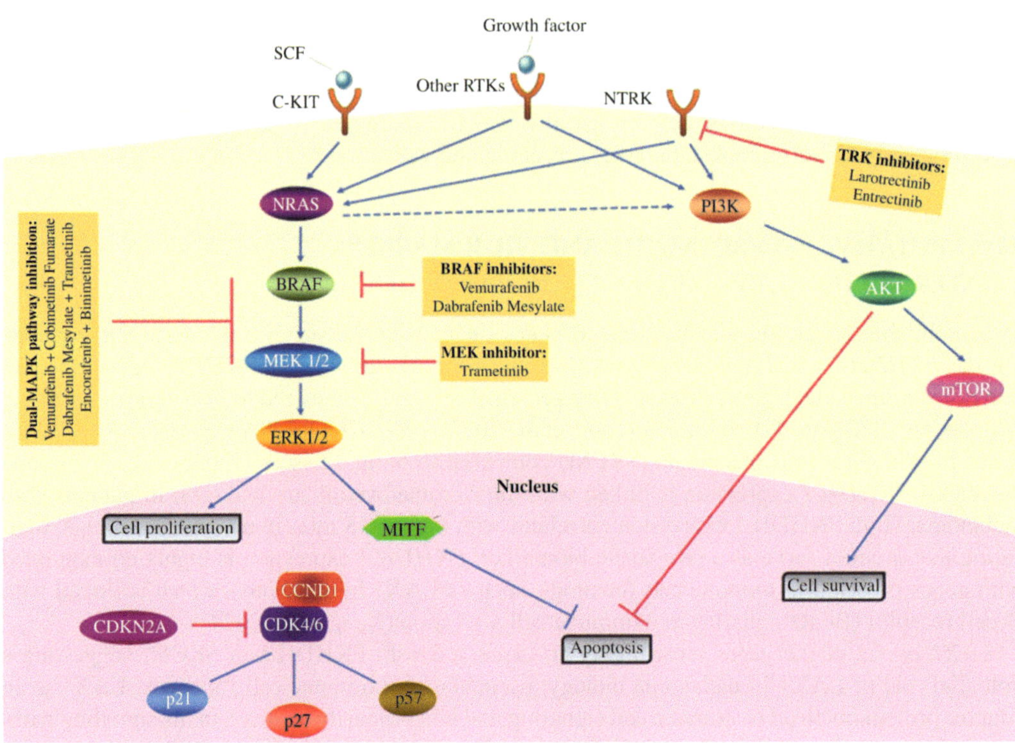

FIGURE 2.3 **US FDA-approved targeted treatment for melanoma.** Most of the targeted drug regimens are cell surface agents acting as Tyrosine Receptor Kinase inhibitors (TRKi), cytoplasmic BRAF inhibitors, and MEK inhibitors, as well as dual-MAPK pathway inhibitors. Various combination therapies assist in overcoming drug resistance. *Abbreviation*: US FDA, United States Food and Drug Administration.

TABLE 2.4
Studies on Targeted Therapy with Implications for Clinical Practice in Melanoma Patients

Trial	Trial Phase	Patients	Treatment Cohorts	Primary Endpoint	*n*	ORR	PFS	OS	References
			Anti-CTLA-4						
MDX010-020 (NCT00094653)	III	Untreated MM	Ipi 3 + gp100 vs. Ipi 3 vs. gp100 (3:1:1)	OS	676	6 vs. 11 vs. 2	2.8 vs. 2.9 vs. 2.8	10.0 vs. 10.1 vs. 6.4	Robert et al., 2011
			Anti-PD-1 +/− Anti-CTLA-4						
CM-066 (NCT01721772)	III	Untreated *BRAF*-wild type MM	Niv 3 q2w + Placebo vs. Placebo + Dacarbazine 1000 q3w (1:1)	OS	418	40 vs. 14	5.1 vs. 2.2	37.5 vs. 11.2	Robert et al., 2015
CM-067 (NCT01844505)	III	Untreated MM	Niv 1 + Ipi 3 (q3w) x4 – Niv 3; Niv 3 alone q2w, vs. Ipi 3 q3w x4 (1:1:1)	PFS and OS co-primary	945	58 vs. 44 vs. 19	11.5 vs. 6.9 vs. 2.9		Larkin et al., 2015
CM-511 (NCT02714218)	III	Untreated MM	Niv 1 + Ipi 3 (q3w) x4 – Niv 3 vs. Niv 3 +Ipi 1 (q3w) x4 – Niv 3 (1:1)	TRAE rate (grade 3–5)	360	48 vs. 34	8.9 vs. 9.9	NR vs. NR	Lebbé et al., 2018
KN-006 (NCT1866319)	III	MM ≤ 1 line (anti-PD-1/ PD-L1+/− anti-CTLA-4 included)	Pem 10 q2w vs. Pem 10 q3w vs. Ipi 3 q3w (1:1:1)	PFS and OS (co-primary)	834	34 vs. 33 vs. 12	8.4 vs. 3.4	32.7 vs. 15.9	Schachter et al., 2017
			BRAFi Monotherapy						
BRIM-3 (NCT01006980)	III	Untreated MM	Vem 960 mg bd vs. DTIC (1:1)	PFS and OS (co-primary)	675	48 vs. 5	5.3 vs. 1.6	13.6 vs. 9.7	Chapman et al., 2011
BREAK3 (NCT01227889)	III	Untreated *BRAF* V600E MM	Dab 150 bd vs. DTIC (3:1)	ORR	250	50 vs. 6	6.9 vs. 2.7	20 vs. 15.6	Hauschild et al., 2012
			Combined BRAFi + MEKi						
COMBI-v (NCT01597908)	III	Untreated *BRAF* V600E/K MM	Dab 150 bd + Tra 2 od vs. Vem 960 bd (1:1)	OS	704	64 vs. 51	11.4 vs. 7.3	NR vs. 17.2	Robert et al., 2015
COMBI-d (NCT01584648)	III	Untreated *BRAF* V600E/K MM	Dab 150 bd + Tra 2 od vs. Dab 150 bd (1:1)	PFS	423	69 vs. 53	11.0 vs. 8.8	25.1 vs. 18.7	Long et al., 2017

(Continued)

TABLE 2.4 *(Continued)*
Studies on Targeted Therapy with Implications for Clinical Practice in Melanoma Patients

Trial	Trial Phase	Patients	Treatment Cohorts	Primary Endpoint	*n*	ORR	PFS	OS	References
CoBRIM (NCT01689519)	III	Untreated *BRAF*V600 MM	Cob 60 od d1-21 + Vem 960 bd vs. Vem 960 bd + Placebo (1:1)	PFS	495	68 vs. 45	12.3 vs. 7.2	22.3 vs. 17.4	Larkin et al., 2014
COLUMBUS (NCT01909453)	III	Untreated *BRAF* V600E/K MM	Enc 450 od + Bin 45 mg bd vs. Enc 300 mg od vs. Vem 960 mg bd (1:1:1)	PFS	577	64 vs. 52 vs. 41	14.9 vs. 9.6 vs. 6.3	33.6 vs. 23.5 vs. 16.9	Dummer et al., 2018
Triplet Therapy (ICI + BRAFi + MEKi)									
IMSpire150 (NCT02908672)	III	Untreated *BRAF*V600 MM	Ate 840 d1,15 + Vem 720 bd + Cob 60 od d1-21 vs. Placebo + Vem 960 bd + Cob 60 od d1-21 (all: q4w)	PFS	514	66 vs. 65	15.1 vs. 10	Not yet reported	Gutzmer et al., 2020
COMBI-I (NCT02967692)	III	Untreated *BRAF*V600 MM	Spa 400 mg + Dab 150 bd + Tra 2 od vs. Placebo + Dab 150 + Tra 2 (q4w)	PFS	532	69 vs. 64	16.2 vs. 12.0	NR vs. NR	Long et al., 2020

Abbreviations: Ate, atezolizumab; bd, twice daily; Bin, binimetinib; Cob, cobimetinib; Dab, dabrafenib; Enc, encorafenib; Ipi, ipilimumab; IT, immunotherapy; MM, metastatic melanoma; Niv, nivolumab; NR, not reached; nr, not reported; od, once daily; ORR, overall response rate; OS, median overall survival; Pem, pembrolizumab; PFS, median progression-free survival; q2w/q3w/q4w, all two/three/four weeks; Spa, spartalizumab; Tra, trametinib; TRAE, treatment-related adverse event; Vem, vemurafenib; vs., versus.

Several molecular targets of therapy have been identified (see **Figure 2.3**), and these include the following.

BRAF AND MEK INHIBITORS

The most recent WHO classification divides melanocytic lesions into 9 groups. They are divided according to CSD, which influences the molecular changes in tumors. It also recognizes the unique genetic factors that contribute to the development of melanoma. The majority of melanomas are classified as superficial spreading or low-CSD, and they frequently exhibit the *BRAF* ^{V600} mutation. High-mutation-burden melanomas, such as desmoplastic melanomas and lentigo/maligna type, are associated with *NRAS*, *BRAF* non-^{V600E}, or *NF1* mutations. Acral and mucosal melanomas, which are not linked with CSD, do not typically exhibit *NRAS*, *BRAF*, or *NF1* mutations (triple wild type). Nonetheless, a small percentage of them may carry *KIT* or *SF3B1* mutations (Ferrara and Argenziano, 2021). Targeted therapy can be used to treat these driver genetic changes and achieve strong antitumor activity, which will enhance survival. ICIs and BRAF/MEK tyrosine kinase inhibitors have been shown to considerably ameliorate the prognosis and survival of individuals with melanoma (Teixido et al., 2021).

BRAF is a prominent target for therapy and the most frequent genetic mutation existing in 40–60% of cutaneous melanoma cases (Davies et al., 2002). About 80% of *BRAF*-mutated melanomas have the most frequent kind of *BRAF* mutation, V600E, whereas only 15% of instances have V600K and the remaining 5% have V600R/M/D/G mutations (Castillo et al., 2020). The *BRAF* ^{V600E} mutation is most commonly found in the superficial spreading subtype, lower patient ages, and non-CSD skin locales, like the proximal and trunk areas of the extremities. However, patients with V600K mutations tend to be older and have skin areas associated with CSD, like the head and neck. *BRAF* mutations in nevi are consistent with the notion that the RAF/MEK pathway activation is an early onset of melanoma, considering that certain nevi, particularly dysplastic nevi, are recognized precursor lesions of melanomas (Menzies et al., 2012; Pollock et al., 2003). Melanoma patients who have *BRAF* ^{V600} mutations have responded remarkably well to treatment when using selective BRAF inhibitors, like vemurafenib, as the first line of treatment (Chapman et al., 2011, Robert et al., 2016).

Based on the BRIM3 phase III study results, patients exposed to vemurafenib had a PFS and an OS of 5.3 and 13.6 months, respectively. This is in comparison to patients treated with dacarbazine, who had 1.6 and 9.7 months, respectively (Dummer et al., 2018). In the BREAK3 phase III trial, individuals exposed to dabrafenib had an OS and PFS of 20 and 6.9 months, respectively, whereas those exposed to the conventional chemotherapy had 15.6 and 2.7 months, respectively (Hauschild et al., 2012). In light of these discoveries, the FDA also authorized dabrafenib as a first-line therapy for *BRAF* ^{V600} mutation-positive metastatic or unresectable melanomas. A combination of BRAF inhibitor (BRAFi) called dabrafenib + MEK inhibitor (MEKi) called trametinib was the first combination of *BRAF*i + *MEK*i approved for treating advanced melanoma in the US and the European Union in 2014 and 2015, respectively. This was based on the findings of the COMBI-v trial (Robert et al., 2015). This trial contrasted dabrafenib + trametinib to vemurafenib, while the COMBI-d trial contrasted dabrafenib + trametinib to dabrafenib monotherapy (Long et al., 2015).

During the phase III COMBI-d trial, the combination had a higher overall response rate (ORR) of 69% than dabrafenib alone (53%). In the phase III COMBI-v study, the combination had an ORR of 64%, compared to 51% for vemurafenib alone. The rates of serious adverse events (AEs) and study drug discontinuation were comparable in both arms (see **Table 2.2**). The 5-year OS rate for both pooled trials was 34% for the combination arm. Furthermore, 19% of patients exposed to *BRAF*i *MEK*i achieved a complete response, while for these patients, the OS rate was 71% at 5 years (Robert et al., 2019). A second potential combination is cobimetinib + vemurafenib. Cobimetinib, another MEKi, was developed to treat metastatic melanoma in conjunction with vemurafenib. In the phase III CoBRIM study, 495 patients with previously untreated advanced melanoma were randomly randomized to receive vemurafenib plus cobimetinib or vemurafenib alone (see **Table 2.2**). ORR was 45% for vemurafenib alone and 68% for vemurafenib with cobimetinib (Larkin et al., 2014). Compared to 17.4 months for vemurafenib, the combination's median OS was 22.3 months. Extended follow-up reported a 4-year OS rate of 35% in the combination group and 29% in the control cohort (Ascierto et al., 2016). The toxicity profile of vemurafenib with cobimetinib is different from that of dabrafenib with trametinib. While pyrexia is more likely to arise with dabrafenib + trametinib, nausea, diarrhea, weariness, liver enzyme abnormalities, rash, and photosensitivity (induced by vemurafenib) are more likely to occur with vemurafenib + cobimetinib (Dreno et al., 2018).

Much more recently, a third combination of BRAFi and MEKi, encorafenib + binimetinib, was authorized. This was based on the results of the three-arm, phase III COLUMBUS experiment. In this trial, 577 patients with *BRAF* ^{V600} mutation-positive metastatic melanoma were randomly subjected to encorafenib and binimetinib, encorafenib alone, or vemurafenib monotherapy. The combination group had the greatest outcomes, with an objective response rate (ORR) of 63% compared to 51% versus 40% and a median OS of 33.6 months versus 23.5 months versus 16.9 months (Table 2.2). The most prevalent grade 3 or 4 treatment-related adverse events (TRAEs) associated with the combination were elevated glutamyltransferase (9%), creatine phosphokinase (7%), and hypertension (6%) (Dummer et al., 2018). The distinction between *BRAF* ^{V600K} and *BRAF* ^{V600E} mutations is that *BRAF* ^{V600K} melanomas exhibited a poorer response rate and a shorter median PFS with BRAFi. This is in contrast to V600E melanomas and two pooled analyses of BRAFi with MEKi in three independent trials, which revealed a shorter PFS in multivariate analysis. Even though no direct comparison was undertaken in individual phase III targeted treatment trials. V600E accounts for 80% of all BRAF V600 mutations, with V600K accounting for 14%. Although phase III targeted therapy trials did not directly compare BRAF V600K and BRAF V600E mutant melanomas, three independent trials found that BRAF V600K melanomas had a worse response rate and a shorter median PFS with BRAFi than V600E melanomas. In contrast, two pooled analyses of BRAFi + MEKi demonstrated a shorter PFS in multivariate analysis (Long et al., 2016; Schadendorf et al., 2017).

Immune Checkpoint Inhibitors

Five decades ago, Lewis Thomas and Frank Macfarlane Burnet introduced the concept of cancer immunosurveillance (Burnet, 1970). In the context of cancer, immunosurveillance plays a critical role in identifying and destroying emerging tumor cells. Nonetheless, some cancer cells can evade detection or suppress the immune response, causing tumor development and spread. This has resulted in the development of immunotherapies aimed at increasing the immune system's ability to recognize and kill cancer cells. Based on this concept and additional study findings, many immune processes' mechanisms for identifying and eliminating cancer have been identified. The year 2018 saw the Nobel Prize awarded to James Allison and Tasuku Honjo for their discoveries of PD-1 and PD-L1, two molecules essential to the inhibition of the immune system's negative regulators (Meng et al., 2024). This led to the discovery of ICIs involved in the inhibition of negative immune modulation to improve immunity against cancer cells (Kraehenbuehl et al., 2022). Immune checkpoints are immune cell surface receptors found on the surface of immune cells and function as gatekeepers (Basudan, 2023). They activate or halt the immune response (Meng et al., 2024). During the past few decades, different types of immune checkpoint molecules were discovered. These comprise, among others, lymphocyte-activation gene 3 (LAG-3), T-cell immunoglobulin, PD-1/PD-L1, CTLA-4, mucin-domain containing-3 (TIM-3), and lymphocyte-activation gene 3 (LAG-3) (Shibru et al., 2021). Due to the complex mechanism of immune checkpoint molecules, the FDA has approved a restricted number of these molecules (Meng et al., 2024). ICIs, including anti-PD-1/PD-L1 drugs, have shown remarkable effectiveness and versatility in treating a wide range of malignancies. Regretfully, not every cancer patient experiences a significant improvement from ICIs, and for the majority of cancer types, the ORRs are still somewhat low. Furthermore, there are significant obstacles to the clinical use of cancer immunotherapy due to primary and acquired resistance to ICIs (Meng et al., 2024).

Cytotoxic T-Lymphocyte-Associated Protein 4 (CTLA-4) Inhibitors

The transmembrane receptor CTLA-4, commonly referred to as CD152, is a co-inhibitory member of the immunoglobulin superfamily. It shares the B7 ligand with the co-stimulatory receptor CD28. The same B7 ligands, CD80 (B7-1) and CD86 (B7-2), are bound by both of them. Only activated conventional T lymphocytes and immunosuppressive T regulatory cells (Tregs) express CTLA-4 on their surface. The induction of T-cell immunological tolerance and the inhibitory control of T-cell activation are the primary functions of CTLA-4. CTLA-4 has been shown to reduce T-cell differentiation and proliferation, trigger cell cycle arrest, and lower interleukin 2 (IL-2) syntheses to play an inhibitory function in T-cell control (Meng et al., 2024). CTLA-4 negatively regulates T-cell responses by deploying phosphatases to the CTLA-4 intracellular domain or attenuating the T-cell receptor (TCR) and CD28 signaling by competitively binding to B7 with CD28, among other methods. Activation of Treg development and function is another mechanism (Buchbinder and Desai, 2016; Zhang et al., 2021). The protein sequences of CD28 and CTLA-4 are similar. Closely related genes can be located on chromosome 2q33. With varying affinities, they both bind the same ligands and form homodimers. T cells begin to signal negatively when CTLA-4 attaches to CD28 with an enhanced affinity and scavenges its ligands. Since antigen-presenting cells (APCs) are the primary site of expression for CTLA-4's ligands, B7-2 (CD86) and B7-1 (CD80), CTLA-4 plays a major role in immunoregulation during the early phases of the T-cell response in lymph nodes. By outbidding the costimulatory receptor CD28 for binding to B7 ligands, this placement enables CTLA-4 to modulate the initial activation of T cells and transmit inhibitory signals that stifle T-cell activity and proliferation.

Absence or blockade of CTLA-4 culminates in unregulated T-cell proliferation due to the lack of inhibitory signaling. This has been a critical insight that suggests that CTLA-4 blockade might enhance antitumor immune responses (Basudan, 2023). By blocking CTLA-4 with monoclonal antibodies, its inhibitory effects on T cells are relieved. This results in the reactivation of T-cell proliferation and differentiation into cytotoxic T lymphocytes (CTLs). These reactivated CTLs are capable of targeting and destroying tumor cells, thus exerting potent antitumor-immune effects (Meng et al., 2024). This therapeutic strategy has resulted in the development and utilization of CTLA-4 blocking antibodies, such as ipilimumab, which have shown significant promise in enhancing the body's immune response against various cancers. CTLA-4 inhibition not only boosts the total T-cell response but also promotes a more robust and prolonged immune onslaught on tumor cells, making it a valuable weapon in cancer immunotherapy. Multiple studies have indicated antitumor response via CTLA-4 inhibition in animal models with various malignancies, such as melanoma, breast, prostate, lymphoma, and colon cancers (Kwon et al., 1997; Van Elsas et al., 1999; Van Ginderachter et al., 2000). At present, ipilimumab, a human IgG1 monoclonal antibody (mAb), is a conventional antibody used as immunotherapy targeting CTLA-4. It was the first CTLA-4 antibody drug approved for the treatment of melanoma in 2010 (Boasberg et al., 2010). Several clinical investigations have found that ipilimumab has a high rate of disease modulation and benefits for improving prognosis (Larkin et al., 2019; Tawbi et al., 2021). Other studies demonstrate that treatment was linked with a considerable survival increase, a long-lasting response (>2.5 years), and perhaps long-run disease management (Hodi et al., 2010; Robert et al., 2011). Furthermore, the majority of current research has mostly focused on ICI combination therapies (Meng et al., 2024).

LAG-3 Inhibitors

LAG-3 (also called CD223) is an inhibitory transmembrane receptor in the immunoglobulin superfamily. It is expressed in activated immune cells, including regulatory T cells, effector T cells, activated B cells, plasmacytoid dendritic cells, and natural killer cells. The LAG-3 gene contains eight exons, and the encoded protein is separated into three domains (transmembrane, extracellular, and intracellular), similar to CD4. LAG-3 has several ligands, including MHC Class II (MHC-II), galactin-3 (Gal-3), LSECtin, and fibrin-as-protein 1 (FGL1). LAG-3 is significantly expressed in several tumor cells, including melanoma, colorectal cancer, and lung cancer cells. Blocking the connection between LAG-3 and FGL1 can restore T cells' ability to fight tumors. The binding of LAG-3 and FGL1 suppresses the immunological response of T cells to certain antigens. Anti-PD-1 resistance and a poor prognosis may also be linked to FGL1 expression upregulation (Meng et al., 2024).

There are various LAG-3 inhibitors available right now, some of which have started clinical studies. When combined with MHC II ligand, they can adversely control and decrease T-cell activation and proliferation. Furthermore, through binding to LSECtin and Galectin-3, LAG-3 inhibitors can also influence T-cell activity. Furthermore, LAG-3 inhibitors can stop the FGL1-LAG-3 connection (Huo et al., 2022). Relatlimab is a human IgG4 anti-LAG-3 antibody that attaches to LAG-3 and restores T-cell activity (Su et al, 2024). According to research, PD-1 and LAG-3 are co-expressed on CD8+ and CD4+ T cells, with tumor-infiltrating T cells showing the highest expression. This emphasizes the need for combined therapy (Okagawa et al., 2018; Tawbi et al., 2022). The FDA has approved the combination therapy of Relatlimab and PD-1 mAb nivolumab for treating metastatic or unresectable melanoma (Basudan, 2023).

PD-1 Inhibitors

PD-1 (also called CD279), a member of the CD28 immunoglobulin superfamily, is required to communicate programmed cell death in response to T-cell-induced processes. PD-1 is found in the TME of a variety of immune cells. T-cell exhaustion and inhibition result from inhibitory signals sent when PD-1 binds to its ligand, PD-L1 (B7-H1) (Meng et al., 2024). The FDA initially authorized pembrolizumab, a humanized IgG4 mAb, for the treatment of non-small-cell lung cancer (NSCLC) and metastatic melanoma (Kang et al., 2017; Raedler, 2015). Later, pembrolizumab was approved for treatment in other tumors, including HNSCC (Burtness et al., 2019), urothelial carcinoma, solid tumors with high microsatellite instability (MSI-H), tumors with high mutational burden (TMB-H), cervical cancer, triple-negative breast cancer (TNBC), advanced gastric cancer, and others. Pembrolizumab has been licensed by the FDA for treating advanced endometrial cancer, MSI-H, or mismatch repair-deficient (dMMR), as informed by the KEYNOTE-158 clinical trial (Basudan, 2023).

The FDA in 2014 approved nivolumab. Nivolumab is a fully human IgG4 mAb for the treatment of melanoma (Raedler, 2015). Later, nivolumab was indicated for the treatment of other cancers, including NSCLC, hepatocellular carcinoma, renal cell carcinoma, pleural mesothelioma, Hodgkin's lymphoma, HNSCC, esophageal squamous cell carcinoma (ESCC), colorectal cancer with dMMR or MSI-H, and others (Basudan, 2023). Additionally, the RELATIVITY-047 trial's outcomes demonstrated that nivolumab with a LAG-3 inhibitor can be combined to treat metastatic or incurable melanoma (Tawbi et al., 2022). Furthermore, nivolumab with chemotherapy was authorized as a neoadjuvant treatment for NSCLC in its early stages (Forde et al., 2022). Furthermore, nivolumab was granted approval for utilization in combination with either ipilimumab or chemotherapy for patients with advanced or metastatic ESCC that was not curable as advised by the CheckMate-648 clinical trial (Doki et al., 2022). In 2018, the FDA authorized cemiplimab, a fully humanized IgG4 mAb, for cutaneous squamous cell carcinoma (CSCC) treatment (Migden et al., 2018). Treatment with cemiplimab showed better PFS and OS with an adequate safety profile in comparison to other treatments like chemotherapy and EGFR inhibitors (Keeping et al., 2021).

PD-L1 Inhibitors

PD-L1, also called CD274 or B7-H1, is a ligand for PD-1 (De Sousa Linhares et al., 2019; Herbst et al., 2014). The FDA first authorized pembrolizumab, a humanized IgG4 mAb, for the treatment of NSCLC (Raedler, 2015). Later, it was approved for other types of tumors. Durvalumab (MEDI4736), a PD-L1 inhibitor, attaches to PD-L1 and inhibits interaction with PD-1. It was authorized in May 2017 by the FDA for use in conjunction with platinum-based chemotherapy for locally advanced or metastatic urothelial carcinoma (Baldini et al., 2019). The FDA authorized nivolumab, a completely human IgG4 mAb, in 2014 for the management of melanoma. Subsequently, nivolumab was approved for treating other solid tumors. A combination treatment of nivolumab + LAG-3 inhibitor has been authorized for treating unresectable or metastatic melanoma according to the RELATIVITY-047 trial findings (Tawbi et al., 2022).

Other Immunotherapy Treatment Strategies: Adoptive Cell Therapy

Adoptive immune therapy, commonly known as adoptive cell transfer (ACT), is a type of sophisticated immunotherapy in which a patient's immune cells are extracted, modified, and reinfused to combat cancer. This method typically uses T cells that are isolated from the patient's blood or tumor, multiplied, and frequently genetically altered in the laboratory to improve their ability to recognize and target cancer cells more efficiently. Common methods include CAR-T-cell therapy, where T cells are modified to express chimeric antigen receptors that specifically target cancer cells, and TIL therapy, where TILs are expanded and reinfused. Once reinfused into the patient, these enhanced T cells seek out and destroy cancer cells, offering a highly targeted and personalized treatment option. ACT has shown significant success in treating certain types of cancer, particularly hematological malignancies, and represents a promising avenue for future cancer therapies.

ACT response is achieved by identifying tumor antigens as potential targets for TILs or genetically modified T cells that target specific receptors (i.e., TCRs or CARs) (Das et al., 2023). ACT is the most effective treatment for metastatic melanoma patients, particularly those who have progressed following anti-PD-1 therapy, anti-PD-1 + anti-CTLA-4 therapy, or targeted drugs. Several papers have shown satisfactory response with increasing lymphodepletion before infusion of autologous TIL (see **Figure 2.4**). ACT uses genetically engineered autologous lymphocytes that express antitumor TCRs to induce tumor regression (Rosenberg and Dudley, 2009).

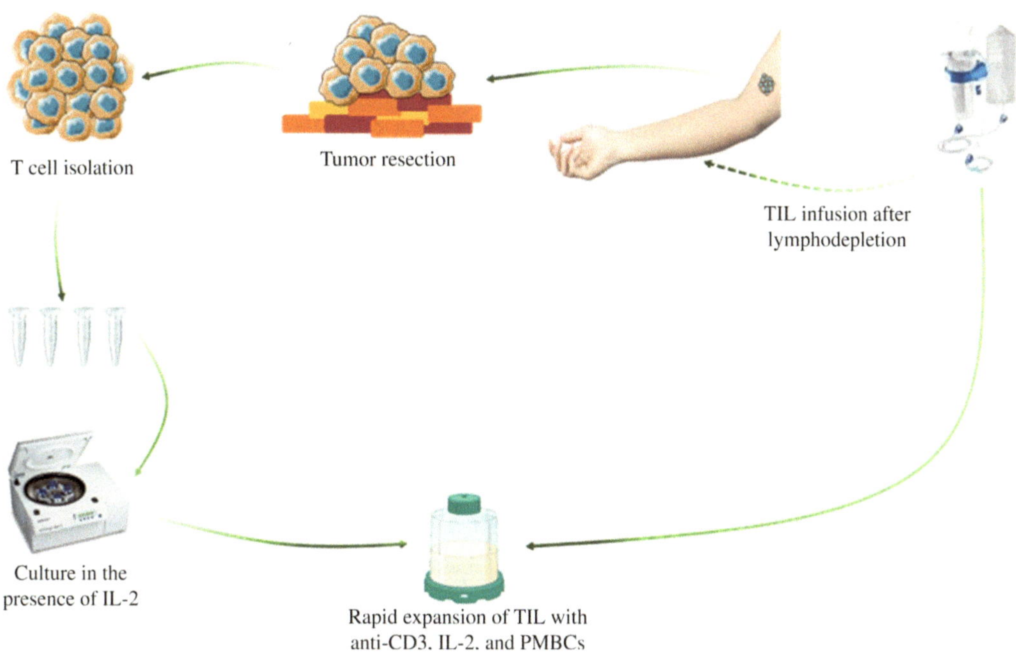

FIGURE 2.4 An illustration showing how TIL therapy is performed after lymphodepletion. T cells are harvested from the host tumor to expand tumor-reactive T-cells *in vitro*. Once this is achieved, reinfusion into the host is done so that immunoreactivity is enhanced *in vivo*.

Tumor-Infiltrating Lymphocytes

TILs are autologous CD8 and CD4 T cells with the capacity to identify antigens unique to tumors. They do, however, reach a condition of "exhaustion" and functional impairment as a result of persistent antigenic stimulation. It has been possible to reawaken these cells with good response rates by expanding them *in vitro* with IL-2 present and isolating autologous TILs from a resected metastatic melanoma (Rosenberg and Dudley, 2009).

T-Cell Receptor-Engineered T Cells

CD3 cells can be modified genetically and shortly expanded *in vitro* and be infused to be immunoreactive to a host of tumor-associated antigens. Some of these antigens include gp100-reactive TCR-T and MART-1 (Sharpe and Mount, 2015).

Chimeric Antigen Receptor T Cells

Since CAR-T cells are equipped with an entirely synthetic antigen receptor, they can specifically target and eliminate cancer cells. Apheresis is used to gather the patient's T cells at the start of the procedure. Then, in the lab, these T cells undergo genetic modification to enable CAR expression on their surface. The components of CAR include a hinge region, a transmembrane domain, an extracellular antigen recognition domain (usually derived from a monoclonal antibody), which enables the T cell to precisely recognize and bind to a target antigen on the surface of tumor cells, and intracellular signaling domains that activate the T cell upon CAR-target antigen binding.

One of the major benefits of CAR-T-cell therapy is that it does not rely on the patient's Human Leukocyte Antigen (HLA) type for targeting, making it broadly applicable. This contrasts with traditional T-cell therapies, which often require matching HLA types between the donor and recipient. CAR-T cells can directly recognize antigens on tumor cells, thereby circumventing some of the processes that tumors utilize to elude the immune system, such as the downregulation of HLA molecules. Once transformed, CAR-T cells are multiplied in the laboratory before being administered back to the patient. Upon infusion, CAR-T cells can adhere to their specific target antigen on the surface of cancer cells, activating and proliferating them, and eventually eliminating cancer cells. This unique approach has demonstrated great effectiveness in the treatment of specific types of blood malignancies, like acute lymphoblastic leukemia (ALL) and diffuse large B-cell lymphoma (DLBCL) and has promise for treating other cancer types as well (June et al., 2018).

LIMITATIONS

Resistance Mechanisms

Resistance Mechanisms to MEK and BRAF Inhibition

Despite promising findings, the majority of *BRAF*-mutated advanced melanoma patients have tumor relapse immediately after starting the BRAFi +/– MEKi treatment regimen. Drug resistance causes disease development through a variety of mechanisms, the majority of which include alternative pathway activation of both the PI3K/AKT and MAPK pathways. Inhibiting BRAF induces the upregulation of RAS activity, in turn stimulating the PI3K-AKT signaling pathway. In addition, melanoma patients having *PTEN* mutation/loss and exposed to dabrafenib have a lower median PFS (Nathanson et al., 2013). Acquired resistance mechanisms highly depend on the *NRAS* and *MAP2K* mutations (Atefi et al., 2011).

NF-1 Inhibition

Since NF-1 suppresses RAS activity in physiological circumstances, there has been much research on how it contributes to therapy resistance targeting BRAF. Constitutive RAS activation, downstream stimulation of the MAPK and PI3K-AKT signaling cascade, and resistance to target therapy are typically caused by NF-1 loss-of-function mutations. Through its interaction with CDKN2A, BRAF causes senescence and cell arrest. This implies that in a BRAF-mutated nevus, blocking CDKN2A may initiate the progression of melanoma. (Kiuru et al., 2018) found that in patients receiving dabrafenib, a decreased copy number of *CDKN2A* was substantially linked to a worse prognosis. On the other side, a larger *CCND1* copy number was significantly related to a worse prognosis and resistance to BRAFi therapy (Nathanson et al, 2013).

Due to its physiological inhibition of *RAS* activity, NF-1 has been extensively researched in resistance to BRAF-targeted therapy. Mutations that cause NF-1 to lose its function frequently result in constitutive RAS activation. This can activate the downstream PI3K-AKT and MAPK signaling pathways and also provide resistance to target therapy. When CDKN2A and BRAF interact, cell arrest and senescence result. This indicates that in a nevus with a *BRAF* mutation, CDKN2A inactivation may cause melanoma to develop. According to research by Nathanson et al., patients receiving dabrafenib had a significantly shorter PFS when their *CDKN2A* copy number was lower, but a greater *CCND1* copy number was strongly linked to an unfavorable prognosis and resistance to BRAFi (Nathanson et al., 2013).

Resistance may also result from several structural alterations in oncogenic BRAF brought on by abnormal splicing. One such example is the p61-BRAF V600E splice variant, which encodes active kinase activity but is incapable of attaching RAS. They decouple from upstream regulation and dimerize independently of the RAS state, causing constitutive signaling to reach ERK (Poulikakos et al., 2011). Tumor heterogeneity in different metastatic sites also offers heterogeneous mechanisms of resistance due to different tumor microenvironments. This heterogeneity and hence different levels of tumor response to therapies often result from variable transcriptional patterns within each tumor and show varying degrees of predicted responsiveness to inhibition of BRAF (Shi et al., 2014; Tirosh et al., 2016).

CONCLUSION

Understanding melanoma molecular mechanisms of function offers an excellent choice for detecting specific molecular biomarkers for treatment and determining melanoma prognosis. Treatment for disseminated melanoma has improved thanks to several molecular melanoma biomarkers, the most significant of which are *BRAF* mutations. The *BRAF* ^{V600} mutant, in particular, shows a significant response rate and OS benefit when combined with BRAF/MEK inhibition. Nevertheless, medication resistance is a prevalent problem even with this positive treatment outcome. In carefully selected patient cohorts, novel therapeutic targets and the development of novel immunotherapeutic medicines may be considered as alternatives, particularly if immunotherapy using anti-CTLA-4 or anti-PD-1 antibodies fails. A potent and cutting-edge therapeutic alternative has been added with ACT, which uses T cells to regulate disease (e.g., TILS, TCR-T, and CAR-T).

Finding alternate, tailored therapy is urgently needed because of the possibility of medication resistance. To choose the most effective combination treatment to overcome medication resistance, more clinical studies and information on OS and response rates are required. It is challenging to effectively treat melanoma due to the difficulty of delivering therapeutics that could penetrate the epidermis. Recent advancements have shown, however, that ionic liquids (ILs) can penetrate the epidermis, providing a new avenue for local treatment. ILs are salts in a liquid state, which consist of a combination of positively charged ions (cations) and negatively charged ions (anions). Using ILs, it is now possible to transfer multiple siRNAs against various mRNAs associated with melanoma. ILs are not only effective but also safe, non-toxic, biodegradable, and cost-effective, making them a promising solution for melanoma therapy. In contrast to classical approaches where antibodies, chemical inhibitors, and T cells are administered systemically, IL-siRNA can be applied locally, minimizing the cytotoxic effects of another systemic delivery (Eakins et al., 2022).

REFERENCES

Alaiwi, S. A. et al. 2020. Mammalian SWI/SNF complex genomic alterations and immune checkpoint blockade in solid tumors, *Cancer Immunology Research*, 8(8), pp. 1075–1084. doi: 10.1158/2326-6066.CIR-19-0866.

Alonso-Curbelo, D. et al. 2014. RAB7 controls melanoma progression by exploiting a lineage-specific wiring of the endolysosomal pathway, *Cancer Cell*, 26(1), pp. 61–76. doi: 10.1016/j.ccr.2014.04.030.

Andersen, L. et al. 1993. Mutations in the neurofibromatosis 1 gene in sporadic malignant melanoma cell lines, *Nature Genetics*, 3, pp. 73–96.

Antonellis, A. et al. 2008. Identification of neural crest and glial enhancers at the mouse Sox10 locus through transgenesis in zebrafish, *PLoS Genetics*, 4(9), p. e1000174. doi: 10.1371/journal.pgen.1000174.

Ascierto, P. A. et al. 2016. Cobimetinib combined with vemurafenib in advanced BRAFV600-mutant melanoma (coBRIM): Updated efficacy results from a randomized, double-blind, phase 3 trial, *Lancet Oncology*, 17(9), pp. 1248–1260. doi: 10.1016/S1470-2045(16)30122-X.

Asnaghi, L. et al. 2012. Notch signaling promotes growth and invasion in uveal melanoma, *Clinical Cancer Research*, 18(3), pp. 654–665. doi: 10.1158/1078-0432.CCR-11-1406.

Atefi, M. et al. 2011. Reversing melanoma cross-resistance to BRAF and MEK inhibitors by co-targeting the AKT/mTOR pathway, *PLOS ONE*, 6(12). doi: 10.1371/journal.pone.0028973.

Ayers, M. et al. 2017. IFN-γ–related mRNA profile predicts clinical response to PD-1 blockade, *Journal of Clinical Investigation*, 127(8). https://doi.org/10.1172/jci91190

Back, P. I. et al. 2023. Targeting immune checkpoint pathways in melanoma: Triumphs and challenges, *Future Drug Discovery*, 5(1). doi: 10.4155/fdd-2022-0010.

Balch, C. M. et al. 2009. Final version of 2009 AJCC melanoma staging and classification, *Journal of Clinical Oncology*, 27(36), pp. 6199–6206. doi: 10.1200/JCO.2009.23.4799.

Baldini, C. et al. 2019. Durvalumab for the management of urothelial carcinoma: A short review on the emerging data and therapeutic potential, *OncoTargets and Therapy*, 12, pp. 2505–2512. doi: 10.2147/OTT.S141040.

Balint, K. et al. 2005. Activation of Notch1 signaling is required for β-catenin-mediated human primary melanoma progression, *Journal of Clinical Investigation*, 115(11), pp. 3166–3176. doi: 10.1172/JCI25001.

Bastian, B. C. et al. 2003. Classifying melanocytic tumors based on DNA copy number changes, *American Journal of Pathology*, 163(5), pp. 1765–1770. doi: 10.1016/S0002-9440(10)63536-5.

Basudan, A. M. 2023. The role of immune checkpoint inhibitors in cancer therapy, *Clinics and Practice*, 13(1), pp. 22–40. doi: 10.3390/clinpract13010003.

Bedogni, B. et al. 2008. Notch1 is an effector of Akt and hypoxia in melanoma development, *Journal of Clinical Investigation*, 118(11), pp. 3660–3670. doi: 10.1172/JCI36157.

Beuret, L. et al. 2011. BRCA1 is a new MITF target gene, *Pigment Cell and Melanoma Research*, 24(4), pp. 725–727. doi: 10.1111/j.1755-148X.2011.00862.x.

Bianchi-Smiraglia, A. et al. 2017. Microphthalmia-associated transcription factor suppresses invasion by reducing intracellular GTP pools, *Oncogene*, 36(1), pp. 84–96. doi: 10.1038/onc.2016.178.

Bishop, D. T. et al. 2009. Genome-wide association study identifies three loci associated with melanoma risk, *Nature Genetics*, 41(8), pp. 920–925. doi: 10.1038/ng.411.

Blochin, E. and Nonaka, D. 2009. Diagnostic value of Sox10 immunohistochemical staining for the detection of metastatic melanoma in sentinel lymph nodes: Correspondence, *Histopathology*, 55(5), pp. 626–628. doi: 10.1111/j.1365-2559.2009.03415.x.

Boasberg, P., Hamid, O. and O'Day, S. 2010. Ipilimumab: Unleashing the power of the immune system through CTLA-4 blockade, *Seminars in Oncology*, 37(5), pp. 440–449. doi: 10.1053/j.seminoncol.2010.09.004.

Buchbinder, E. I. and Desai, A. 2016. CTLA-4 and PD-1 pathways similarities, differences, and implications of their inhibition, *American Journal of Clinical Oncology: Cancer Clinical Trials*, 39(1), pp. 98–106. doi: 10.1097/COC.0000000000000239.

Burnet, F. M. 1970. The concept of immunological surveillance against neoplasia, *Progress in Experimental Tumor Research*, 13, pp. 1–27.

Burtness, B. et al. 2019. Pembrolizumab alone or with chemotherapy versus cetuximab with chemotherapy for recurrent or metastatic squamous cell carcinoma of the head and neck (KEYNOTE-048): A randomised, open-label, phase 3 study, *Lancet*, 394(10212), pp. 1915–1928. doi: 10.1016/S0140-6736(19)32591-7.

Carreira, S. et al. 2005. Mitf cooperates with Rb1 and activates p21Cip1 expression to regulate cell cycle progression, *Nature*, 433(7027), pp. 764–769. doi: 10.1038/nature03269.

Carreira, S. et al. 2006. Mitf regulation of Dia1 controls melanoma proliferation and invasiveness, *Genes and Development*, 20(24), pp. 3426–3439. doi: 10.1101/gad.406406.

Castillo, P. et al. 2020. Implementation of an NGS panel for clinical practice in paraffin-embedded tissue samples from locally advanced and metastatic melanoma patients, *Exploration of Targeted Anti-Tumor Therapy*, 1(2), pp. 101–108. doi: 10.37349/etat.2020.00006.

Chapman, P. B. et al. 2011. Improved survival with vemurafenib in melanoma with BRAF V600E mutation, *New England Journal of Medicine*, 364(26), pp. 2507–2516. doi: 10.1056/nejmoa1103782.

Chien, A. J. et al. 2009. Activated Wnt/β-catenin signaling in melanoma is associated with decreased proliferation in patient tumors and a murine melanoma model, *Proceedings of the National Academy of Sciences of the United States of America*, 106(4), pp. 1193–1198. doi: 10.1073/pnas.0811902106.

Cronin, J. C. et al. 2013. SOX10 ablation arrests cell cycle, induces senescence, and suppresses melanomagenesis, *Cancer Research*, 73(18), pp. 5709–5718. doi: 10.1158/0008-5472.CAN-12-4620.

Damsky, W. E. et al. 2011. β-catenin signaling controls metastasis in Braf-activated Pten-deficient melanomas, *Cancer Cell*, 20(6), pp. 741–754. doi: 10.1016/j.ccr.2011.10.030.

Das, A. et al. 2023. Advances in adoptive T-cell therapy for metastatic melanoma, *Current Research in Translational Medicine*, 71(3), p. 103404. doi: 10.1016/j.retram.2023.103404.

Davies, H. et al. 2002. Mutations of the BRAF gene in human cancer, *Nature*, 417(6892), pp. 949–954. doi: 10.1038/nature00766.

Davis, L. E., Shalin, S. C. and Tackett, A. J. 2019. Current state of melanoma diagnosis and treatment, *Cancer Biology and Therapy*, 20(11), pp. 1366–1379. doi: 10.1080/15384047.2019.1640032.

De Sousa Linhares, A. et al. 2019. Therapeutic PD-L1 antibodies are more effective than PD-1 antibodies in blocking PD-1/PD-L1 signaling, *Scientific Reports*, 9(1), pp. 1–9. doi: 10.1038/s41598-019-47910-1.

Deacon, D. C., Smith, E. A. and Judson-Torres, R. L. 2021. Molecular biomarkers for melanoma screening, diagnosis and prognosis: Current state and future prospects, *Frontiers in Medicine*, 8(April). doi: 10.3389/fmed.2021.642380.

Delmas, V. et al. 2007. β-Catenin induces immortalization of melanocytes by suppressing p16INK4a expression and cooperates with N-Ras in melanoma development, *Genes and Development*, 21(22), pp. 2923–2935. doi: 10.1101/gad.450107.

Dilshat, R., et al. 2021. MITF reprograms the extracellular matrix and focal adhesion in melanoma, *Elife*, 10, p. e63093. doi: 10.7554/eLife.63093.

Doki, Y. et al. 2022. Nivolumab combination therapy in advanced esophageal squamous-cell carcinoma, *New England Journal of Medicine*, 386(5), pp. 449–462. doi: 10.1056/nejmoa2111380.

Douglass, S. M. et al. 2021. Myeloid-derived suppressor cells are a major source of Wnt5A in the melanoma microenvironment and depend on Wnt5A for full suppressive activity, *Cancer Research*, 81(3), pp. 658–670. doi: 10.1158/0008-5472.CAN-20-1238.

Dreno, B. et al. 2018. Efficacy and safety of cobimetinib (C) combined with vemurafenib (V) in patients (pts) with BRAFV600 mutation–positive metastatic melanoma: Analysis from the 4-year extended follow-up of the phase 3 coBRIM study, *Journal of Clinical Oncology*, 36(15). doi: https://doi.org/10.1200/JCO.2018.36.15_suppl.9522.

Duarte, A. F. et al. 2021. Clinical ABCDE rule for early melanoma detection, *European Journal of Dermatology*, 31(6), pp. 771–778. doi: 10.1684/ejd.2021.4171.

Dummer, R. et al. 2018. Encorafenib plus binimetinib versus vemurafenib or encorafenib in patients with BRAF-mutant melanoma (COLUMBUS): A multicentre, open-label, randomised phase 3 trial, *Lancet Oncology*, 19(5), pp. 603–615. doi: 10.1016/S1470-2045(18)30142-6.

Eakins, R. A. et al. 2022. Chemical complementarity between tumor resident, T-cell receptor CDR3s and MAGEA3/6 correlates with increased melanoma survival: Potential relevance to MAGE vaccine autoreactivity, *Molecular Immunology*, 150, pp. 58–66, ISSN 0161-5890.

Ebbelaar, C. F. et al. 2021. Genome-wide copy number variations as molecular diagnostic tool for cutaneous intermediate melanocytic lesions: A systematic review and individual patient data meta-analysis, *Virchows Archiv*, 479(4), pp. 773–783. doi: 10.1007/s00428-021-03095-5.

Elmore, J. G. et al. 2017. Pathologists' diagnosis of invasive melanoma and melanocytic proliferations: Observer accuracy and reproducibility study, *BMJ (Online)*, 357. doi: 10.1136/bmj.j2813.

Ertekin, S. S. et al. 2021. Initial stage of cutaneous primary melanoma plays a key role in the pattern and timing of disease recurrence, *Acta Dermato-Venereologica*, 101(7). doi: 10.2340/00015555-3832.

Ferrara, G. and Argenziano, G. 2021. The WHO 2018 classification of cutaneous melanocytic neoplasms: Suggestions from routine Practice, *Frontiers in Oncology*, 11(July), pp. 1–16. doi: 10.3389/fonc.2021.675296.

Forde, P. M. et al. 2022. Neoadjuvant nivolumab plus chemotherapy in resectable lung cancer, *New England Journal of Medicine*, 386(21), pp. 1973–1985. doi: 10.1056/nejmoa2202170.

Forschner, A. et al. 2020. MDM2, MDM4 and EGFR amplifications and hyperprogression in metastatic acral and mucosal melanoma, *Cancers*, 12(3), pp. 1–17. doi: 10.3390/cancers12030540.

Gallagher, S. J. et al. 2013. Beta-catenin inhibits melanocyte migration but induces melanoma metastasis, *Oncogene*, 32(17), pp. 2230–2238. doi: 10.1038/onc.2012.229.

García-Borrón, J. C., Sánchez-Laorden, B. L. and Jiménez-Cervantes, C. 2005. Melanocortin-1 receptor structure and functional regulation, *Pigment Cell Research*, 18(6), pp. 393–410. doi: 10.1111/j.1600-0749.2005.00278.x.

Garraway, L. A. et al. 2005. Integrative genomic analyses identify MITF as a lineage survival oncogene amplified in malignant melanoma, *Nature*, 436(7047), pp. 117–122. doi: 10.1038/nature03664.

Gerami, P. et al. 2012. A highly specific and discriminatory FISH assay for distinguishing between benign and malignant melanocytic neoplasms, *American Journal of Surgical Pathology*, 36(6), pp. 808–817. doi: 10.1097/PAS.0b013e31824b1efd.

Girard, M. and Goossens, M. 2006. Sumoylation of the SOX10 transcription factor regulates its transcriptional activity, *FEBS Letters*, 580(6), pp. 1635–1641. doi: 10.1016/j.febslet.2006.02.011.

Goding, C. R. and Arnheiter, H. 2019. MITF—The first 25 years, pp. 983–1007. doi: 10.1101/gad.324657.119. ness.

Graf, S. A. et al. 2014. SOX10 promotes melanoma cell invasion by regulating melanoma inhibitory activity, *Journal of Investigative Dermatology*, 134(8), pp. 2212–2220. doi: 10.1038/jid.2014.128.

Grumolato, L. et al. 2010. Canonical and noncanonical Wnts use a common mechanism to activate completely unrelated coreceptors, *Genes and Development*, 24(22), pp. 2517–2530. doi: 10.1101/gad.1957710.

Guo, W., Wang, H. and Li, C. 2021. Signal pathways of melanoma and targeted therapy, *Signal Transduction and Targeted Therapy*, 6(1). doi: 10.1038/s41392-021-00827-6.

Gutzmer, R. et al. 2020. Atezolizumab, vemurafenib, and cobimetinib as first-line treatment for unresectable advanced BRAFV600 mutationpositive melanoma (IMspire150): Primary analysis of the randomised, double-blind, placebo-controlled, Phase 3 trial, *Lancet*, 395, pp. 1835–1844.

Han, S. et al. 2018. ERK-mediated phosphorylation regulates SOX10 sumoylation and targets expression in mutant BRAF melanoma, *Nature Communications*, 9(1), pp. 1–14. doi: 10.1038/s41467-017-02354-x.

Han, S. et al. 2021. LncRNA SAMMSON mediates adaptive resistance to RAF inhibition in BRAF-mutant melanoma cells, *Cancer Research*, 81(11), pp. 2918–2929. doi: 10.1158/0008-5472.CAN-20-3145.

Handolias, D. et al. 2010. Mutations in KIT occur at low frequency in melanomas arising from anatomical sites associated with chronic and intermittent sun exposure, *Pigment Cell and Melanoma Research*, 23(2), pp. 210–215. doi: 10.1111/j.1755-148X.2010. 00671.x.

Haq, R. et al. 2013. BCL2A1 is a lineage-specific antiapoptotic melanoma oncogene that confers resistance to BRAF inhibition, *Proceedings of the National Academy of Sciences of the United States of America*, 110(11), pp. 4321–4326. doi: 10.1073/pnas.1205575110.

Harris, M. L. et al. 2010. Sox proteins in melanocyte development and melanoma, *Pigment Cell and Melanoma Research*, 23(4), pp. 496–513. doi: 10.1111/j.1755-148X.2010.00711.x.

Hartman, M. L. and Czyz, M. 2015. Pro-survival role of MITF in melanoma, *Journal of Investigative Dermatology*, 135(2), pp. 352–358. doi: 10.1038/jid.2014.319.

Harvey, N. T. et al. 2021. Correlation of FISH and PRAME immunohistochemistry in ambiguous superficial cutaneous melanocytic proliferations, *American Journal of Dermatopathology*, 43(12), pp. 913–920. doi: 10.1097/DAD.0000000000001951.

Hauschild, A. et al. 2012. Dabrafenib in BRAF-mutated metastatic melanoma: A multicentre, open-label, phase 3 randomised controlled trial, *Lancet*, 380(9839), pp. 358–365. doi: 10.1016/S0140-6736(12)60868-X.

Hawryluk, E. B. and Tsao, H. 2014. Melanoma: Clinical features and genomic insights, *Cold Spring Harbor Perspectives in Medicine*, 4(9), pp. 1–18. doi: 10.1101/cshperspect.a015388.

Herbst, R. S. et al. 2014. Predictive correlates of response to the anti-PD-L1 antibody MPDL3280A in cancer patients, *Nature*, 515(7528), pp. 563–567. doi: 10.1038/nature14011.

Hodi, F. S. et al. 2010. Improved survival with ipilimumab in patients with metastatic melanoma. Improved survival with ipilimumab in patients with metastatic melanoma, *New England Journal of Medicine*, 363(8), pp. 711–723.

Horn, S. et al. 2013. TERT promoter mutations in familial and sporadic melanoma, *Science*, 339(February), pp. 959–961.

Howard, J. D. et al. 2013. Notch signaling mediates melanoma-endothelial cell communication and melanoma cell migration, *Pigment Cell and Melanoma Research*, 26(5), pp. 697–707. doi: 10.1111/pcmr.12131.

Huo, J. L. et al. 2022. The promising immune checkpoint LAG-3 in cancer immunotherapy: From basic research to clinical application, *Frontiers in Immunology*, 13(July), pp. 1–10. doi: 10.3389/fimmu.2022.956090.

Jönsson, G. et al. 2007. Genomic profiling of malignant melanoma using tiling-resolution arrayCGH, *Oncogene*, 26(32), pp. 4738–4748. doi: 10.1038/sj.onc.1210252.

June, C. H. et al. 2018. CAR T cell immunotherapy for human cancer, *Science*, 359(6382), pp. 1361–1365. doi: 10.1126/science.aar6711.

Kageshita, T. et al. 2001. Loss of β-catenin expression associated with disease progression in malignant melanoma, *British Journal of Dermatology*, 145(2), pp. 210–216. doi: 10.1046/j.1365-2133.2001.04336.x.

Kang, J. Y., Yang, J., Lee, H., Park, S., Gil, M., Kim, K. E. 2023. Systematic multiomic analysis of *PKHD1L1* gene expression and its role as a predicting biomarker for immune cell infiltration in skin cutaneous melanoma and lung adenocarcinoma, *International Journal of Molecular Sciences*, 25(1), p.359. doi: 10.3390/ijms25010359. PMID: 38203530, PMCID: PMC10778817.

Kang, S. P. et al. 2017. Pembrolizumab KEYNOTE-001: An adaptive study leading to accelerated approval for two indications and a companion diagnostic, *Annals of Oncology*, 28(6), pp. 1388–1398. doi: 10.1093/annonc/mdx076.

Kaur, A. et al. 2016. SFRP2 in the aged microenvironment drives melanoma metastasis and therapy resistance, *Nature*, 532(7598), pp. 250–254. doi: 10.1038/nature17392.

Keeping, S. et al. 2021. Comparative efficacy of cemiplimab versus other systemic treatments for advanced cutaneous squamous cell carcinoma, *Future Oncology*, 17(5), pp. 611–627. doi: 10.2217/fon-2020-0823.

Kim, H. and Ronai, Z. A. 2016. HIV drug to aid melanoma therapies? *Cancer Cell*, 29(3), pp. 245–246. doi: 10.1016/j.ccell.2016.02.014.

Kiuru, M. et al. 2018. Improving classification of melanocytic nevi: Association of BRAF V600E expression with distinct histomorphologic features, *Journal of the American Academy of Dermatology*, 79(2), pp. 221–229. doi: 10.1016/j.jaad.2018.03.052.

Knight, A., Karapetyan, L. and Kirkwood, J. M. 2023. Immunotherapy in melanoma: Recent advances and future directions, *Cancers*, 15(4), pp. 1–18. doi: 10.3390/cancers15041106.

Knispel, S. et al. 2021. Outcome of melanoma patients with elevated LDH treated with first-line targeted therapy or PD-1-based immune checkpoint inhibition, *European Journal of Cancer*, 148, pp. 61–75. doi: 10.1016/j.ejca.2021.01.034.

Kong, Y. et al. 2017. Frequent genetic aberrations in the CDK4 pathway in acral melanoma indicate the potential for CDK4/6 inhibitors in targeted therapy, *Clinical Cancer Research*, 23(22), pp. 6946–6957. doi: 10.1158/1078-0432.CCR-17-0070.

Kraehenbuehl, L. et al. 2022. Enhancing immunotherapy in cancer by targeting emerging immunomodulatory pathways, *Nature Reviews Clinical Oncology*, 19, pp. 37–50. https://doi.org/10.1038/s41571-021-00552-7

Krauthammer, M. et al. 2015. Exome sequencing identifies recurrent mutations in NF1 and RASopathy genes in sun-exposed melanomas, *Nature Genetics*, 47(9), pp. 996–1002. doi: 10.1038/ng.3361.

Kwon, E. D. et al. 1997. Manipulation of T cell costimulatory and inhibitory signals for immunotherapy of prostate cancer, *Proceedings of the National Academy of Sciences of the United States of America*, 94(15), pp. 8099–8103. doi: 10.1073/pnas.94.15.8099.

Kyrgidis, A. 2017. Chapter 1 - Melanoma Epidemiology. In: Argenziano, G., Lallas, A., Longo, C., Moscarella, E., Kyrgidis, A. and Ferrara, G. (eds.) *Cutaneous Melanoma*. Academic Press, 1–9. Available at: https://www.sciencedirect.com/science/article/pii/B9780128040003000016

Larkin, J. et al. 2014. Combined vemurafenib and cobimetinib in BRAF-mutated melanoma, *New England Journal of Medicine*, 371(20), pp. 1867–1876. doi: 10.1056/nejmoa1408868.

Larkin, J. et al. 2015. Combined nivolumab and ipilimumab or monotherapy in untreated melanoma, *New England Journal of Medicine*, 373(1), pp. 23–34. doi: 10.1056/NEJMoa1504030. Erratum in: *New England Journal of Medicine*, 2018;379(22), p. 2185. doi: 10.1056/NEJMx180040.

Larkin, J. et al. 2019. Five-year survival with combined nivolumab and ipilimumab in advanced melanoma, *New England Journal of Medicine*, 381(16), pp. 1535–1546. doi: 10.1056/nejmoa1910836.

Lebbé, C. et al. 2019. Evaluation of two dosing regimens for nivolumab in combination with ipilimumab in patients with advanced melanoma: Results from the Phase IIIb/IV CheckMate 511 Trial, *Journal of Clinical Oncology*, 37(11), pp. 867–875. doi: 10.1200/JCO.18.01998.

Lazar, I. et al. 2012. The clinical effect of the inhibitor of apopotosis protein livin in melanoma, *Oncology*, 82(4), pp. 197–204. doi: 10.1159/000334234.

Leucci, E. et al. 2016. Melanoma addiction to the long non-coding RNA *SAMMSON*, *Nature*, 531(7595), pp. 518–522. doi: 10.1038/nature17161.

Liu, Z. J. et al. 2006. Notch1 signaling promotes primary melanoma progression by activating mitogen-activated protein kinase/phosphatidylinositol 3-kinase-Akt pathways and up-regulating N-cadherin expression, *Cancer Research*, 66(8), pp. 4182–4190. doi: 10.1158/0008-5472.CAN-05-3589.

Loercher, A. E. et al. 2005. MITF links differentiation with cell cycle arrest in melanocytes by transcriptional activation of INK4A, *Journal of Cell Biology*, 168(1), pp. 35–40. doi: 10.1083/jcb.200410115.

Long, G. V. et al. 2011. Prognostic and clinicopathologic associations of oncogenic BRAF in metastatic melanoma, *Journal of Clinical Oncology*, 29(10), pp. 1239–1246. doi: 10.1200/JCO.2010.32.4327.

Long, G. V. et al. 2015. Dabrafenib and trametinib versus dabrafenib and placebo for Val600 BRAF-mutant melanoma: A multicentre, double-blind, phase 3 randomised controlled trial, *Lancet*, 386(9992), pp. 444–451. doi: 10.1016/S0140-6736(15)60898-4.

Long, G. V. et al. 2016. Factors predictive of response, disease progression, and overall survival after dabrafenib and trametinib combination treatment: A pooled analysis of individual patient data from randomised trials, *Lancet Oncology*, 17(12), pp. 1743–1754. doi: 10.1016/S1470-2045(16)30578-2.

Long, G. V. et al. 2017. Standard-dose pembrolizumab in combination with reduced-dose ipilimumab for patients with advanced melanoma (KEYNOTE-029): An open-label, phase 1b trial, *Lancet Oncology*, 18(9), pp. 1202–1210. doi: 10.1016/S1470-2045(17)30428-X.

Long, G. V. et al. 2020. The anti–PD-1 antibody spartalizumab in combination with dabrafenib and trametinib in advanced *BRAF* V600–mutant melanoma: Efficacy and safety findings from parts 1 and 2 of the Phase III COMBI-i trial, *Journal of Clinical Oncology*, 8,(15_suppl).

Lovly, C. M. et al. 2012. Routine multiplex mutational profiling of melanomas enables enrollment in genotype-driven therapeutic trials, *PLOS ONE*, 7(4), p. e35309. doi: 10.1371/journal.pone.0035309.

Lv, X. B. et al. 2015. Regulation of SOX10 stability via ubiquitination-mediated degradation by Fbxw7α modulates melanoma cell migration, *Oncotarget*, 6(34), pp. 36370–36382. doi: 10.18632/oncotarget.5639.

Mælandsmo, G. M. et al. 2003. Reduced β-catenin expression in the cytoplasm of advanced-stage superficial spreading malignant melanoma, *Clinical Cancer Research*, 9(9), pp. 3383–3388.

Makoto, I. et al. 1997. Wnt signalling required for expansion of neural crest and CNS progenitors, *Nature*, 389(6654), pp. 966–970. doi: 10.1038/40146.

Mann, G. J. et al. 2013. BRAF mutation, NRAS mutation, and the absence of an immune-related expressed gene profile predict poor outcome in patients with stage III melanoma, *Journal of Investigative Dermatology*, 133(2), pp. 509–517. doi: 10.1038/jid.2012.283.

Maresca, V., Flori, E. and Picardo, M. 2015. Skin phototype: A new perspective, *Pigment Cell and Melanoma Research*, 28(4), pp. 378–389. doi: 10.1111/pcmr.12365.

Martín-Lluesma, S. et al. 2024. Efficacy of TIL therapy in advanced cutaneous melanoma in the current immuno-oncology era: updated systematic review and meta-analysis, *Annals of Oncology*, 35(10), pp. 860–872. doi: 10.1016/j.annonc.2024.07.723. Epub 2024 Jul 23. PMID: 39053767.

McGill, G. G. et al. 2002. Bcl2 regulation by the melanocyte master regulator Mitf modulates lineage survival and melanoma cell viability, *Cell*, 109(6), pp. 707–718. doi: 10.1016/S0092-8674(02)00762-6.

Meng, L. et al. 2024. Mechanisms of immune checkpoint inhibitors: Insights into the regulation of circular RNAS involved in cancer hallmarks, *Cell Death and Disease*, 15(1). doi: 10.1038/s41419-023-06389-5.

Menzies, A. M. et al. 2012. Distinguishing clinicopathologic features of patients with V600E and V600K BRAF-mutant metastatic melanoma, *Clinical Cancer Research*, 18(12), pp. 3242–3249. doi: 10.1158/1078-0432.CCR-12-0052.

Migden, M. R. et al. 2018. PD-1 blockade with cemiplimab in advanced cutaneous squamous-cell carcinoma, *New England Journal of Medicine*, 379(4), pp. 341–351. doi: 10.1056/nejmoa1805131.

Müller, J. et al. 2014. Low MITF/AXL ratio predicts early resistance to multiple targeted drugs in melanoma, *Nature Communications*, 5. doi: 10.1038/ncomms6712.

Murtas, D. et al. 2015. Activated Notch1 expression is associated with angiogenesis in cutaneous melanoma, *Clinical and Experimental Medicine*, 15(3), pp. 351–360. doi: 10.1007/s10238-014-0300-y.

Nassar, K. W. and Tan, A. C. 2020. The mutational landscape of mucosal melanoma, *Seminars in Cancer Biology*, 61, pp. 139–148. doi: 10.1016/j.semcancer.2019.09.013.

Nathanson, K. L. et al. 2013. Tumor genetic analyses of patients with metastatic melanoma treated with the BRAF inhibitor dabrafenib (GSK2118436), *Clinical Cancer Research*, 19(17), pp. 4868–4878. doi: 10.1158/1078-0432.CCR-13-0827.

Newell, F. et al. 2019. Whole-genome landscape of mucosal melanoma reveals diverse drivers and therapeutic targets, *Nature Communications*, 10(1). doi: 10.1038/s41467-019-11107-x.

Newell, F. et al. 2020. Whole-genome sequencing of acral melanoma reveals genomic complexity and diversity, *Nature Communications*, 11(1), pp. 1–14. doi: 10.1038/s41467-020-18988-3.

Nissan, M. H. et al. 2014. Loss of NF1 in cutaneous melanoma is associated with RAS activation and MEK dependence, *Cancer Research*, 74(8), pp. 2340–2350. doi: 10.1158/0008-5472.CAN-13-2625.

Nonaka, D., Chiriboga, L. and Rubin, B. P. 2008. Sox10: A pan-Schwannian and melanocytic marker, *American Journal of Surgical Pathology*, 32(9), pp. 1291–1298. doi: 10.1097/PAS.0b013e3181658c14.

Okagawa, T. et al. 2018. Cooperation of PD-1 and LAG-3 in the exhaustion of CD4+ and CD8+ T cells during bovine leukemia virus infection, *Veterinary Research*, 49(1), p. 50. doi: 10.1186/s13567-018-0543-9.

Pavlidis, E. T. and Pavlidis, T. E. 2022. Diagnostic biopsy of cutaneous melanoma, sentinel lymph node biopsy and indications for lymphadenectomy, *World Journal of Clinical Oncology*, 13(10), pp. 861–865. doi: 10.5306/wjco.v13.i10.861.

Pollock, P. M. et al. 2003. High frequency of BRAF mutations in nevi, *Nature Genetics*, 33(1), pp. 19–20. doi: 10.1038/ng1054.

Porcelli, L. et al. 2021. Active notch protects MAPK activated melanoma cell lines from MEK inhibitor cobimetinib, *Biomedicine and Pharmacotherapy*, 133(October 2020). doi: 10.1016/j.biopha.2020.111006.

Poulikakos, P. I. et al. 2011. RAF inhibitor resistance is mediated by dimerization of aberrantly spliced BRAF(V600E), *Nature*, 480(7377), pp. 387–390. doi: 10.1038/nature10662.

Puckett, Y. et al. 2022. Melanoma Pathology. *StatPearls [Internet].* Treasure Island (FL): StatPearls Publishing; 1–9. doi: 10.1093/med/9780199971015.003.0002.

Rabbie, R. et al. 2019. Melanoma subtypes: Genomic profiles, prognostic molecular markers and therapeutic possibilities, *Journal of Pathology*, 247(5), pp. 539–551. doi: 10.1002/path.5213.

Raedler, L. 2015. Keytruda (pembrolizumab): First PD-1 inhibitor approved for previously treated unresectable or metastatic melanoma, *American Health & Drug Benefits*, 8(March), pp. 96–100.

Raedler, L. A. 2015. Opdivo (nivolumab): Second PD-1 inhibitor receives FDA approval for unresectable or metastatic melanoma, *American Health & Drug Benefits*, 8(March), pp. 180–183.

Randic, T. et al. 2021. NRAS mutant melanoma: Towards better therapies, *Cancer Treatment Reviews*, 99, p. 102238. doi: 10.1016/j.ctrv.2021.102238.

Rausch, M. P. and Hastings, K. T. 2017. Immune Checkpoint Inhibitors in the Treatment of Melanoma: From Basic Science to Clinical Application. In: Ward, W. and Farma, J. (eds.) *Cutaneous Melanoma: Etiology and Therapy.* Brisbane: Codon Publications. doi: 10.15586/codon.cutaneousmelanoma.2017.ch9.

Robert, C. et al. 2011. Improved survival with ipilimumab in patients with metastatic melanoma. Improved survival with ipilimumab in patients with metastatic melanoma, *New England Journal of Medicine*, 363(26), pp. 2517–2526. doi: 10.1056/nejmoa1104621.

Robert, C. et al. 2015. Nivolumab in previously untreated melanoma without BRAF mutation, *New England Journal of Medicine*, 372(4), pp. 320–330. doi: 10.1056/nejmoa1412082.

Robert, C. et al. 2016. Three-year estimate of overall survival in COMBI-v, a randomized phase 3 study evaluating first-line dabrafenib (D) + trametinib (T) in patients (pts) with unresectable or metastatic BRAF V600E/K–mutant cutaneous melanoma, *Annals of Oncology*, 27(April), p. vi575. doi: 10.1093/annonc/mdw435.37.

Robert, C. et al. 2019. Five-year outcomes with dabrafenib plus trametinib in metastatic melanoma, *New England Journal of Medicine*, 381(7), pp. 626–636. doi: 10.1056/nejmoa1904059.

Robertson, G. P. 2005. Functional and therapeutic significance of Akt deregulation in malignant melanoma, *Cancer and Metastasis Reviews*, 24(2), pp. 273–285. doi: 10.1007/s10555-005-1577-9.

Rodriguez-Hernandez, I. et al. 2020. WNT11-FZD7-DAAM1 signalling supports tumour initiating abilities and melanoma amoeboid invasion, *Nature Communications*, 11(1). doi: 10.1038/s41467-020-18951-2.

Rosenberg, S. A. and Dudley, M. E. 2009. Adoptive cell therapy for the treatment of patients with metastatic melanoma, *Current Opinion in Immunology*, 21(2), pp. 233–240. doi: 10.1016/j.coi.2009.03.002.

Rubinstein, J. C. et al. 2010. Incidence of the V600K mutation among melanoma patients with BRAF mutations, and potential therapeutic response to the specific BRAF inhibitor PLX4032, *Journal of Translational Medicine*, 8(67), pp. 2–4.

Sauter, E. R. et al. 2002. Cyclin D1 is a candidate oncogene in cutaneous melanoma, *Cancer Research*, 62(11), pp. 3200–3206.

Schadendorf, D. et al. 2017. Three-year pooled analysis of factors associated with clinical outcomes across dabrafenib and trametinib combination therapy phase 3 randomised trials, *European Journal of Cancer*, 82, pp. 45–55. doi: 10.1016/j.ejca.2017.05.033.

Schachter, J. et al. 2017. Pembrolizumab versus ipilimumab for advanced melanoma: Final overall survival results of a multicentre, randomised, open-label phase 3 study (KEYNOTE-006). *Lancet*, 390(10105), pp. 1853–1862. doi: 10.1016/S0140-6736(17)31601-X.

Scherer, D. and Kumar, R. 2010. Genetics of pigmentation in skin cancer – A review, *Mutation Research – Reviews in Mutation Research*, 705(2), pp. 141–153. doi: 10.1016/j.mrrev.2010.06.002.

Shakhova, O. et al. 2012. Sox10 promotes the formation and maintenance of giant congenital naevi and melanoma, *Nature Cell Biology*, 14(8), pp. 882–889. doi: 10.1038/ncb2535.

Sharma, A. et al. 2009. Targeting Akt3 signaling in malignant melanoma using isoselenocyanates: *Clinical Cancer Research*, 15 (5): 1674–1685. doi: 10.1158/1078-0432.CCR-08-2214.

Sharpe, M. and Mount, N. 2015. Genetically modified T cells in cancer therapy: Opportunities and challenges, *DMM Disease Models and Mechanisms*, 8(4), pp. 337–350. doi: 10.1242/dmm.018036.

Shi, H. et al. 2014. Acquired resistance and clonal evolution in melanoma during BRAF inhibitor therapy, *Cancer Discovery*, 4(1), pp. 80–93. doi: 10.1158/2159-8290.CD-13-0642.

Shibru, B. et al. 2021. Detection of immune checkpoint receptors – A current challenge in clinical flow cytometry, *Frontiers in Immunology*, 12(July), pp. 1–32. doi: 10.3389/fimmu.2021.694055.

Sinnberg, T. et al. 2018. Wnt-signaling enhances neural crest migration of melanoma cells and induces an invasive phenotype, *Molecular Cancer*, 17(1), pp. 1–19. doi: 10.1186/s12943-018-0773-5.

Smith, M. P. et al. 2016. Inhibiting drivers of non-mutational drug tolerance is a salvage strategy for targeted melanoma therapy, *Cancer Cell*, 29(3), pp. 270–284. doi: 10.1016/j.ccell.2016.02.003.

Spranger, S., Bao, R. and Gajewski, T. F. 2015. Melanoma-intrinsic β-catenin signalling prevents anti-tumour immunity, *Nature*, 523(7559), pp. 231–235. doi: 10.1038/nature14404.

Stahl, J. M. et al. 2004. Deregulated Akt3 activity promotes development of malignant melanoma, *Cancer Research*, 64(19), pp. 7002–7010. doi: 10.1158/0008-5472.CAN-04-1399.

Stark, M. and Hayward, N. 2007. Genome-wide loss of heterozygosity and copy number analysis in melanoma using high-density single-nucleotide polymorphism arrays, *Cancer Research*, 67(6), pp. 2632–2642. doi: 10.1158/0008-5472.CAN-06-4152.

Su, J. et al. 2024. Relatlimab: A novel drug targeting immune checkpoint LAG-3 in melanoma therapy. *Frontiers in Pharmacology*, 14, p. 1349081. doi: 10.3389/fphar.2023.1349081.

Sun, C. et al. 2014. Reversible and adaptive resistance to BRAF(V600E) inhibition in melanoma, *Nature*, 508(1), pp. 118–122. doi: 10.1038/nature13121.

Swoboda, A. et al. 2021. STAT3 promotes melanoma metastasis by CEBP-induced repression of the MITF pathway, *Oncogene*, 40(6), pp. 1091–1105. doi: 10.1038/s41388-020-01584-6.

Szumera-Ciećkiewicz, A. et al. 2020. SOX10 is as specific as S100 protein in detecting metastases of melanoma in lymph nodes and is recommended for sentinel lymph node assessment, *European Journal of Cancer*, 137, pp. 175–182. doi: 10.1016/j.ejca.2020. 06.037.

Takeda, K. et al. 2000. Induction of melanocyte-specific microphthalmia-associated transcription factor by Wnt-3a, *Journal of Biological Chemistry*, 275(19), pp. 14013–14016. doi: 10.1074/jbc.C000113200.

Tawbi, H. A. et al. 2021. Safety and efficacy of the combination of nivolumab plus ipilimumab in patients with melanoma and asymptomatic or symptomatic brain metastases (CheckMate 204), *Neuro-Oncology*, 23(11), pp. 1961–1973. doi: 10.1093/neuonc/noab094.

Tawbi, H. A. et al. 2022. Relatlimab and nivolumab versus nivolumab in untreated advanced melanoma, *New England Journal of Medicine*, 386(1), pp. 24–34. doi: 10.1056/nejmoa2109970.

Taylor, K. M. and LaBonne, C. 2005. SoxE factors function equivalently during neural crest and inner ear development and their activity is regulated by SUMOylation, *Developmental Cell*, 9(5), pp. 593–603. doi: 10.1016/j.devcel.2005.09.016.

Teixido, C. et al. 2021. Molecular markers and targets in melanoma, *Cells*, 10(9), pp. 1–31. doi: 10.3390/cells10092320.

Tirosh, I. et al. 2016. Dissecting the multicellular ecosystem of metastatic melanoma by single-cell RNA-seq, *Science*, 352(6282), pp. 189–196. doi: 10.1126/science.aad0501.

Tsoi, J. et al. 2018. Multi-stage differentiation defines melanoma subtypes with differential vulnerability to drug-induced iron-dependent oxidative stress, *Cancer Cell*, 33(5), pp. 890–904.e5. doi: 10.1016/j.ccell.2018.03.017.

Uka, R. et al. 2020. Temporal activation of WNT/β-catenin signaling is sufficient to inhibit SOX10 expression and block melanoma growth, *Oncogene*, 39(20), pp. 4132–4154. doi: 10.1038/s41388-020-1267-7.

Van Elsas, A., Hurwitz, A. A. and Allison, J. P. 1999. Combination immunotherapy of B16 melanoma using Anti-Cytotoxic T Lymphocyte-associated antigen 4 (CTLA-4) and Granulocyte/Macrophage colony-stimulating factor (GM-CSF)-producing vaccines induces rejection of subcutaneous and metastatic tumors accompanied, *Journal of Experimental Medicine*, 190(3), pp. 355–366.

Van Ginderachter, J. et al. 2000. B7-1, IFN gamma and anti-CTLA-4 co-operate to prevent T-cell tolerization during immunotherapy against a murine T-lymphoma, *International Journal of Cancer*, 87(4), pp. 539–547.

Van Raamsdonk, C. D. et al. 2009. Frequent somatic mutations of GNAQ in uveal melanoma and blue naevi, *Nature*, 457(7229), pp. 599–602. doi: 10.1038/nature07586.

Van Raamsdonk, C. D. et al. 2010. Mutations in GNA11 in uveal melanoma catherine, *New England Journal of Medicine*, 363(23), pp. 2191–2199.

Vivas-García, Y. et al. 2020. Lineage-restricted regulation of SCD and fatty acid saturation by MITF controls melanoma phenotypic plasticity, *Molecular Cell*, 77(1), pp. 120–137.e9. doi: 10.1016/j.molcel.2019.10.014.
Waninger, J. J. et al. 2021. Validation of the American Joint Committee on Cancer Eighth Edition staging of patients with metastatic cutaneous melanoma treated with immune checkpoint inhibitors, *JAMA Network Open*, 4(3), p. E210980. doi: 10.1001/jamanetworkopen.2021.0980.
Ward, K. A., Lazovich, D. and Hordinsky, M. K. 2012. Germline melanoma susceptibility and prognostic genes: A review of the literature, *Journal of the American Academy of Dermatology*, 67(5), pp. 1055–1067. doi: 10.1016/j.jaad.2012.02.042.
Waseh, S. and Lee, J. B. 2023. Advances in melanoma: Epidemiology, diagnosis, and prognosis, *Frontiers in Medicine*, 10(November), pp. 1–14. doi: 10.3389/fmed.2023.1268479.
Webster, M. R. and Weeraratna, A. T. 2013. A Wnt-er migration: The confusing role of β-catenin in melanoma metastasis, *Science Signaling*, 6(268), pp. 10–12. doi: 10.1126/scisignal.2004114.
Wessely, A. et al. 2021. How neural crest transcription factors contribute to melanoma heterogeneity, cellular plasticity, and treatment resistance, *International Journal of Molecular Sciences*, 22(11). doi: 10.3390/ijms22115761.
Widlund, H. R. et al. 2002. β-Catenin-induced melanoma growth requires the downstream target microphthalmia-associated transcription factor, *Journal of Cell Biology*, 158(6), pp. 1079–1087. doi: 10.1083/jcb.200202049.
Wieland, E. et al. 2017. Endothelial Notch1 activity facilitates metastasis, *Cancer Cell*, 31(3), pp. 355–367. doi: 10.1016/j.ccell.2017.01.007.
Willsmore Z. N. et al. 2021. B cells in patients with melanoma: Implications for treatment with checkpoint inhibitor antibodies. *Frontiers in Immunology*, 11, p. 622442. doi: 10.3389/fimmu.2020.622442. PMID: 33569063; PMCID: PMC7868381.
Worm, J. et al. 2004. Genetic and epigenetic alterations of the APC gene in malignant melanoma, *Oncogene*, 23(30), pp. 5215–5226. doi: 10.1038/sj.onc.1207647.
Xu, L. et al. 2019. Frequent genetic aberrations in the cell cycle related genes in mucosal melanoma indicate the potential for targeted therapy, *Journal of Translational Medicine*. BioMed Central, 17(1), pp. 1–15. doi: 10.1186/s12967-019-1987-z.
Yeh, I. and Bastian, B. C. 2021. Melanoma pathology: New approaches and classification, *British Journal of Dermatology*, 185(2), pp. 282–293. doi: 10.1111/bjd.20427.
Yeh, I. et al. 2019. Targeted genomic profiling of acral melanoma, *Journal of the National Cancer Institute*, 111(10), pp. 1068–1077. doi: 10.1093/jnci/djz005.
Yin, C. et al. 2019. Pharmacological targeting of STK19 inhibits oncogenic NRAS-driven melanomagenesis, *Cell*, 176(5), pp. 1113–1127.e16. doi: 10.1016/j.cell.2019.01.002.
Zhang, A. et al. 2021. Dual targeting of CTLA-4 and CD47 on T_{reg} cells promotes immunity against solid tumors, *Science Translational Medicine*, 13(605), pp. 1–15. doi: 10.1126/scitranslmed.abg8693.
Zhang, G. and Herlyn, M. 2014. Linking SOX10 to a slow-growth resistance phenotype, *Cell Research*, 24(8), pp. 906–907. doi: 10.1038/cr.2014.67.
Zhou, S. et al. 2021. Epigenetic regulation of melanogenesis, *Ageing Research Reviews*, 69(May). doi: 10.1016/j.arr.2021.101349.

3 Artificial Intelligence in Melanoma Diagnostics
Revolutionizing Detection and Diagnosis

Sikhumbuzo Z. Mbatha
University of Pretoria, Pretoria, South Africa

Anil Madaree
University of KwaZulu-Natal, Nelson R. Mandela School of Medicine, Durban, South Africa

Ravi Mehrotra
Indian Cancer Genome Atlas, Pune, Maharashtra, India
Centre for Health Innovation and Policy (CHIP) Foundation, Noida, Uttar Pradesh, India

Zodwa Dlamini
SAMRC Precision Oncology Research Unit (PORU), DSTI/NRF SARChI Chair in Precision Oncology and Cancer Prevention (POCP), Pan African Cancer Research Institute (PACRI), University of Pretoria, Pretoria, South Africa

INTRODUCTION

Skin cancer prevalence has significantly increased over the past decades, particularly keratinocyte carcinomas (KC), such as squamous cell carcinoma and basal cell carcinoma, with melanoma also increasing significantly amongst fair-skinned individuals. Melanoma arises from melanocytes (melanin-producing cells) and is predominantly found in the skin; however, rarely, it can involve other epithelial surfaces such as the gastrointestinal mucosa and uveal tract (Rabbie et al., 2019). It is a heterogeneous malignancy composed of various histological variants that have different clinical behavior and prognosis. These variants include mucosal melanoma, desmoplastic melanoma, nevoid melanoma, lentigo maligna melanoma, nodular melanoma, acral lentiginous melanoma, and superficial spreading melanoma (Davis et al., 2019). It was estimated that, in 2022, there were 331,647 new instances of cutaneous malignant melanoma (MM) with 58,645 mortalities (Bray et al., 2024). There are wide geographic variations in the incidence rates of melanoma, with the highest incidence rates seen in countries populated by fair-skinned individuals in Europe, North America, and Australia, whilst the lowest incidence rates are seen in darker-skinned populations (Arnold et al., 2022). This is a result of low levels of the black/brown pigment eumelanin, which is abundant in darker-skinned individuals, and higher levels of red/yellow pigment pheomelanin seen in lighter-skinned people. Whilst eumelanin offers a more

 DOI: 10.1201/9781003511625-3

effective ultraviolet (UV) shield, pheomelanin confers poorer protection against UV radiation, and its production is associated with carcinogen production and UV-A-induced reactive oxygen species (ROS) production. These ROS facilitate greater DNA damage in skin cells in response to UV radiation (Davis et al., 2019).

Although constituting only approximately 2–5% of all cutaneous malignancies, melanoma is the most perilous and lethal form of skin cancer, accounting for 75–80% of all deaths related to the disease (Esteva et al., 2017; Urban et al., 2021). It's critical to diagnose melanoma early to be able to achieve favorable outcomes, and therefore the best form of management will be to identify early lesions that have excellent prognosis following appropriate curative surgical resection. The management and prognosis of melanoma are largely guided by the staging of the tumor. The Breslow depth classification has long been used to stage the tumor. This is the measurement of the tumor depth from the granular layer of the epidermis. The stages are T1s (no penetration into the dermis), T2 (<1 mm), T3 (1–2 mm), T4 (2–4 mm), and T5 (>4 mm). The American Joint Committee on Cancer (AJCC) staging system is the current standard for staging. The AJCC system assigns a stage based on the tumor (depth and presence of ulceration), node, and metastasis (TNM) scores. Enough research has conclusively confirmed that thin early melanomas have the best prognosis, with a 10-year survival rate of 99.5% seen in patients with lesions that are thinner than 0.76 mm (Friedman et al., 1985). Early recognition of melanoma is associated with an overall 5-year survival of over 99% for stage 1–2 disease, whilst delayed diagnosis with stage 4 disease is linked to a poor prognosis; in America, the 5-year overall survival rate is less than 30% (Saginala et al., 2021). The ultimate diagnosis of melanoma is reached using a series of steps that include the patient's self-examination with identification of a suspicious new lesion, an evaluation by a primary care physician, who subsequently refers the patient to a specialist dermatologist for assessment of the lesion, and finally a biopsy for histopathological confirmation of the diagnosis. Strategies to improve diagnostic accuracy can be implemented during any of the above steps (Phillips et al., 2019). A reasonably reliable diagnosis of melanoma still relies on obtaining a histopathological diagnosis via a biopsy, which is laborious, expensive, time-consuming, and leads to significant discomfort for the patient. Computer-based technologies involving artificial intelligence (AI) promise to help us arrive at diagnosis timeously whilst avoiding unnecessary biopsies (Singh et al., 2024).

AI in healthcare systems has been successfully utilized in multiple phases of healthcare delivery, such as in diagnostics, perioperative planning, drug development and drug delivery, prognostication, and robotic applications (Bellini et al., 2022). Over the past 2–3 decades, the amount of big data that is currently available in the medical field has increased exponentially, driven largely by the advent of multi-omic studies (i.e., pathomics, radiomics, etc.); this increase in available data has fortunately been accompanied by a notable increase in the computational abilities of computer science and AI capabilities. Big data analytics, which uses AI algorithms, has been demonstrated to greatly increase diagnostic speed and accuracy. It also offers clinical decision support tools that assist physicians in improving cancer treatment outcomes for patients (Borges Do Nascimento et al., 2021). The number needed for biopsy to identify a single melanoma showed wide variance between different health regions and amongst clinicians resulting in a large number of unnecessary biopsies with the attendant consequences of increased healthcare costs and patient morbidity, which highlights the difficulties associated with melanoma diagnosis (Nelson et al., 2019). Strategies to improve the NNB can include the incorporation of AI in the melanoma diagnostic armamentarium. AI algorithms have been used successfully in the evaluation of multiple cancers, including MM. The AI models used to evaluate the dermoscopic images of melanoma include machine learning processes such as convolutional neural network (CNN), neural network classifiers, and support vector machines, all of which can process medical images with high sensitivity, specificity, and accuracy (Zhang et al., 2022).

Skin cancer represents one of the most common malignancies globally and is associated with increasing incidence amongst the white population, with both melanoma and non-melanoma skin cancers accounting for the majority of cancer cases found in people with fair skin (Leiter et al., 2020). Previously, accurate classification and diagnosis of skin cancer by clinicians relied on experience gained from seeing a large number of patients over several years. AI in skin cancer promises to provide a reliable and novel diagnostic tool that will facilitate early, prompt diagnosis and a quick bridge between primary, secondary, and tertiary care. In dermatology, machine learning algorithms have made considerable advancements in image categorization and visual pattern detection of diverse skin lesions (Du-Harpur et al., 2020). Incorporating AI tools as part of diagnostic activities will most likely lead to a more standardized diagnostic accuracy at the primary care level with subsequent improvements in earlier diagnosis, more appropriate referrals to specialists, and fewer unnecessary invasive procedures leading to decreased morbidity and improved healthcare costs (**Figure 3.1**). In addition, AI can be quite critical during the targeted surveillance of high-risk individuals when it is integrated with high-resolution total-body imaging and serial imaging, especially for those patients who require life-long surveillance (Mar and Soyer, 2019). The most common AI application for cancer prediction seems to be supervised learning. This includes using methods such as support vector machines (SVMs), convolutional neural networks (CNNs), k-nearest neighbors (KNNs), and decision trees (Singh et al., 2024).

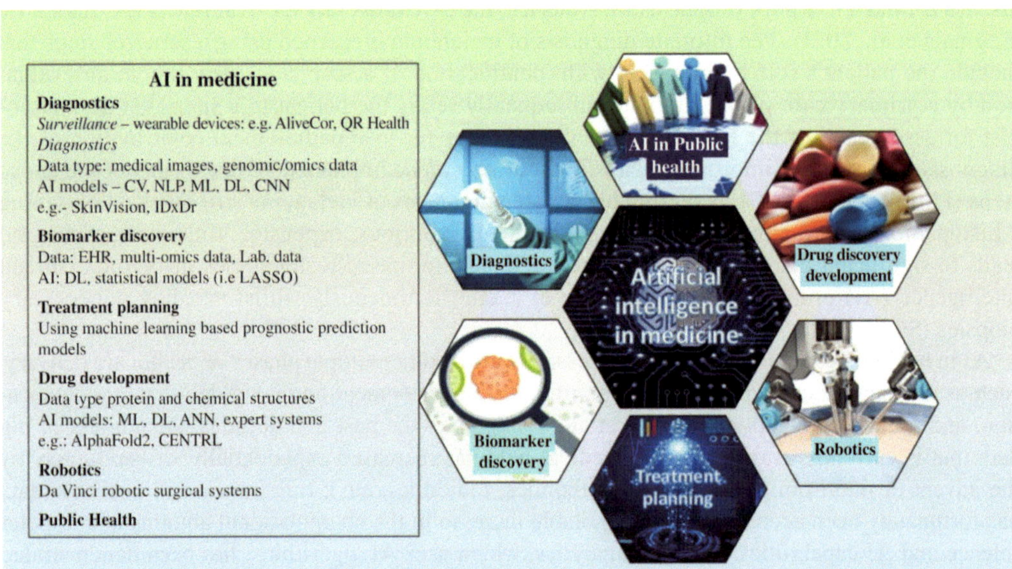

FIGURE 3.1 **AI in medicine.** AI has been applied in various areas of medicine and healthcare delivery, such as AI-enabled diagnostics and computer vision-based AI, which helps in image diagnosis and screening tests, AI-enhanced robots to surgical procedures, and computer vision-based AI to improve actual surgical procedures by providing intraoperative guidance, pharma robots that assist with drug preparation and delivery, fast-tracking and significantly shortening the drug development process, machine learning, and deep learning algorithms that are used as clinical decision support systems, algorithm that can help predict response to chemotherapy, and can even assist, in public health. AI techniques were used during the SARS-CoV-19 epidemic to analyze trends and improve diagnosis, etc. *Abbreviations*: AliveCor developed an algorithm that can detect atrial fibrillation; AlphaFold2 is an AI algorithm created by DeepMind that predicts three-dimensional (3D) protein structure and can be used in drug discovery; CNN, convolutional neural network; CV, computer vision; DL, deep learning; IDx-DR is an AI tool used to predict diabetic neuropathy; LASSO (least absolute shrinkage and selection operator) statistical method used in AI; ML, machine learning; NLP, natural language processing; SkinVision, smartphone app used to detect melanoma. (Data extracted from Bellini et al., 2022; Xu et al., 2021; Yang et al., 2023.)

DETECTING AND DIAGNOSING MELANOMA

Clinical Diagnosis

An increased ability to diagnose melanoma in the early stages is crucial if we are to achieve favorable clinical outcomes. A medical professional must have a high degree of suspicion, be knowledgeable about the various clinical manifestations observed in pigmented skin lesions, particularly those that may signal melanoma, and be aware of the risk factors for melanoma to effectively identify pigmented skin lesions at an early stage. Friedman and colleagues suggested that the clinical features of melanoma can be easily detected using the ABCD (asymmetry, border irregularity, color variegation, and diameter larger than 6 mm) criterion (Friedman et al., 1985). Later, an E was added to the mnemonic to represent rapid Evolution as another feature that might suggest melanoma. The publication of Friedman and colleagues was aimed at enhancing the comprehension of pigmented skin lesions and early detection of melanoma by both primary care physicians and the public. This ABCD(E) criterion has been the bedrock of basic teaching of clinical diagnosis of melanoma since 1985. However, though it has good clinical diagnostic accuracy in typical melanomas, more especially when employed by a dermatologist, its sensitivity and utility are diminished in atypical lesions such as small lesions (<6 mm), nodular melanoma, melanocytic melanoma, and desmoplastic melanoma (Tsao et al., 2015).

Imaging Technologies to Detect Melanoma

Because of the poor prognosis associated with late-stage thick melanoma, the focus to improve outcomes has been on early detection and diagnosis (Oliveria et al., 2003). In an attempt to enhance the early identification of melanoma and decrease the rate of needless biopsies, several noninvasive image-based technologies have been developed, such as electrical impedance spectroscopy, confocal scanning laser microscopy, dermoscopy, digital photography, and computerized image analysis systems, as well as smartphone applications aimed at self-evaluation by the general public and hand-held scanners of varying light wavelengths, such as MelaFind and Spectrophotometric intracutaneous analysis (SIAscope) (Knackstedt et al., 2018; Oliveria et al., 2003). Dermoscopy and total-body photography have emerged as the most important and more widely accepted noninvasive techniques in the assessment and surveillance of dysplastic nevi among clinicians (Terushkin et al., 2010).

Dermoscopy

Dermoscopy is a noninvasive imaging procedure that is conducted utilizing a portable device called a dermatoscope or dermoscope, which has standard magnifying optics and a transilluminating light source (Holmes et al., 2018). The dermatoscope helps to visualize skin characteristics beneath the surface in the epidermis, dermo-epidermal junction, and papillary dermis, which are typically imperceptible to the unaided human eye. It assesses the color patterns and structural arrangement to differentiate between the different characteristics. Provided adequate training has been received, dermoscopy has been demonstrated to enhance the specificity, sensitivity, and diagnostic accuracy of melanoma and the diagnostic accuracy of other nonpigmented and pigmented lesions (Marghoob et al., 2013). During dermoscopic assessments, shining white structures, pseudopods, uneven coloration, blue-white veil, and peppering were the patterns and structures that yielded the highest odds ratio for melanoma, each of which produced a risk for melanoma that was more than six times higher. However, the overall pattern of color and structures offers better overall diagnostic accuracy than individual features in isolation (Williams et al., 2021).

Total-Body Photography

Whilst clinical skin examination is helpful in the early detection of melanoma or atypical lesions, its utility, sensitivity, and specificity are affected by the experience and memory of the examining clinician and the ability to identify lesions that are in hidden areas of the skin surface. Capturing photographic images of the lesions facilitates objective record-keeping of the lesion, thereby allowing assessment by other clinicians (i.e., specialist dermatologists) and follow-up monitoring of the lesion (Dengel et al., 2015; Helfand et al., 2001). This is referred to as "mole mapping." Total-body photography (TBP) comprises the capture and storage of high-resolution images of the full skin surface area and has been found particularly useful in individuals with atypical nevi and in individuals with five or more nevi. The baseline TBP images are used in subsequent total-body skin examinations to track or identify lesions that are changing or to detect new lesions. It reduces the number of unnecessary biopsies, thereby reducing healthcare costs, patient morbidity, and patient anxiety, and improving well-being (Fried et al., 2020). The TBP's utility in monitoring pigmented skin lesions arises from the understanding that the natural history of benign nevis is long-term senescence without change in its character, whereas melanomas are characterized by changes in the lesion's features that occur over time (Navarrete-Dechent et al., 2020). TBP images can be obtained as two-dimensional (2D) images or three-dimensional (3D) images with the creation of the digital body avatar. Besides decreasing over-biopsy, TBP improves the early identification of melanoma and increases the detection of *in situ* lesions and thin Breslow lesions in high-risk populations when compared to normal follow-up without TBP (Hornung et al., 2021).

While 2D TBP applies skin photos that are collected to generate a 2D map of the body, 3D TBP merges a succession of high-resolution macroscopic images of the whole skin surface into a 3D avatar format. The 3D avatar allows the clinician to see the number, color distribution, and border irregularity of nevi and other skin lesions, which can then be followed up using tracking software, making it easier to compare the appearance of nevi over time (Horsham et al., 2022).

Computer-Aided Multispectral Digital Analysis

This requires more sophisticated tools and is more appropriate for evaluating a smaller number of more atypical, preselected lesions than for conducting comprehensive skin cancer screening exams. An example is MelaFind which is an imaging system used to evaluate melanocytic lesions with a suspicious melanoma feature. It exposes the skin to ten different spectral wavelengths ranging from blue (430 nm) to near-infrared (950 nm), subsequently engages in computer analysis, and provides a diagnostic probability score (Fink and Haenssle, 2017).

Reflectance Confocal Microscopy

Reflectance confocal microscopy (RCM) entails real-time, nonintrusive skin tissue imaging with a resolution that is remarkably comparable to histological resolution. It allows *in vivo* visualization of the human skin down to a depth of 200 μm from the superficial epidermis to the papillary dermis and can provide sufficient diagnostic information without requiring a biopsy (Mehrabi et al., 2021). The RCM device uses a point laser light source to illuminate the tissue and utilizes a scanning mode for lesions up to 8 mm in diameter; the light reflected from lesion structures allows morphological evaluation of the skin lesion. This technology is typically found in highly specialized centers, operated by highly trained experts using very expensive microscopy machines (Fink and Haenssle, 2017). However, it has been shown that RCM, either by itself or in conjunction with dermoscopy, improves the accuracy of diagnosis for equivocal lesions on clinical examination and dermoscopy and dramatically reduces the number of unneeded biopsies and benign lesion excisions (Alarcon et al., 2014).

Histopathological Diagnosis

The crucial diagnostic step in melanoma involves biopsy for histopathological or cytological evaluation. Biopsy provides a definitive diagnostic method that aids in distinguishing melanoma from other pigmented lesions that may resemble melanoma on clinical evaluation (Holmes et al., 2018). Despite advances in the fields of immunohistochemistry and molecular biology, comprehensive histological analyses still form the basis of the diagnosis of MM by evaluating the pattern of growth, microscopic levels of invasion, and the thickness of the primary lesion. This comprehensive histological study of the initial lesion allows for the morphological classification of the tumor and the identification of criteria utilized in diagnosis and prognostication (Piris and Mihm, 2009).

Unfortunately, the histological diagnosis of melanoma is associated with interobserver variability and misdiagnoses even among expert dermatopathologists. The biggest professional liability insurance provider owned by physicians in America reported that 11% of their biopsy-related claims between 1995 and 1997, and 16% between 1998 and 2001 involved misdiagnoses of melanoma, second only to breast cancer misdiagnosis (Troxel, 2003).

The histological characteristics of melanoma tend to resemble feature characteristics of various other malignancies, encompassing sarcomas, poorly differentiated carcinomas, lymphomas, neuroendocrine tumors, and germ cell cancers. Immunohistochemistry has emerged as a useful tool that can be used to distinguish melanoma from these other tumors and continues to be the most often used diagnostic technique for melanocytic skin lesions (Knackstedt et al., 2018; Ohsie et al., 2008).

ARTIFICIAL INTELLIGENCE AND MELANOMA DIAGNOSIS

Significant advancements have been made in the field of dermatology regarding the use of AI for the detection and diagnosis of skin cancer. Deep learning CNNs have been employed in dermatology, demonstrating skin cancer classification capabilities that are comparable to those of board-certified dermatologists. AI allows models to incorporate clinical data, such as patient demographics and past medical history, in addition to picture data analysis (Wei et al., 2024). Some of the applications in skin cancer diagnostics are shown in **Table 3.1**. **Figure 3.2** illustrates the schematic representation of the CNN.

TABLE 3.1
Artificial Intelligence Applications in Skin Cancer

Applications	Utility, Pros and Cons	Examples	References
	Patients/Lay Public		
Patients can directly screen to identify and monitor their skin spots using their cellphones, which have AI applications embedded within them.	The lack of generalizability and the scarcity of well-curated, high-quality photographs used in training are the main limitations of smartphone applications. Biases may be introduced by limited lesion variability and skin color. These apps are plagued by low sensitivity and specificity.	SkinVision 2D FotoFinder ATBM®	Jahn et al. (2022)
	Primary Healthcare Practitioners		
Usually, the first professional assessing skin lesions is a primary healthcare practitioner. Due to the shortage of dermatologists, applications to improve diagnostic accuracy among PCP are needed.	Teledermatology – digital images of affected skin areas are submitted to a dermatologist with additional medical data. Deep learning algorithms are being developed to help general practitioners detect skin diseases more accurately.	A Deep Learning System (DLS) was developed to recognize 26 of the most prevalent skin diseases in adults. The DLS outperformed primary care physicians with a 0.67 top-1 accuracy, which was also non-inferior to the top-1 accuracy of board-certified dermatologists of 0.63.	Liu et al. (2020)

(Continued)

TABLE 3.1 *(Continued)*
Artificial Intelligence Applications in Skin Cancer

Applications	Utility, Pros and Cons	Examples	References
		Dermatology Practice	
In dermatology practices, artificial intelligence risk prediction models to improve diagnostic accuracy.	Self-assessed risk variables (age, sex, country of birth, city of recruitment, ethnicity, skin color, eye color, natural hair color at age 18, skin reaction to sunlight, and nevus density) were used to build the melanoma risk prediction model.	Researchers created an unconditional logistic regression model. In external validation, utilizing the risk prediction model to categorize individuals as high-risk resulted in a higher net benefit than classifying all persons as high-risk.	Vuong et al. (2016)
Augmented Intelligence (AuI) – using AI algorithms in decision-making.	Assist dermatologists in more effectively managing teledermatology, evaluating and monitoring lesion change.	Dermatologists who also included CNN results in their decision-making noticed significant improvements in diagnostic sensitivity and specificity (mean sensitivity increased from 84.2% to 100.0% and mean specificity from 72.1% to 83.7%); the addition of AuI led to a 19.2% decrease in unwarranted excisions of benign lesions.	Winkler et al. (2023)
Imaging in dermatology (Lesion and Body imaging) – using AI-enhanced technologies to capture skin images.	Emerging AI-enabled imaging technologies can detect, track, analyze, and predict the diagnosis of various skin lesions.	3D Vectra® WB360 — whole-body imaging system — takes 2D images of the whole body from a patient standing in a certain anatomical position using 92 cameras. The images are uploaded into automated software that creates a 3D avatar and automatically denotes lesion features.	Marchetti et al. (2023b)
		Dermatopathology	
AI has the ability to assist dermatopathologists in multiple ways by creating models based on whole-slide imaging (WSI).	These models can facilitate the creation of decision support systems for pathologists and be deployed in clinical settings.	A framework for deep learning was created that used a MIL approach and integrated CNNs and RNNs. The researchers assembled an immense dataset that included 44,732 slides from 15,187 patients with three distinct cancer forms, including BCC. When used in a clinical setting, pathologists will be able to eliminate 65–75% of slides to be assessed, while maintaining 100% sensitivity.	Campanella et al. (2019)

This table denotes some examples of artificial intelligence employment in the detection of skin lesions.
Abbreviations: ATMB, automated total-body mapping; CNN, convolutional neural networks; MIL, multiple instances learning, which is a form of supervised machine learning; PCP, primary care physicians; RNN, recurrent neural networks.

Dermoscopy and AI in Melanoma

The use of AI to evaluate skin images possesses the capacity to increase diagnostic accuracy of melanoma without a biopsy to the same degree as diagnosis confirmed by biopsy (Marchetti et al., 2023a). Image analysis using a computer-aided dermatological image classification has largely depended on limited, insufficient, and uniform data sets obtained from dermoscopy and histology images, and as such lacks the generalization capacity that healthcare professionals may possess. Deep learning algorithms, on the other hand, can be trained on variable, multiple, and large datasets acquired from different image formats to develop melanoma classification and diagnostic capabilities that can outperform dermatologists (Esteva et al., 2017). Accurate classification of skin lesions based on photographic and dermoscopic images will assist in decreasing the number of unnecessary biopsies whilst providing early identification of suspicious lesions (Seiverling et al., 2023). Amongst the deep learning models, the CNNs have emerged as the best-performing models in terms of image analysis, recognition, and accurate classification. It can be trained using large datasets of millions of images from thousands of categories as long as there is enough memory and computing power in the graphical processing units (GPUs) that are used in the implementation of the convolution operation and sufficient time is allowed to complete the training (Krizhevsky et al., 2017). Accessible datasets are the most important element in building a successful network. Through transfer learning, CNNs can be trained on massive datasets using well-known software frameworks like TensorFlow and PyTorch. Fortunately, pretraining an algorithm can be easily conducted using a variety of publicly available validated training datasets, including ImageNet, International Skin Imaging Collaboration (ISIC), DermQuest, and Dermofit Image Library (Stiff et al., 2022). Several novel CNNs trained on large image datasets have been developed by large tech companies and are publicly available for further training on specific datasets through transfer learning. These CNNs encompass the "Inception" from Google and "ResNet" from Microsoft (Du-Harpur et al., 2020).

Marchetti and colleagues prospectively evaluated the capability of an open-source AI algorithm called "All Data Are Ext" (ADAE) to accurately predict melanoma from dermoscopy images of skin lesions when compared to an expert dermatologist. The ADAE was trained solely on publicly accessible dermoscopy images. They assessed 435 patients selected by 11 dermatologists and included 603 lesions from these participants. All the included participants had consented to biopsies of the lesions. The study's intended principal objective was to evaluate the performance of the algorithm at a predetermined 95% sensitivity threshold (for biopsied lesions). They observed that the ADAE exhibited a 37.4% (95% CI: 33.3–41.7%) specificity and a 96.8% (95% CI: 91.1–98.9%) sensitivity. Additionally, they discovered that after reviewing the ADAE data, the dermatologists' AUC, which was determined using their projected melanoma probability, increased from 0.7798 to 0.8161, and they concluded that the exposure to ADAE was associated with consistent improvement in the dermatologist's ability to differentiate melanomas from the benign lesions (Marchetti et al., 2023a).

Esteva and colleagues constructed a CNN that modeled dermatologists' performance in three main diagnostic domains: melanoma classification, melanoma classification using dermoscopy, and keratinocyte carcinoma classification. They used GoogleNet Inception v3 CNN architecture that had been previously trained on an estimated 1.28 million images and trained it on their own sets of data composed of 127,463 clinical and dermoscopic images of skin lesions using transfer learning. When validating the effectiveness of the model by utilizing a three-class disease division system (benign, malignant, and non-neoplastic lesions), the CNN achieved an overall accuracy of 72.1 ± 0.9% (mean ± s.d.) compared to two dermatologists who achieved 65.56% and 66.0% accuracy on a subset of the validation, respectively. Furthermore, the CNN matched or outperformed the sensitivity and specificity performance of ≥21 board-certified dermatologists in the image-based classification of skin lesions and deciding on further course of action (i.e., continue to biopsy or reassure patient). For the classifications of carcinoma, melanoma, and dermoscopy melanoma, the CNN's image classification AUCs were 0.96, 0.94, and 0.91, respectively (Esteva et al., 2017).

Brinker and colleagues trained a ResNet50 CNN algorithm using only 12,378 dermoscopic images of melanomas and atypical nevi obtained from the ISIC image bank and the HAM10000 dataset. They compared the algorithm's performance against the capacity of 145 dermatologists from 12 German university hospitals in the classification of 100 clinical images composed of 80 nevi and 20 biopsy-proven melanomas. The dermatologists achieved an average sensitivity and specificity of 89.4% (range 55.0%–100%) and 64.4% (range 22.5%–92.5%) with clinical images, respectively. At the same sensitivity level, the CNN obtained an average specificity of 68.2%. Dermatologists achieved the highest average sensitivity of 92.8% and the lowest average specificity of 57.7%, whilst the CNN achieved an average specificity of 61.1% at the same high sensitivity of 92.8%. This study also demonstrated that a CNN model trained on high-resolution dermoscopic images can be successfully utilized in low-resolution clinical image classification tasks (Brinker et al., 2019).

Philips and colleagues engaged in a prospective, multicenter, single arm, masked diagnostic study to assess the capability of Deep Ensemble for Recognition of Malignancy algorithm to identify melanoma from images of multiple pigmented skin lesions and contrast its accuracy to that of clinical diagnosis by specialist dermatologists. This algorithm was developed by Skin Analytics Ltd as a decision support system for the diagnosis of skin cancer from dermoscopic pictures of pigmented skin lesions. To conduct the trial, they took photographs of suspicious-looking lesions using three different cameras (Apple iPhone 6s, Samsung Galaxy S6, and Nikon digital single-lens reflex [DSLR] camera D5500). The algorithm was retrained with 289 images from this study, and 1550 images were subsequently analyzed by the algorithm, of which 551 were biopsied suspicious lesions and 999 were control lesions. Melanoma was confirmed with histopathology. The algorithm achieved an AUROC of 90.1% for biopsied lesions and 95.8% for all lesions using iPhone 6s images; an AUROC of 85.8% for biopsied lesions and 93.8% for all lesions using Galaxy S6 images; and an AUROC of 86.9% for biopsied lesions and 91.8% for all lesions using DSLR camera pictures. Specialists achieved an AUROC of 77.8% (95% CI: 72.5%–81.9%) and a specificity of 69.9% at 100% sensitivity, whereas the algorithm obtained a specificity of 64.8% with iPhone 6s images at 100% sensitivity. The AUROC for clinical diagnosis was 90.8%. The overall accuracy level of the algorithm was similar to that of a specialist (Phillips et al., 2019). The study reveals the enormous potential of AI in enhancing access and efficacy of detection and clinical therapy of skin cancer in general and melanoma in particular, despite certain limitations that the scientists have observed.

An Australian study investigated the point prevalence of actinic keratosis (AK), KC, and MM in people with high exposure to UV radiation, such as surfers, swimmers, and walkers/runners. In order to determine the probable risk of MM, they performed whole-body screening under the supervision of a skin cancer physician and evaluated the accuracy, sensitivity, and specificity of a high-resolution, commercial dermatoscope that integrated AI in a primary care context. They found that the prevalence of skin cancer was much higher than in the general population, with melanoma rate being higher in surfers (who have longer high UVR peak exposure). In terms of the AI-enabled device (FotoFinder Vexia) performance, they found a sensitivity of 53.33%, specificity of 54.44%, and accuracy of 54.17% for MM risk prediction, which were all significantly lower than the values that had previously been documented in the literature. They speculated that the poor performance was due to the device's lack of training in sun-damaged skin and exposure to clinical settings. FotoFinder is reported to be using CNN algorithms for skin examinations (Miller et al., 2023).

Whilst CNN models seem to perform well when used individually, hybrid models that combine and interconnect at least two CNNs, which are then fed into SVM classifier algorithm, may perform even better in accurately predicting benign and melanoma lesions. For example, Keerthana and colleagues analyzed ten publicly available CNN models that were pre-trained on datasets of dermoscopy images. They created two hybrid models that were trained and tested using the ISBI 2016 datasets, namely (a) DenseNet-201 and MobileNet-v2 and (b) DenseNet-201 and ResNet-50. They concatenated the CNN models extracted and combined valuable features, which were then submitted into the SVM classifier from which the final classified output was acquired. The hybrid model combining DenseNet-201 and MobileNet-v2 with SVM classifier and RMSProp optimizer achieved an accuracy of 88.02% for 25 epochs, and the hybrid model using DenseNet-201 and ResNet-50 with SVM classifier and RMSProp optimizer achieved an accuracy of 87.43% for 30 epochs (Keerthana et al., 2023).

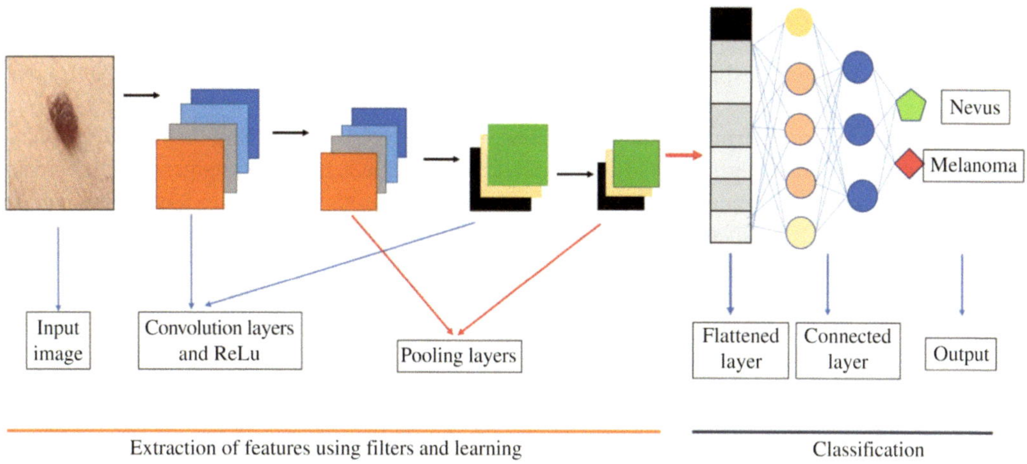

FIGURE 3.2 **Schematic representation of a convolutional neural network.** CNN is a form of deep learning approach for analyzing data that is presented in a grid structure, such as images. It has since been extensively utilized in various computer vision tasks. It is meant to learn spatial feature hierarchies autonomously and adaptively, from low-level patterns to high-level ones. The basic structure is made up of three fundamental layers that can be regarded as the building blocks, namely the convolutional, pooling, and fully connected layers. The function of the initial two layers, convolution and pooling, is to extract features from images, while the third layer, a fully connected layer, functions similarly to a standard artificial neural network, mapping the extracted features into an output, such as classification. Each network can consist of multiple convolutional layers, which may be in series with each subsequent layer extracting more complex features. The rectified linear unit (ReLu) is applied to introduce nonlinearity; the flattened layer is the flattening of the final stacked pooling layer. (Data extracted from O'Shea and Nash, 2015; Yamashita et al., 2018.)

Photography and AI in Melanoma

The existing melanoma diagnostic activities usually involve the identification of an individual suspicious lesion by the patient or healthcare practitioner, which then gets assessed further. Unfortunately, this strategy is susceptible to missing other significant lesions. Techniques that offer simultaneous whole-body assessment will improve the early detection of melanocytic, changing, and new lesions (Fried et al., 2020). Marchetti et al. (2023b) evaluated the ability of an AI-based prediction model to discriminate melanoma from non-melanoma lesions using automated data generated from the VECTRA WB360 Whole Body 3D Imaging System (Canfield Scientific). This imaging system captures skin surface images that are subsequently converted to a 3D whole-body avatar of the patient. The technology's software, the Vectra DermaGraphix software, automatically identifies and characterizes the clinical appearance of all lesions on a person's body that are visible and larger than 2 mm. Thirty-five patients with histologically confirmed melanomas were used in the study. The researchers discovered that the 15-variable prediction model's area under the receiver operating characteristic curve was 0.94 (95% CI: 0.92–0.96). They also came to the conclusion that melanoma may be accurately distinguished from other skin lesions using automated analysis of whole-body 3D images (Marchetti et al., 2023b).

Another systemic review analyzed 38 studies that included 20,126 melanomas and found that approximately only 29.1% of melanomas were nevus-associated melanomas that developed from preexisting nevi, whereas *de novo* melanomas arising as new lesions constituted the majority of the melanomas at 70.9% (Pampena et al., 2017). Thus, total skin photography is essential for tracking the progress of pigmented skin lesions as well as for detecting new lesions. In fact, the European consensus-based melanoma guidelines recommend using TBP in conjunction with sequential digital dermoscopy (SSDI) to improve early detection and diagnosis of melanoma, especially in individuals who have an increased risk profile (Garbe et al., 2022).

An observational study from Basel, Switzerland, was conducted to compare the diagnostic accuracy between the dermatologist, 2D TBP, and 3D TBP CNNs in relation to augmented intelligence (where augmented intelligence was described as a decision based on dermatologist assessment in concert with 2D and 3D CNNs) in the real-world setting. Participants were first evaluated by clinical assessment and dermoscopy (using two dermatoscopes, Medicam 1000 and VISIOMED D200Evo), conducted by a dermatologist, and they then completed TBP utilizing the 3D imaging system Vectra WB360 and the 2D FotoFinder automatic total-body mapping (ATBM Master) device. The study assessed 1690 melanocytic lesions found in 143 high-risk individuals and discovered that while dermatologists and augmented intelligence achieved similar sensitivity (90%) and comparable classification ROC-AUC (0.91 [CI: 0.80–1.00], 0.88 [CI: 0.77–1.00]) with 3D-CNN, their specificity was much better at 92.3% and 86.2%, respectively. The 2D-CNN was outclassed by both the 3D CNN and dermatologists; it only achieved a sensitivity of 70%, with 40% specificity and ROC-AUC of 0.68 [CI: 0.46–0.90]). The shortcomings of the CNNs are the low specificities, which may lead to a high number of unnecessary biopsies/excisions (Cerminara et al., 2023). Augmented intelligence (AuI) is an emerging concept in dermatology characterized by the use of AI models created from clinical and image data to assist and enhance decision-making in the delivery of healthcare by treating physicians (Kovarik et al., 2019).

One of the shortcomings of previously developed algorithms is the use of images only to develop the AI models without taking into consideration other clinical data that is typically available to clinicians. In an effort to address these limitations, Primerio and colleagues recently developed a study protocol that seeks to integrate comprehensive patient metadata (which includes demographics, medical history, sun exposure behavior, skin phenotype, and genetic risk factors) with total-body imaging and dermoscopy to develop machine learning and deep learning algorithms that will analyze skin images for identification of skin lesions, classification, segmentation, 3D mapping, change detection, and risk assessment for patients. The proposed approach will be a multidisciplinary collaboration between physicians, software engineers, medical data annotation experts, data management specialists, bioethics experts, and patient advocates. The stated purpose of this work will be to propose a holistic method for AI-driven computer-aided diagnostic tools that can be used for the early identification of melanoma (Primiero et al., 2024).

Reflectance Confocal Microscopy and AI

RCM allows noninvasive *in vivo* appraisal of skin lesions with a cellular level resolution that is comparable to histopathology, thereby essentially allowing a virtual diagnosis of skin lesions. However, it requires extensive training, and the results are affected by the clinical expertise (Narayanamurthy et al., 2018). Moreover, RCM images are prone to having artifacts that make accurate image interpretation difficult. These artifacts include relics resulting from surface reflections, artifacts caused by patient movements during image acquisition (including breathing, heartbeats, and talking), and artifacts from air and oil bubbles on the skin surfaces. The application of AI to RCM images can potentially limit the number of artifacts affecting image analysis, improve the ease of interpretation, and streamline skin lesion detection (Malciu et al., 2022). Wodzinski and colleagues developed a CNN that was pre-trained on ResNet architecture using the ImageNet dataset and then fine-tuned on RCM mosaics. They aimed to assist in the automatic skin lesion diagnosis using raw RCM mosaics. The RCM dataset contained 429 mosaics that were divided into three classes: Melanoma malignum (MM), Basal Cell Carcinoma (BCC), and naevus (NE). Their network achieved an overall classification accuracy of 0.89 and 0.87 in the validation set and test set, respectively, which was better than the medical experts. For melanoma, they achieved precision rates of 0.89 in the test set (Wodzinski et al., 2019).

Histopathology and AI

The gold standard for diagnosing cancer has consistently been histopathological confirmation of malignancy; nevertheless, observer variability remains a significant issue with this method. Fortunately, the clinical impact of this observer variability is still minimal at the population level. However, in the modern age of precision healthcare, where personalized treatment plans are tailored based on accurate individual patient diagnoses, this variability could have disastrous consequences (Tizhoosh et al., 2021). The diagnosis of skin cancer is also affected by discrepancies between pathologists who examine Hematoxylin and Eosin (H&E) stained slides, which serve as the basis for biopsy-based diagnosis of benign and malignant skin lesions. As a result, there is a high degree of intra- and interobserver variability in the assessment of melanocytic skin lesions. A study by Shoo and colleagues found a discrepancy rate of 14.3% in melanoma diagnosis among pathologists (Shoo et al., 2010). This observer variability and discrepancy leads to either overestimation or underestimation of melanoma. AI might assist with the creation of new techniques for the identification of skin malignancies from histopathological images, allowing pathologists to standardize diagnoses and efficiently organize personalized care (unsupervised training machine learning algorithms and deep learning networks seem to offer more promise in this regard) (De Logu et al., 2020; Tizhoosh et al., 2021). The application of AI in pathology has been described as the third revolution that will advance tissue analysis and diagnostics. The initial baseline was, of course, the H&E staining with the first revolution being the introduction of immunohistochemistry and the second revolution being the recent rise in genomics and molecular pathology. And now with recent improvements in the field of digital pathology and digital capture of whole slide images, the integration of AI techniques in histopathological analysis can be realized. AI has the capacity to combine complex diagnostic data sets and create new, highly integrated diagnostic signatures that allow for the merging of enormous data sets and the provision of insights that are not achievable with the human eye or intellect working alone (Salto-Tellez et al., 2018). Besides the digital pathology advances, recent improvements and advances in multiplexed immunohistochemistry and single-cell technologies also lend themselves to easy AI integration and particularly deep learning techniques. The diagnostic accuracy of digitalized whole slide images for melanocytic lesions is comparable to that of traditional microscopy. Additionally, digitization offers the benefit of enabling virtual image sharing between pathologists located in different locations and computational platforms (Van Herck et al., 2021).

De Logu and colleagues built a CNN-based algorithm that analyzed whole slide images to identify areas of healthy and diseased tissue even in poor samples with minimal tumor tissue that might be difficult for the pathologist to analyze. The CNN was developed using a pre-trained Inception-ResNet-v2, which they retrained using whole-slide digital images from 100 formalin-fixed paraffin-embedded primary cutaneous melanomas. The training and validation datasets consisted of 1377 patches representing healthy tissue and 2141 patches representing melanoma, all derived from 60 regions of interest (ROI); the test dataset consisted of 791 patches representing healthy tissue and 1122 patches representing melanoma, all derived from 40 ROIs. The model demonstrated the ability to differentiate between segments of diseased and healthy tissues when tested on independent datasets, achieving the accuracy, sensitivity, specificity, and F1 score of 96.5%, 95.7%, 97.7%, and 97.0%, respectively (De Logu et al., 2020).

Ba and colleagues developed a deep learning algorithm using 781 whole slide images (86 melanomas, 695 nevi) for training and validation, and 104 WSIs (29 melanomas, 75 nevi) were used to test the classification performance of the algorithm, classifying the images into melanoma and nevus. Their framework integrated three modules: a region of interest tissue (RIT) extraction module, a

CNN-based melanoma patch detection module, and a slide-level classification module based on a random forest classifier. Their algorithm achieved a specificity of 97.3%, which was similar to the mean specificity of 96.0% achieved by the seven participating dermatopathologists who evaluated the WSI, and the sensitivity was also similar at 96.5% and mean sensitivity of 95.1% for the algorithm and dermatopathologist, respectively. When evaluating the diagnostic accuracy of melanoma, the algorithm obtained a *Jaccard index* of 77.78%, therefore correctly identifying the majority of melanoma regions (Ba et al., 2021).

AI and Melanoma Molecular Profiling

Melanoma may develop in response to mutational changes in DNA sequences; these mutations are commonly seen following DNA damage by external factors such as UV radiation. The mutations may induce proliferation of oncogenes or suppression of tumor suppressor elements, resulting in cancer development and progression. The ability to assess and predict these DNA cancer driver mutations timeously can improve the detection and diagnosis of melanoma at its initial stages. Shah and colleagues developed a blended ensemble-based deep learning model, a deep neural network made up of multiple layers, to detect melanoma driver mutation in a balanced dataset of aberrant and normal sequences. Their dataset included 2608 human samples, 6450 normal gene sequences procured from the *asia.ensembl.org* websites, and 6778 mutated gene sequences procured from the *intogen.org.* database. For the study, they employed three forms of deep learning recurrent neural network (RNN) methods, namely: Long Short-Term Memory (LSTM), Gated Recurrent Units (GRU), and Bidirectional LSTM. These deep learning (DL) methods were validated for performance in detecting cutaneous melanoma using three tests: self-consistency (SCT), independent set (IST), and tenfold cross-validation (10-FCVT). The model demonstrated high accuracy levels in predicting cutaneous melanoma of 94%, 93%, and 97% accuracy in SCT, 10-FCVT, and IST, respectively. Additionally, the BLSTM model predicted cutaneous melanoma with an incredible 99% accuracy (Ali Shah et al., 2023).

AI and Cross-Sectional Images: Radiomics

Radiomics is becoming a more significant method for the identification, diagnosis, and staging of several malignancies, including cutaneous melanoma. It is a technique of extracting quantitative data from radiology images and other cross-sectional images, such as nuclear medicine images. It employs data analysis processes using features generated using ML algorithms to predict the type of lesion or malignancy being imaged. Currently, cross-sectional imaging platforms that can be used to detect and diagnose malignant cutaneous melanoma are still in the investigational stages. They entail the utilization of targeted molecular imaging employing PET/CT with biomarkers, such as FAP-targeted PET imaging, PD-L1-targeted PET imaging, and melanin imaging. Melanin imaging appears effective in the early diagnosis of cutaneous melanoma. However, these techniques do have certain constraints for the early identification of melanoma that can be overcome or improved by the application of advanced AI algorithms. These constraints include tracer availability, histotype, and resolution limits (Higgins et al., 2023).

LIMITATIONS

Maybe as a prelude to this section on the limitations of AI in melanoma diagnostics and healthcare in general, I should share a quote from John McArthur from his paper on the "Problems and Projections in Computer Sciences for the Next 49 Years" where he states, "We shouldn't exaggerate. The computer has caused big changes in society, but these probably aren't as great as those caused by the automobile" (Mccarthy, 2003); maybe not yet.

Despite advances in the computational power of GPUs and an increase in available image data, the best available algorithms are still a long way from approximating the inferotemporal pathway of the human visual system., especially since current training is on static images without the additional information that can be gleaned from temporal effects that may be seen on videos (Krizhevsky et al., 2017).

Other important factors to consider as far as image-based CNN is concerned are (1) the performance of CNN is directly linked to the labeled input data used to train the model, which implies that any biases in the training data sets will directly influence outcomes, for example fewer validated images from non-Caucasian people have been incorporated into CNN models (Charalambides and Singh, 2020) and (2) image-based CNN models only evaluate a single aspect of the disease (i.e., medical images); whereas clinicians and dermatologists assess lesions in the context of full patient evaluation and as such their clinical decisions (i.e., to biopsy or not) may be motivated by other factors besides lesion appearance, for example a clinician may decide to biopsy a lesion based on a strong history of a particular risk factor. (3) The black box effect of deep learning neural pathways has not been resolved; with current technology, the full explanation of the network's decision-making process is not achievable (Du-Harpur et al., 2020). (4) The performance of AI in accurately diagnosing atypical melanoma is uncertain, which ironically is the area where perhaps it is most needed. This is influenced by the difficulty associated with imaging these lesions and the low number of these lesions that are available to adequately train AI models (Mar and Soyer, 2019). The prognosis and treatment of melanoma are largely related to the staging of the disease, and one of the key factors for this is measuring the depth of the tumor. Whilst this is readily available in an incision biopsy, further AI technology must be investigated to see if this can be mimicked.

CONCLUSION

The incorporation of AI when evaluating noninvasive dermatological imaging techniques could completely change the way melanomas are identified and treated. Machine learning algorithms have the potential to fast-track the process of diagnosis and decrease the number of times patients visit the clinic (Patel et al., 2023). Deep learning CNNs have emerged as the most feasible machine algorithms that can be employed to improve the accuracy of the diagnostic modalities utilized in melanoma detection and can help decrease the number of unnecessary biopsies. The CNNs are probably the best deep learning networks that are employed in image recognition, including photographic images, dermoscopy, radiomics, and histopathology images. In some studies, their diagnostic accuracy was found to be similar to that of experienced dermatologists. Moreover, AI applications offer the advantage of the ease of simultaneous monitoring and surveillance of multiple lesions.

REFERENCES

Alarcon, I., Carrera, C., Palou, J., Alos, L., Malvehy, J. and Puig, S. 2014. Impact of in vivo reflectance confocal microscopy on the number needed to treat melanoma in doubtful lesions, *British Journal of Dermatology*, 170, pp. 802–808.

Ali Shah, A., Shaker, A. S. A., Jabbar, S., Abbas, Q., Al-Balawi, T. S. and Celebi, M. E. 2023. An ensemble-based deep learning model for detection of mutation causing cutaneous melanoma, *Scientific Reports*, 13, p. 22251.

Arnold, M., Singh, D., Laversanne, M., Vignat, J., Vaccarella, S., Meheus, F., Cust, A. E., De Vries, E., Whiteman, D. C. and Bray, F. 2022. Global burden of cutaneous melanoma in 2020 and projections to 2040, *JAMA Dermatology*, 158, pp. 495–503.

Ba, W., Wang, R., Yin, G., Song, Z., Zou, J., Zhong, C., Yang, J., Yu, G., Yang, H., Zhang, L. and Li, C. 2021. Diagnostic assessment of deep learning for melanocytic lesions using whole-slide pathological images, *Translational Oncology*, 14, p. 101161.

Bellini, V., Cascella, M., Cutugno, F., Russo, M., Lanza, R., Compagnone, C. and Bignami, E. G. 2022. Understanding basic principles of artificial intelligence: A practical guide for intensivists, *Acta Biomedica*, 93, p. e2022297.

Borges Do Nascimento, I. J., Marcolino, M. S., Abdulazeem, H. M., Weerasekara, I., Azzopardi-Muscat, N., Gonçalves, M. A. and Novillo-Ortiz, D. 2021. Impact of big data analytics on People's health: Overview of systematic reviews and recommendations for future studies, *Journal of Medical Internet Research*, 23, p. e27275.

Bray, F., Laversanne, M., Sung, H., Ferlay, J., Siegel, R. L., Soerjomataram, I. and Jemal, A. 2024. Global cancer statistics 2022: GLOBOCAN estimates of incidence and mortality worldwide for 36 cancers in 185 countries, *CA: A Cancer Journal for Clinicians*, 74, pp. 229–263.

Brinker, T. J., Hekler, A., Enk, A. H., Klode, J., Hauschild, A., Berking, C., Schilling, B., Haferkamp, S., Schadendorf, D., Fröhling, S., Utikal, J. S. and Von Kalle, C. 2019. A convolutional neural network trained with dermoscopic images performed on par with 145 dermatologists in a clinical melanoma image classification task, *European Journal of Cancer*, 111, pp. 148–154.

Campanella, G., Hanna, M. G., Geneslaw, L., Miraflor, A., Werneck Krauss Silva, V., Busam, K. J., Brogi, E., Reuter, V. E., Klimstra, D. S. and Fuchs, T. J. 2019. Clinical-grade computational pathology using weakly supervised deep learning on whole slide images, *Nature Medicine*, 25, pp. 1301–1309.

Cerminara, S. E., Cheng, P., Kostner, L., Huber, S., Kunz, M., Maul, J.-T., Böhm, J. S., Dettwiler, C. F., Geser, A., Jakopović, C., Stoffel, L. M., Peter, J. K., Levesque, M., Navarini, A. A. and Maul, L. V. 2023. Diagnostic performance of augmented intelligence with 2D and 3D total body photography and convolutional neural networks in a high-risk population for melanoma under real-world conditions: A new era of skin cancer screening? *European Journal of Cancer*, 190, p. 112954.

Charalambides, M. and Singh, S. 2020. Artificial intelligence and melanoma detection: Friend or foe of dermatologists? *British Journal of Hospital Medicine (London)*, 81, pp. 1–5.

Davis, L. E., Shalin, S. C. and Tackett, A. J. 2019. Current state of melanoma diagnosis and treatment, *Cancer Biology & Therapy*, 20, pp. 1366–1379.

De Logu, F., Ugolini, F., Maio, V., Simi, S., Cossu, A., Massi, D., Italian Association for Cancer Research (AIRC) Study Group, Nassini, R., and Laurino, M. 2020. Recognition of cutaneous melanoma on digitized histopathological slides via artificial intelligence algorithm, *Frontiers in Oncology*, 10.

Dengel, L. T., Petroni, G. R., Judge, J., Chen, D., Acton, S. T., Schroen, A. T. and Slingluff, C. L., Jr. 2015. Total body photography for skin cancer screening, *International Journal of Dermatology*, 54, pp. 1250–1254.

Du-Harpur, X., Watt, F. M., Luscombe, N. M. and Lynch, M. D. 2020. What is AI? Applications of artificial intelligence to dermatology, *British Journal of Dermatology*, 183, pp. 423–430.

Esteva, A., Kuprel, B., Novoa, R. A., Ko, J., Swetter, S. M., Blau, H. M. and Thrun, S. 2017. Dermatologist-level classification of skin cancer with deep neural networks, *Nature*, 542, pp. 115–118.

Fink, C. and Haenssle, H. A. 2017. Non-invasive tools for the diagnosis of cutaneous melanoma, *Skin Research and Technology*, 23, pp. 261–271.

Fried, L., Tan, A., Bajaj, S., Liebman, T. N., Polsky, D. and Stein, J. A. 2020. Technological advances for the detection of melanoma: Advances in diagnostic techniques, *Journal of the American Academy of Dermatology*, 83, pp. 983–992.

Friedman, R. J., Rigel, D. S. and Kopf, A. W. 1985. Early detection of malignant melanoma: The role of physician examination and self-examination of the skin, *CA: A Cancer Journal for Clinicians*, 35, pp. 130–151.

Garbe, C., Amaral, T., Peris, K., Hauschild, A., Arenberger, P., Basset-Seguin, N., Bastholt, L., Bataille, V., Del Marmol, V., Dréno, B., Fargnoli, M. C., Forsea, A.-M., Grob, J.-J., Höller, C., Kaufmann, R., Kelleners-Smeets, N., Lallas, A., Lebbé, C., Lytvynenko, B., Malvehy, J., Moreno-Ramirez, D., Nathan, P., Pellacani, G., Saiag, P., Stratigos, A. J., Van Akkooi, A. C. J., Vieira, R., Zalaudek, I. and Lorigan, P. 2022. European consensus-based interdisciplinary guideline for melanoma. Part 1: Diagnostics: Update 2022, *European Journal of Cancer*, 170, pp. 236–255.

Helfand, M., Mahon, S. M., Eden, K. B., Frame, P. S. and Orleans, C. T. 2001. Screening for skin cancer, *American Journal of Preventive Medicine*, 20, pp. 47–58.

Higgins, H., Nakhla, A., Lotfalla, A., Khalil, D., Doshi, P., Thakkar, V., Shirini, D., Bebawy, M., Ammari, S., Lopci, E., Schwartz, L. H., Postow, M. and Dercle, L. 2023. Recent advances in the field of artificial intelligence for precision medicine in patients with a diagnosis of metastatic cutaneous melanoma, *Diagnostics (Basel)*, 13, p. 3483.

Holmes, G. A., Vassantachart, J. M., Limone, B. A., Zumwalt, M., Hirokane, J. and Jacob, S. E. 2018. Using dermoscopy to identify melanoma and improve diagnostic discrimination, *Federal Practitioner*, 35, pp. S39–S45.

Hornung, A., Steeb, T., Wessely, A., Brinker, T. J., Breakell, T., Erdmann, M., Berking, C., and Heppt, M. V. 2021. The value of total body photography for the early detection of melanoma: A systematic review, *International Journal of Environmental Research and Public Health*, 18.

Horsham, C., O'hara, M., Sanjida, S., Ma, S., Jayasinghe, D., Green, A. C., Schaider, H., Aitken, J. F., Sturm, R. A., Prow, T., Soyer, H. P., and Janda, M. 2022. The experience of 3D total-body photography to monitor Nevi: Results from an Australian general population-based cohort study, *JMIR Dermatology*, 5, p. e37034.
Jahn, A. S., Navarini, A. A., Cerminara, S. E., Kostner, L., Huber, S. M., Kunz, M., Maul, J.-T., Dummer, R., Sommer, S., Neuner, A. D., Levesque, M. P., Cheng, P. F. and Maul, L. V. 2022. Over-detection of melanoma-suspect lesions by a CE-certified smartphone app: Performance in comparison to dermatologists, 2D and 3D convolutional neural networks in a prospective data set of 1204 pigmented skin lesions involving Patients' perception, *Cancers*, 14, p. 3829.
Keerthana, D., Venugopal, V., Nath, M. K. and Mishra, M. 2023. Hybrid convolutional neural networks with SVM classifier for classification of skin cancer, *Biomedical Engineering Advances*, 5, p. 100069.
Knackstedt, T., Knackstedt, R. W., Couto, R. and Gastman, B. 2018. Malignant melanoma: Diagnostic and management update, *Plastic and Reconstructive Surgery*, 142, pp. 202e–216e.
Kovarik, C., Lee, I., Ko, J., Adamson, A., Otley, C., Kvedar, J., Vedak, P., Huang, S., Fitzgerald, M. and Chaudhari, R. 2019. Commentary: Position statement on augmented intelligence (AuI), *Journal of the American Academy of Dermatology*, 81, pp. 998–1000.
Krizhevsky, A., Sutskever, I. and Hinton, G. E. 2017. ImageNet classification with deep convolutional neural networks, *Communications of the ACM*, 60, pp. 84–90.
Leiter, U., Keim, U. and Garbe, C. 2020. Epidemiology of skin cancer: Update 2019, *Advances in Experimental Medicine and Biology*, 1268, pp. 123–139.
Liu, Y., Jain, A., Eng, C., Way, D. H., Lee, K., Bui, P., Kanada, K., De Oliveira Marinho, G., Gallegos, J. and Gabriele, S. 2020. A deep learning system for differential diagnosis of skin diseases, *Nature Medicine*, 26, pp. 900–908.
Malciu, A. M., Lupu, M. and Voiculescu, V. M. 2022. Artificial intelligence-based approaches to reflectance confocal microscopy image analysis in dermatology. *Journal of Clinical Medicine*, 11, p. 429.
Mar, V. J. and Soyer, H. P. 2019. Artificial intelligence for melanoma diagnosis: How can we deliver on the promise? *Annals of Oncology*, 30, pp. e1–e3.
Marchetti, M. A., Cowen, E. A., Kurtansky, N. R., Weber, J., Dauscher, M., Defazio, J., Deng, L., Dusza, S. W., Haliasos, H., Halpern, A. C., Hosein, S., Nazir, Z. H., Marghoob, A. A., Quigley, E. A., Salvador, T. and Rotemberg, V. M. 2023a. Prospective validation of dermoscopy-based open-source artificial intelligence for melanoma diagnosis (PROVE-AI study), *NPJ Digital Medicine*, 6, p. 127.
Marchetti, M. A., Nazir, Z. H., Nanda, J. K., Dusza, S. W., D'alessandro, B. M., Defazio, J., Halpern, A. C., Rotemberg, V. M. and Marghoob, A. A. 2023b. 3D whole-body skin imaging for automated melanoma detection, *Journal of the European Academy of Dermatology and Venereology*, 37, pp. 945–950.
Marghoob, A. A., Usatine, R. P., and Jaimes, N. 2013. Dermoscopy for the family physician, *American Family Physician*, 88, pp. 441–450.
Mccarthy, J. 2003. Problems and projections in CS for the next 49 years, *Journal of the ACM*, 50, pp. 73–79.
Mehrabi, J. N., Baugh, E. G., Fast, A., Lentsch, G., Balu, M., Lee, B. A. and Kelly, K. M. 2021. A clinical perspective on the automated analysis of reflectance confocal microscopy in dermatology, *Lasers in Surgery and Medicine*, 53, pp. 1011–1019.
Miller, I. J., Stapelberg, M., Rosic, N., Hudson, J., Coxon, P., Furness, J., Walsh, J. and Climstein, M. 2023. Implementation of artificial intelligence for the detection of cutaneous melanoma within a primary care setting: Prevalence and types of skin cancer in outdoor enthusiasts, *PeerJ*, 11, p. e15737.
Narayanamurthy, V., Padmapriya, P., Noorasafrin, A., Pooja, B., Hema, K., Firus Khan, A. Y., Nithyakalyani, K. and Samsuri, F. 2018. Skin cancer detection using non-invasive techniques, *RSC Advances*, 8, pp. 28095–28130.
Navarrete-Dechent, C., Liopyris, K., Rishpon, A., Marghoob, N. G., Monnier, J. and Marghoob, A. A. 2020. Total Body Photography as an Aid for the Early Detection of Skin Cancer. In: Pasquali, P. (ed.) *Photography in Clinical Medicine*. Cham: Springer International Publishing.
Nelson, K. C., Swetter, S. M., Saboda, K., Chen, S. C. and Curiel-Lewandrowski, C. 2019. Evaluation of the number-needed-to-biopsy metric for the diagnosis of cutaneous melanoma: A systematic review and meta-analysis, *JAMA Dermatology*, 155, pp. 1167–1174.
O'Shea, K. and Nash, R. 2015. An introduction to convolutional neural networks. *arXiv preprint arXiv:1511.08458*.
Ohsie, S. J., Sarantopoulos, G. P., Cochran, A. J. and Binder, S. W. 2008. Immunohistochemical characteristics of melanoma, *Journal of the Cutaneous Pathology*, 35, pp. 433–444.
Oliveria, S. A., Sachs, D., Belasco, K. T. and Halpern, A. C. 2003. Adoption of new technologies for early detection of melanoma in dermatologic practice, *Journal of the American Academy of Dermatology*, 49, pp. 955–959.

Pampena, R., Kyrgidis, A., Lallas, A., Moscarella, E., Argenziano, G. and Longo, C. 2017. A meta-analysis of nevus-associated melanoma: Prevalence and practical implications, *Journal of the American Academy of Dermatology*, 77, pp. 938–945.e4.

Patel, R. H., Foltz, E. A., Witkowski, A. and Ludzik, J. 2023. Analysis of artificial intelligence-based approaches applied to non-invasive imaging for early detection of melanoma: A systematic review. *Cancers (Basel)*, 15, pp. 4694.

Phillips, M., Marsden, H., Jaffe, W., Matin, R. N., Wali, G. N., Greenhalgh, J., Mcgrath, E., James, R., Ladoyanni, E., Bewley, A., Argenziano, G. and Palamaras, I. 2019. Assessment of accuracy of an artificial intelligence algorithm to detect melanoma in images of skin lesions, *JAMA Network Open*, 2, p. e1913436.

Piris, A. and Mihm, M. C. 2009. Progress in melanoma histopathology and diagnosis, *Hematology/Oncology Clinics of North America*, 23, pp. 467–480.

Primiero, C. A., Betz-Stablein, B., Ascott, N., D'alessandro, B., Gaborit, S., Fricker, P., Goldsteen, A., González-Villà, S., Lee, K., Nazari, S., Nguyen, H., Ntouskos, V., Pahde, F., Pataki, B. E., Quintana, J., Puig, S., Rezze, G. G., Garcia, R., Soyer, H. P. and Malvehy, J. 2024. A protocol for annotation of total body photography for machine learning to analyze skin phenotype and lesion classification, *Frontiers in Medicine (Lausanne)*, 11, p. 1380984.

Rabbie, R., Ferguson, P., Molina-Aguilar, C., Adams, D. J. and Robles-Espinoza, C. D. 2019. Melanoma subtypes: Genomic profiles, prognostic molecular markers and therapeutic possibilities, *Journal of Pathology*, 247, pp. 539–551.

Saginala, K., Barsouk, A., Aluru, J. S., Rawla, P. and Barsouk, A. 2021. Epidemiology of melanoma, *Medical Sciences (Basel)*, 9, p. 63.

Salto-Tellez, M., Maxwell, P., and Hamilton, P. W. 2018. Artificial intelligence-the third revolution in pathology, *Histopathology*.

Seiverling, E. V., Prentiss, M. A., Stevens, K., Stoddard, H., Cyr, P. R. and Ahrns, H. 2023. Impact of dermoscopy training for primary care practitioners on number needed to biopsy to detect melanoma, *PRiMER*, 7, p. 276659.

Shoo, B. A., Sagebiel, R. W., and Kashani-Sabet, M. 2010. Discordance in the histopathologic diagnosis of melanoma at a melanoma referral center, *Journal of the American Academy of Dermatology*, 62, pp. 751–756.

Singh, V., Sultanpure, K. A. and Patil, H. 2024. Frontier machine learning techniques for melanoma skin cancer identification and categorization: An in-depth review, *Oral Oncology Reports*, 9, p. 100217.

Stiff, K. M., Franklin, M. J., Zhou, Y., Madabhushi, A. and Knackstedt, T. J. 2022. Artificial intelligence and melanoma: A comprehensive review of clinical, dermoscopic, and histologic applications, *Pigment Cell & Melanoma Research*, 35, pp. 203–211.

Terushkin, V., Oliveria, S. A., Marghoob, A. A. and Halpern, A. C. 2010. Use of and beliefs about total body photography and dermatoscopy among US dermatology training programs: An update, *Journal of the American Academy of Dermatology*, 62, pp. 794–803.

Tizhoosh, H. R., Diamandis, P., Campbell, C. J. V., Safarpoor, A., Kalra, S., Maleki, D., Riasatian, A., and Babaie, M. 2021. Searching images for consensus: Can AI remove observer variability in pathology? *The American Journal of Pathology*, 191, pp. 1702–1708.

Troxel, D. B. 2003. Pitfalls in the diagnosis of malignant melanoma: Findings of a risk management panel study, *The American Journal of Surgical Pathology*, 27, pp. 1278–1283.

Tsao, H., Olazagasti, J. M., Cordoro, K. M., Brewer, J. D., Taylor, S. C., Bordeaux, J. S., Chren, M.-M., Sober, A. J., Tegeler, C., Bhushan, R. and Begolka, W. S. 2015. Early detection of melanoma: Reviewing the ABCDEs, *Journal of the American Academy of Dermatology*, 72, pp. 717–723.

Urban, K., Mehrmal, S., Uppal, P., Giesey, R. L. and Delost, G. R. 2021. The global burden of skin cancer: A longitudinal analysis from the Global Burden of Disease Study, 1990–2017, *JAAD International*, 2, pp. 98–108.

Van Herck, Y., Antoranz, A., Andhari, M. D., Milli, G., Bechter, O., De Smet, F., and Bosisio, F. M. 2021. Multiplexed immunohistochemistry and digital pathology as the foundation for next-generation pathology in melanoma: Methodological comparison and future clinical applications, *Frontiers in Oncology*, 11.

Vuong, K., Armstrong, B. K., Weiderpass, E., Lund, E., Adami, H.-O., Veierod, M. B., Barrett, J. H., Davies, J. R., Bishop, D. T., Whiteman, D. C., Olsen, C. M., Hopper, J. L., Mann, G. J., Cust, A. E., Mcgeechan, K. and Investigators, A. T. A. M. F. S. 2016. Development and external validation of a melanoma risk prediction model based on self-assessed risk factors, *JAMA Dermatology*, 152, pp. 889–896.

Wei, M. L., Tada, M., So, A. and Torres, R. 2024. Artificial intelligence and skin cancer, *Frontiers in Medicine*, 11, p. 1331895.

Williams, N. M., Rojas, K. D., Reynolds, J. M., Kwon, D., Shum-tien, J., and Jaimes, N. 2021. Assessment of diagnostic accuracy of dermoscopic structures and patterns used in melanoma detection: A systematic review and meta-analysis, *JAMA Dermatology*, 157, pp. 1078–1088.

Winkler, J. K., Blum, A., Kommoss, K., Enk, A., Toberer, F., Rosenberger, A. and Haenssle, H. A. 2023. Assessment of diagnostic performance of dermatologists cooperating with a convolutional neural network in a prospective clinical study: Human with machine, *JAMA Dermatology*, 159, pp. 621–627.

Wodzinski, M., Skalski, A., Witkowski, A., Pellacani, G. and Ludzik, J. Convolutional neural network approach to classify skin lesions using reflectance confocal microscopy. 2019 41st Annual International Conference of the IEEE Engineering in Medicine and Biology Society (EMBC), 2019. IEEE, 4754–4757.

Xu, Y., Liu, X., Cao, X., Huang, C., Liu, E., Qian, S., Liu, X., Wu, Y., Dong, F., Qiu, C.-W., Qiu, J., Hua, K., Su, W., Wu, J., Xu, H., Han, Y., Fu, C., Yin, Z., Liu, M., Roepman, R., Dietmann, S., Virta, M., Kengara, F., Zhang, Z., Zhang, L., Zhao, T., Dai, J., Yang, J., Lan, L., Luo, M., Liu, Z., An, T., Zhang, B., He, X., Cong, S., Liu, X., Zhang, W., Lewis, J. P., Tiedje, J. M., Wang, Q., An, Z., Wang, F., Zhang, L., Huang, T., Lu, C., Cai, Z., Wang, F. and Zhang, J. 2021. Artificial intelligence: A powerful paradigm for scientific research, *The Innovation*, 2, p. 100179.

Yamashita, R., Nishio, M., Do, R. K. G. and Togashi, K. 2018. Convolutional neural networks: An overview and application in radiology, *Insights into Imaging*, 9, pp. 611–629.

Yang, Z., Zeng, X., Zhao, Y. and Chen, R. 2023. AlphaFold2 and its applications in the fields of biology and medicine, *Signal Transduction and Targeted Therapy*, 8, p. 115.

Zhang, S., Wang, Y., Zheng, Q., Li, J., Huang, J. and Long, X. 2022. Artificial intelligence in melanoma: A systematic review, *Journal of Cosmetic Dermatology*, 21, pp. 5993–6004.

4 Immunotherapy Advancements

Harnessing the Immune System with Technological Precision

Botle Precious Damane, Thanyani Mulaudzi, Tania Maphoso, Dakalo Ramali, and Cebo Beja
Department of Surgery, Steve Biko Academic Hospital, Faculty of Health Sciences, University of Pretoria, Pretoria, South Africa

Carmen Besliu and Jose Espinoza
Fortrea Inc., Durham, North Carolina, USA

Kamal S. Saini
Fortrea Inc., Durham, North Carolina, USA
Addenbrooke's Hospital, Cambridge University Hospitals NHS Foundation Trust, Cambridge, UK

Talent Chipiti, Thabiso Victor Miya, and Zodwa Dlamini
SAMRC Precision Oncology Research Unit (PORU), DSTI/NRF SARChI Chair in Precision Oncology and Cancer Prevention (POCP), Pan African Cancer Research Institute (PACRI), University of Pretoria, Pretoria, South Africa

INTRODUCTION

Cancer immunotherapy has emerged as a transformative approach in the fight against cancer through a series of stepwise events that must be carried out for an effective anticancer immune response called the cancer immunity cycle. A single step within the cycle can limit the immune response's effectiveness, but a successful response can be self-reinforcing. Even synthetic immunity strategies brought about by immunotherapies must work within this cycle to be effective (Mellman et al., 2023). Immunotherapy can combat cancer cells and prevent their recurrence by harnessing the immune system's power. Significant advancements have been made in this field, leading to novel immunotherapeutic strategies and the approval of numerous cancer-specific immunotherapeutic drugs (Yang, 2015). The application of immunotherapy in treating advanced and high-risk melanoma has significantly enhanced patient outcomes. For instance, median survival for patients with inoperable stage IV disease has increased from around six months to nearly six years, despite the rising incidence of melanoma (Knight et al., 2023).

In recent decades, there has been significant advancement in comprehending how cancer avoids detection by the immune system. This knowledge has spurred the development of innovative strategies

 DOI: 10.1201/9781003511625-4

to counteract these mechanisms, aiming to enhance the body's ability to eradicate cancerous cells. Notably, the success of immune checkpoint therapy, which involves using antibodies to block programmed cell death-1 (PD-1), programmed death ligand-1 (PD-L1), and cytotoxic T lymphocyte-associated antigen-4 (CTLA-4), as well as utilizing genetically modified oncolytic immunotherapy, tumor infiltrating lymphocytes (TILs), and chimeric antigen receptor (CAR) T cells, demonstrates the potential to shift the balance in favor of the immune system for cancer elimination (Li et al., 2019; Yang, 2015) (**Figure 4.1**). These breakthroughs emphasize the crucial role of decoding fundamental immunological processes to translate findings into clinical cancer treatments effectively.

However, despite these achievements, challenges persist in optimizing vaccine compositions, overcoming immune resistance, and refining combination therapies (Szeto and Finley, 2019). Addressing these challenges necessitates a concerted effort toward refining antigen selection and optimizing vaccine design, alongside implementing therapies that mitigate immunosuppressive mechanisms, such as PD-1 blockade (Yang, 2015). Additionally, exploring the potential of nanoparticle-based drug delivery systems can enhance the specificity and efficacy of immunotherapy (Amreddy et al., 2018). This chapter aims to explore recent advancements in cancer immunotherapy, focusing on immune system augmentation, precision vaccines, immunomodulation devices, synthetic biology and immunogenetics, immunocomputing, and the existing gaps in the literature. By addressing these gaps, further progress in cancer treatment can be achieved. Integrating these advancements can help develop personalized and effective cancer immunotherapies that target individual patient profiles and tumor characteristics (Abbott and Ustoyev, 2019).

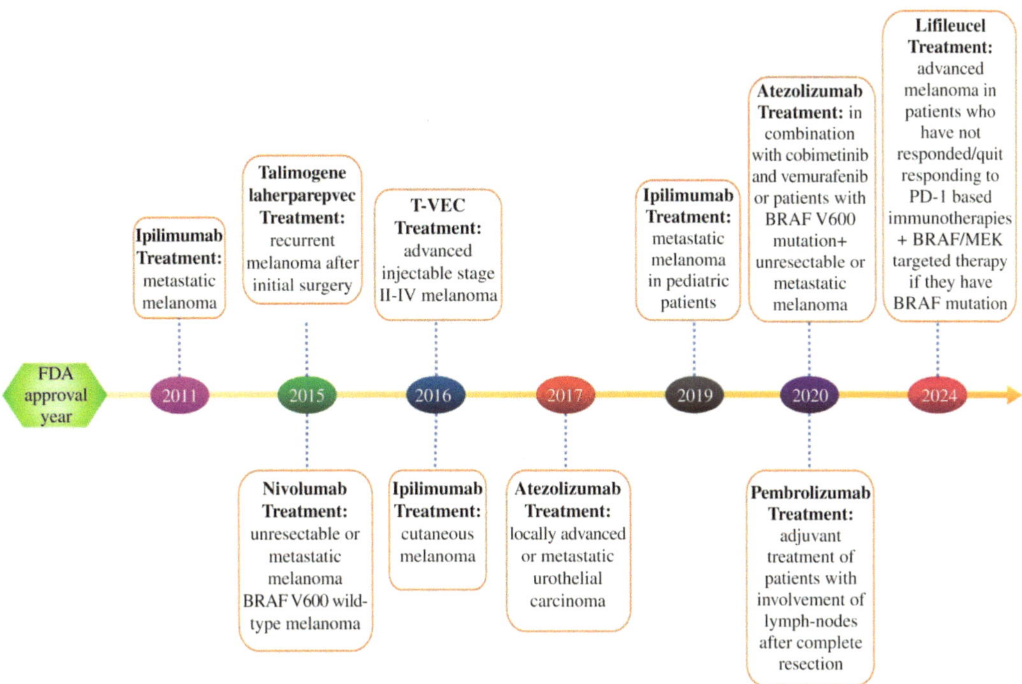

FIGURE 4.1 Treatment of melanoma using FDA-approved immunotherapy drugs. In 2011, ipilimumab, the first CTLA-4 immune checkpoint inhibitor (ICI), was approved to treat advanced inoperable metastatic melanoma. Talimogene laherparepvec, a first-in-class oncolytic immunotherapy, was approved by the FDA in 2015 for the local treatment of patients with melanoma recurrent after the initial surgery. In February 2024, Lifileucel (TILs) was approved by the FDA for patients with advanced melanoma through an accelerated approval process, becoming the first cellular therapy approved for cancer treatment. *Abbreviations*: Food and Drug Administration (FDA), cytotoxic T lymphocyte-associated antigen-4 (CTLA-4).

IMMUNOTHERAPY ADVANCEMENTS

There have been significant advancements in cancer immunotherapy, especially with the progress made in immune checkpoint blockade, oncolytic immunotherapy, and CAR-T-cell therapy. CTLA-4, discovered in 1987, was identified as an inhibitory receptor, leading to the development of anti-CTLA-4 antibodies, such as ipilimumab, which was approved for melanoma treatment in 2011 (Yang, 2015). This has marked a new era in cancer immunotherapy. Similarly, PD-1 blockade has emerged from a series of basic scientific discoveries, culminating in the development of antibodies that block the PD-1/PD-L1 interaction, significantly improving the treatment of advanced solid tumors (Yang, 2015). These treatments have shown notable efficacy also in patients suffering from some types of recurrent or resistant B-cell malignancies (Yang, 2015).

While sparing normal cells, genetically modified herpes simplex virus type 1 (HSV-1) with the insertion of gene-encoding hGM-CSF was discovered to selectively destroy tumor cells and led to the development of talimogene laherparepvec, which produces a direct oncolytic effect in injected lesions by replication of the virus in tumor cells and producing a systemic antitumor immune response enhanced by the local expression of granulocyte-macrophage colony-stimulating factor (GM-CSF). Based on this unique dual mechanism of action, talimogene laherparepvec is considered an oncolytic immunotherapy (Garnock-Jones, 2016; Hoffner et al., 2016). Furthermore, integrating ICIs, such as PD-1/PD-L1 system and CTLA-4 inhibitors, has shown remarkable efficacy in various cancers. As a result, ICIs have led to durable remission in some patients (**Figure 4.2**), significantly improving overall survival and providing long-lasting responses, particularly in cases where traditional treatments have been less effective (Szeto and Finley, 2019).

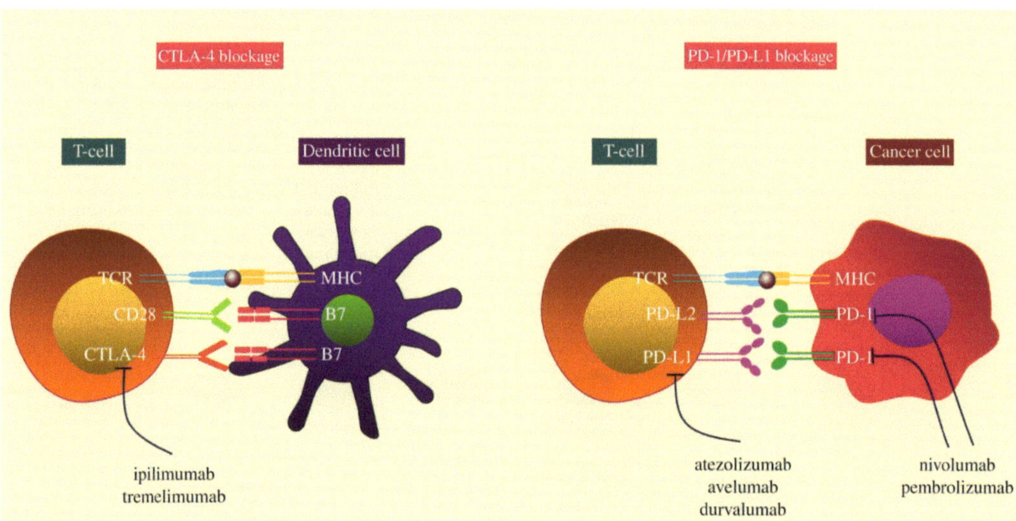

FIGURE 4.2 **CTLA-4 and PD-1/PD-L1 inhibitor action mechanisms.** T cells are the primary cells that express CTLA-4, which modulates the immune system by downregulating T-cell responses, ultimately blocking immune activation. By competing with CD28, the T-cell co-stimulatory receptor, for the binding of the same ligands (CD80, also known as B7.1, and CD86, also known as B7.2), CTLA-4 inhibits the activity of CD28 at the level of T-cell growth and proliferation. Whereas CTLA-4 plays a function in the initial stages of the cancer-immunity cycle, PD-1 and its ligands are essential for the elimination of cancer cells. From a physiological standpoint, PD-1/PD-L1 is responsible for suppressing T-cell activation in peripheral tissues during an inflammatory response to infection, which in turn suppresses autoimmunity. Like CTLA-4, PD-1 is expressed on activated T cells and works by obstructing the signaling pathways of T-cell receptors to suppress T-cell responses. There are two ligands for PD-1: PD-L1 (B7-H1), which is expressed on macrophages, fibroblasts, T cells, and antigen-presenting cells (APCs); and PD-L2 (B7-DC), which are mostly found on APCs. While PD-L2 is expressed comparatively seldomly, PD-L1 is also overexpressed in several solid malignancies. (From Wojtukiewicz et al., 2021.)

The exploration of combination therapies aims to enhance the effectiveness of immunotherapy and improve patient outcomes (Abbott and Ustoyev, 2019). Nanoparticle-based drug delivery systems have shown promise for enhancing the efficacy and specificity of immunotherapy. Nanoparticles can deliver immunotherapeutic agents, such as ICIs or cancer vaccines, thereby improving the immune response against cancer cells (Amreddy et al., 2018). However, optimizing the delivery of these agents, overcoming immune resistance, and enhancing combination therapies are critical challenges that must be addressed to unlock the full potential of nanoparticle-based immunotherapy.

IMMUNE SYSTEM AUGMENTATION

The role of the immune system in cancer control is multifaceted, involving both the recognition and elimination of transformed malignant cells and the suppression of tumor progression. This dual role, known as cancer immunoediting, includes three phases: elimination, equilibrium, and escape. The elimination phase is the protective phase, during which the innate and adaptive immune systems work together to detect and destroy tumor cells (Yang, 2015). If tumor cells survive antitumor immune attacks during the elimination phase, they enter the equilibrium phase, where the tumor cells remain in a dormant state and are unable to grow in number. Tumor cells enter the escape phase once they gain the capability to evade immune recognition and grow progressively (Chen and Mellman, 2013). Understanding these phases and the tumor microenvironment is crucial for developing therapies that target endogenous antitumor responses. Persistent inflammation can foster an immunosuppressive environment within tumors, facilitating tumor progression. Conversely, acute inflammation can bolster antitumor immune responses by promoting dendritic cell maturation and initiating T-cell activation (Yang, 2015).

Intralesional delivery of oncolytic immunotherapy involves the use of a genetically engineered virus that selectively replicates in tumor tissue with minimal toxicity to healthy cells. Malignant cells have characteristics that favor oncolytic virus replication, including an immunosuppressive environment, dysfunctional type 1 interferon (IFN) signaling, uncontrolled proliferation, and resistance to apoptosis. Unlike chemotherapy, the viral genome can be modified by deleting or limiting the expression of virulence genes to reduce or eliminate pathogenicity or by arming the virus with genes encoding, for example, cytokines to enhance antitumor activity (Deweese et al., 2001; Toda et al., 2000). The genetically engineered HSV-1, talimogene laherparepvec, has functionally deleted the neurovirulence factor infected cell protein 34.5 (ICP34.5) and the infected cell protein 47 (ICP47)-encoding gene, while the gene for GM-CSF is inserted into the viral genome. ICP47 blocks antigen presentation to major histocompatibility complex (MHC) class-I. This deletion allows increased expression of the US11 gene, which promotes virus growth in cancer cells (Ferrucci et al., 2021). GM-CSF is a pleiotropic cytokine involved in the stimulation of cellular immune responses by promoting the generation of dendritic cells from blood monocytes. These dendritic cells have the ability to capture antigens, migrate in response to chemotactic stimuli, and induce proliferative responses in $CD4^+$ and $CD8^+$ T-lymphocytes (Demir et al., 2003).

Recent advancements have highlighted the importance of targeting tumor-associated macrophages (TAMs), which play a crucial role in maintaining the suppressive tumor microenvironment and can affect clinical outcomes (Yang, 2015). Augmenting the immune system through T-cell-based immunotherapies involves using tumor-infiltrated or genetically modified T cells to mediate antitumor immune responses. These therapies are classified into adoptive transfer of tumor-infiltrating lymphocytes (TILs), T cells engineered with T-cell receptors (TCR-Ts), and CAR-T cells. This represents a cutting-edge approach to bolster the immune system's ability to recognize and destroy melanoma cells effectively (Rohaan et al., 2019; Szeto and Finley, 2019).

TILs isolated from resected from tumors are expanded *ex vivo* and infused back into patients following lymphodepletion preconditioning. This preconditioning depletes endogenous lymphocytes and removes immunosuppressive cells to disrupt a suppressive microenvironment and maintain TIL function (Robbins et al., 2011, 2015). Adoptive cell therapy with TILs focuses on harnessing the antitumor activity of tumor-resident T cells, while CAR-T-cell therapies require gene engineering to enhance the antitumor T-cell activity. The TILs are not engineered before being expanded *in vitro*. TIL therapy supported by IL2 administration showed consistent efficacy in heavily pretreated patients with metastatic melanoma (Sarnaik et al., 2021). His study contributed to the body of evidence supporting the efficacy of Lifileucel later leading to the FDA's accelerated approval of the first cellular therapy for metastatic melanoma patients in 2024.

Although T-cell receptors (TCRs) and CAR-T cells use different mechanisms of tumor antigen recognition, both involve the modification of T lymphocytes from cancer patients *ex vivo*. These T cells are genetically engineered with a non-viral vector to target melanoma-specific antigens, expanded, and then infused back into the cancer patient. CAR-T cells recognize extracellular antigens in an MHC-restricted fashion, representing about 25% of all antigens and exhibiting high binding strength. In contrast, TCRs recognize both extra- and intracellular antigens, thus representing a broader range of antigens with low-to-medium binding strength, resulting in a wider breadth of targetable antigens (Robbins et al., 2011, 2015). Multiple generations of CAR-T cells have been produced as of now, mainly classified based on their intracellular signaling domain responsible for T-cell activation and activity and T-cell persistence (**Figure 4.3**).

Several clinical trials have tested TCRs restricted to the human lymphocyte antigen (HLA)-A1 or A2 genotypes and directed against various antigens, including differentiation antigens (e.g., gp100, MART-1, p53, and CEA), cancer germline antigens (e.g., MAGE-A3 and NY-ESO-1), and viral antigens. While adoptive TCR therapy has shown promising results, further optimization of safety is needed, particularly for high-affinity TCRs directed against antigens that are overexpressed in both tumors and healthy tissues (Kunert et al., 2013).

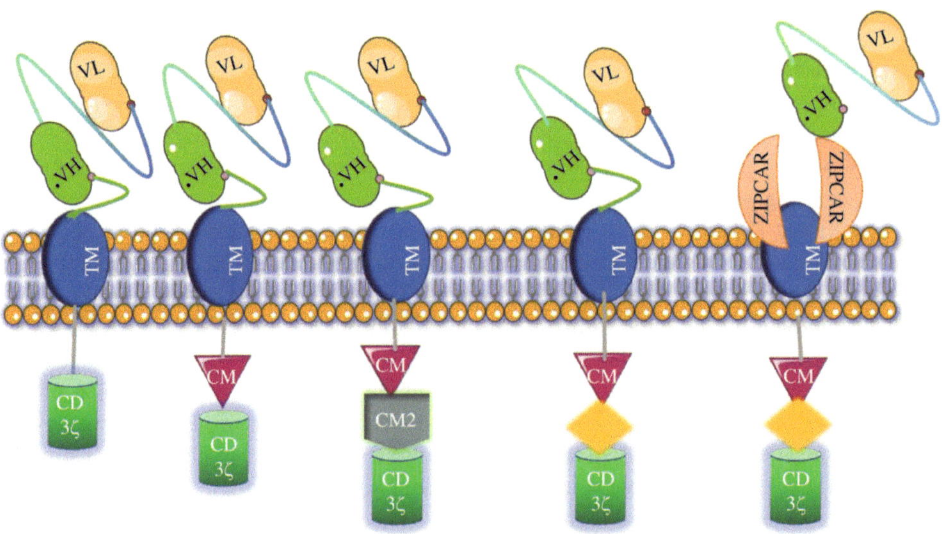

FIGURE 4.3 **CAR-T-cell receptor generations.** The 1G CAR features a single CD3ζ domain without co-stimulatory molecules (CMs), representing the simplest form of CAR design. The 2G CAR introduces one CM alongside the CD3ζ domain, enhancing signaling through dual pathways. The 3G CAR further advances by incorporating multiple CMs (e.g., two or more) with the CD3ζ domain, facilitating multiple signaling pathways for increased efficacy. The 4G CAR adds complexity with the inclusion of a nuclear factor of activated T-cells-responsive cassette along with the CD3ζ domain and one CM, enabling triple-signaling mechanisms from CD3ζ, the CM, and transgenic cytokines or proteins. Finally, the 5G CAR integrates the CD3ζ domain, one CM, and ZIP CAR domain, showcasing a sophisticated design with synergistic triple signaling that combines CD3ζ and the CM components to maximize CAR-T-cell activation and function. The external membrane domain consists of the variable region of the heavy chain and the variable region of the light chain.

Following the outstanding outcomes achieved in different types of leukemia, lymphomas, and multiple myeloma, CAR-T-cell therapies turned toward the treatment of solid tumors as well, including melanoma, where several tumor antigens are currently used as targets for CAR-T cells in clinical studies. However, the hostile tumor microenvironment and the difficulty of CAR-T cells to infiltrate the solid tumors, as well as the tumor antigen heterogenicity, are challenges that need to be circumvented during CAR-T-cell development. Moreover, the use of biomimetic particle coatings to reduce opsonization and uptake by the mononuclear phagocyte system (MPS) enhances the circulation time of nanoparticles and improves treatment efficacy (Blanco et al., 2015).

PRECISION VACCINE+

Despite the achievements in immune checkpoint blockade, innovative HSV-1-based oncolytic immunotherapy, TILs and CAR-T-cell therapies, therapeutic cancer vaccines have yielded suboptimal outcomes, largely due to deficiencies in vaccine design and the immunosuppressive tumor microenvironment (Yang, 2015). Enhancements in selecting antigens and refining vaccine architecture, coupled with strategies that counteract immunosuppression like PD-1 blockade, are essential for improving clinical efficacy. Neoantigens, arising from tumor-specific mutations, are particularly promising for cancer control through vaccination, as T cells targeting these antigens evade central tolerance mechanisms (Yang, 2015). Recent progress in next-generation sequencing and epitope prediction enables rapid identification of neoantigens, informing and facilitating personalized cancer immunotherapies (Yang, 2015).

To address these challenges, researchers are exploring novel vaccine platforms to enhance antigen presentation and immune activation. Novel strategies for producing vaccinations against melanoma using DNA and mRNA vaccines to stimulate the immune system and target tumor cells effectively are highlighted in **Figure 4.4**.

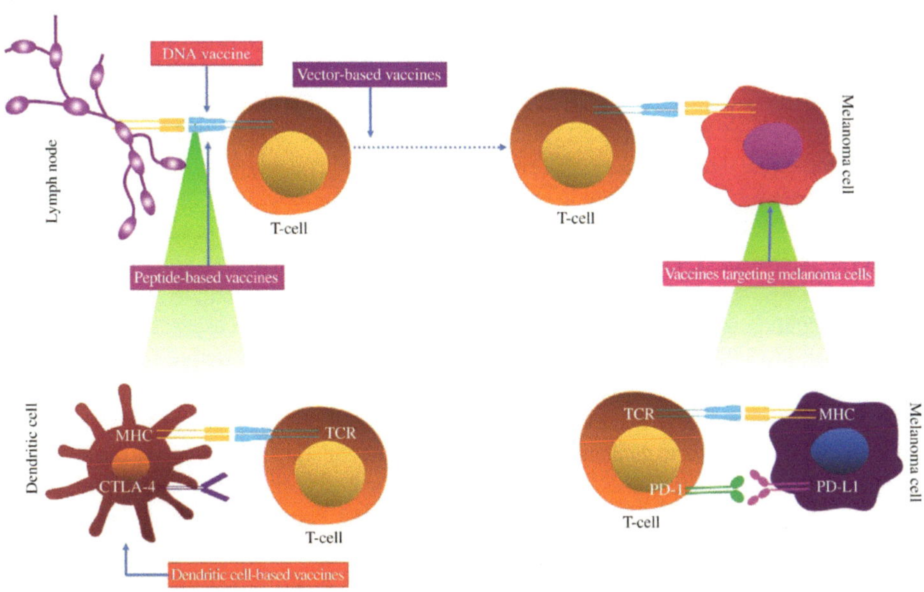

FIGURE 4.4 **Novel strategies for producing vaccinations against melanoma.** Several innovative vaccine strategies aimed at targeting melanoma cells include DNA, peptide, vector-based, and dendritic cell-based vaccines. These vaccines stimulate an immune response that involves lymph nodes, where antigens are presented to immune cells. DNA vaccines deliver plasmid DNA encoding melanoma antigens; peptide vaccines use synthesized epitopes specific to melanoma; vector-based vaccines employ viral or bacterial vectors to introduce melanoma-associated genes; and dendritic cell-based vaccines involve the extraction, loading, and reinfusion of patient-derived dendritic cells with melanoma antigens. These approaches are designed to activate anti-cancer immunity for the elimination of melanoma cells, providing a focused and personalized approach.

Precision vaccines tailored for melanoma aim to induce targeted immune responses against tumor-specific antigens. These vaccines leverage neoantigens derived from individual tumors to stimulate a robust and specific immune reaction against melanoma cells while minimizing collateral damage to healthy tissues and with a low risk of inducing autoimmunity (Szeto and Finley, 2019). The integration of nanoparticle-based radiosensitizers can further enhance the efficacy of radiotherapy by improving the radiosensitivity of the melanoma cells (Boateng and Ngwa, 2019).

IMMUNOMODULATION DEVICES

Devices that modulate the immune system, such as implants or wearable devices, play a crucial role in advancing melanoma immunotherapy. Implants and wearables designed for immunomodulation hold promise for enhancing therapeutic outcomes in melanoma by fine-tuning immune responses against cancer cells (Mariani et al., 2019). **Table 4.1** illustrates the types of immunomodulatory devices that are either being developed or utilized. Thus, this section explores the mechanisms, types, applications, and future potential of these devices in melanoma immunotherapy, highlighting their role in personalized treatment approaches and their impact on improving patient outcomes.

Immunotherapy systems use biomaterials to regulate immune cell function, exert enzyme-like activity, and neutralize cytokines (Dai et al., 2022). One way immunomodulation devices work is through the use of biomaterials in the form of nanoparticle-based devices (Khatun et al., 2023). These devices control the immune system using nanoparticles engineered to deliver particles directly to targeted cells or tissues (Toy and Roy, 2016). Therapeutic nanoparticles are loaded with drugs, proteins, or genes that modulate immune responses (Malachowski and Hassel, 2020). These nanoparticles are designed to navigate biological barriers at both systemic and cellular levels, serving as precision therapeutics focusing on optimizing delivery (Mitchell et al., 2021). Their small size allows them to penetrate tissues and cells, enabling precise treatment and diagnosis (Kong et al., 2023). They are ideal for drug delivery because they are biodegradable, water-soluble, stable during storage, and able to mimic biochemical processes (Valcourt et al., 2020). Nanomaterials exhibit specific optical absorption spectra and biocompatibility features crucial for effective melanoma treatment (Doughty et al., 2019).

Nanoparticles have also shown promising results in melanoma through various mechanisms of action, including encapsulating therapeutic agents for photodynamic therapy (PDT), inducing heat damage using photothermal therapy (PTT), modifying activation and phenotype in immunomodulation, and enhancing drug delivery and penetration in chemotherapy (Diaz et al., 2023). However, research on using nanomaterial-based techniques to target skin cancers is relatively recent compared to other types of cancers (Farhana, 2023). One treatment option involved in melanoma is utilizing thermal energy to target cancer cells, relying on the sensitivity of cancer cells to heat (Doughty et al., 2019). In PTT, nanoparticle excitation is utilized to induce a controlled temperature increase, resulting in irreversible damage to cancerous cells while minimizing harm to nontarget tissues (Chatterjee et al., 2011). In a study by Zhang et al. (2018), the role of necroptosis in the efficacy of PTT using gold nanorods utilized with a targeting adaptor in melanoma treatment was investigated. They demonstrated that the induction of PTT at varying temperatures leads to distinct patterns of cell death, with necroptosis emerging as a significant mechanism at moderate temperatures, alongside apoptosis and necrosis (Zhang et al., 2018). A study by Sobhani et al. (2017) demonstrated the use of PTT in melanoma, combining polyethylene glycol-coated oxidized carbon nanotubes with laser irradiation, noting a significantly reduced melanoma tumor size, highlighting the potential efficacy in cancer therapy (Sobhani et al., 2017).

Bear et al. (2013) also investigated the dual effects of PTT on local tumor debulking and immune response modulation. Their study demonstrated that while PTT induces proinflammatory cytokines and dendritic cell maturation in tumor-draining lymph nodes, a combined approach of PTT with T cells effectively prevents primary tumor recurrence, inhibits distant metastases, and optimizes overall tumor control, offering a promising strategy for clinical application (Bear et al., 2013). Photothermal hydrogels have also been applied in post-chemotherapy and radiotherapy treatment against bacterial infections, as well as in enhancing wound healing (Liu et al., 2024). This hydrogel is developed with nanomaterials that induce photon therapy when induced (Ding et al., 2022). This mode of treatment is especially useful in melanoma because of the high rate of recurrence, and traditional therapies often result in damaged surrounding tissue.

Additionally, their highly hydrophilic three-dimensional (3D) network structure provides a moist environment that offers strong biocompatibility and adhesion for promoting wound healing (Liu et al., 2024). A study by Yang et al. (2024) also utilized smart DNA hydrogel systems designed to improve the efficacy of immunotherapy in melanoma. This localized therapeutic approach achieved a significant tumor suppression rate, demonstrating the hydrogel's capability to synergistically enhance immunotherapy and PDT, highlighting its potential in advancing biomedical applications of DNA materials (Yang et al., 2024). In conclusion, the rapid advancements in immunomodulatory devices offer exciting prospects for refining melanoma therapy through precise immune manipulation and targeted therapeutic delivery. Moving forward, this chapter explores various types of devices, including implants, wearable technologies, and novel biomaterial-based systems, each poised to revolutionize personalized treatment approaches and improve outcomes for melanoma patients.

TYPES OF IMMUNOMODULATORY DEVICES

Nanoparticle devices can be used as wearable gadgets capable of detecting cancer cell conditions, vitals, and other infectious diseases (**Table 4.1**) (Haleem et al., 2023). Nanobots are utilized for *in vitro* diagnosis through smart tablets that transmit data on cancer, enabling noninvasive diagnosis and providing information on treatment effectiveness (Giri et al., 2021). Another innovative approach to nanorobotics is the use of viral capsids, which are more resilient and able to withstand environmental pressures using their proteinaceous shells, safeguarding viral nucleic acids from external denaturation (Kong et al., 2023). These structures are typically developed as organic, inorganic, and carbon-based chemical structures (Anu Mary Ealia and Saravanakumar, 2017). Organic nanocarriers are further grouped into polymer-based smart nanocarriers, including dendrimers and micelles (Sabit et al., 2022). Additionally, organic chemicals are developed as biomimetic-based smart nanocarriers, including liposomes, protein nanoparticles, and cell membrane particles (Farhoudi et al., 2023). Inorganics include metallic, metal oxides, and quantum dots (Krishna et al., 2013). Lastly, carbon-based nanoparticles are grouped into nanotubes or fullerenes (Rahmati and Mozafari, 2019). A study by Wang et al. (2023) addressed the challenge of initiating an adaptive immune response in the immunosuppressive tumor microenvironment within melanoma tumors by developing nanorobots as a dynamic antigen delivery system. This approach effectively boosts the interaction of the antigens, leading to significant immunotherapeutic effects against melanoma, particularly through the activation of cytotoxic T lymphocytes (CTLs) (Wang et al., 2023).

TABLE 4.1
An Overview of Various Types of Immunomodulatory Devices Used in the Context of Melanoma Therapy

Type of Device	Description	References
Nanoparticle-based devices	Use nanoparticles for targeted drug delivery and immune system modulation	Fang and Zhang (2016)
Photothermal hydrogels	Hydrogels incorporating nanomaterials that induce photothermal effects for localized therapy	Ahmadian et al. (2022)
Electromagnetic devices	Devices employing electromagnetic fields to influence immune cell behavior and therapeutic outcomes	Ross et al. (2016)
Bioelectronic devices	Devices interfacing with the nervous system to modulate immune responses and deliver therapeutic agents	Cracchiolo et al. (2021)
Implants and wearables	Devices implanted or worn on the body to continuously monitor and modulate immune responses	Rodrigues et al. (2020)

Electromagnetic devices are other examples of immunomodulatory devices, which utilize electromagnetic fields to influence immune cell behavior and function (Piszczek et al., 2021). Devices utilizing these fields are being explored for their potential to treat inflammatory and autoimmune diseases. Radiofrequency ablation targets specific tissues to modify immune responses, often used in cancer treatments. A study by Souiade et al. (2023) investigated the efficacy of different alternating magnetic field waveforms to induce localized heating. They compared their ability to cause cell death in B16F10 and CT2A cell lines. Non-harmonic waveforms demonstrated superior efficacy over the sinusoidal waveform in enhancing treatment efficiency against melanoma tumor cells. This study highlights the potential of electromagnetic waveforms to improve therapeutic outcomes in cancer treatment (Souiade et al., 2023). These magnetic devices can also be used for noninvasive diagnosis. A study by Shafi et al. (2023) proposed an alternative skin cancer screening method using electromagnetic waves and radio frequency technology with a device. This approach enhanced diagnostic accuracy by differentiating between cancerous and non-cancerous lesions with over 92% sensitivity and 81.4% specificity, potentially improving patient comfort and enabling instantaneous diagnosis (Shafi et al., 2023).

Bioelectronic devices interface with the nervous system to modulate immune responses (Carnevale et al., 2021). In addition, neuromodulation devices control immune responses through neural pathways, offering non-pharmacological options for managing immune-related conditions (Won et al., 2020). These devices can be implanted or used externally to provide real-time adjustments to immune activity. These devices provide a physical structure that can release immunomodulatory agents over time or recruit immune cells to a specific site, facilitating localized immune modulation (Stabler et al., 2019). Three-dimensional (3D)-printed scaffolds are customized to fit patient-specific needs and deliver precise immunomodulatory treatments (Abdelaziz et al., 2023).

In summary, immunomodulatory devices represent a transformative step forward in melanoma therapy; the exploration of implants, wearable technologies, and biomaterial-based systems will play a pivotal role in advancing personalized treatment approaches, offering new avenues for optimizing patient care in the fight against melanoma. Moving forward, the next section of this chapter delves into emerging trends in synthetic biology and immunogenetics.

SYNTHETIC BIOLOGY AND IMMUNOGENETICS

Advances in synthetic biology could enable the engineering of immune cells with enhanced functionalities, such as improved antigen recognition or resistance to immunosuppression (Brenner et al., 2018). Similarly, insights from immunogenetics could inform the development of personalized therapies that target specific genetic variations affecting immune function (Gunter et al., 2019). The genetic and immunological interplay in melanoma plays a significant role in understanding diagnostic and treatment profiles for these cancers (Davis et al., 2019). Although the development of melanoma is complex, understanding this will be essential for early detection and treatment development (Eddy et al., 2021).

The introduction of immunotherapy to melanoma treatment has had exponential results, allowing for molecular and cellular intervention utilizing the understanding of the immune function to ultimately create personalized therapies (Zhu et al., 2016). Connecting synthetic biology and immunogenetics creates a unique opportunity to design therapies that are able to target specific cells, with limited side effects either at a cellular or molecular level (Jain and Jain, 2021). In melanoma, immunogenetics is being utilized to understand the genes involved in the immune response as well as how cancer cells are able to evade immune mechanisms (Queirolo et al., 2019). This research revolves around the characterization of immune cells such as B and T cells, and how they interact with specific receptors. Melanoma tumor cells also have the capacity to evade the immune response through the following mechanisms: modifications of surface molecules, absence of CMs, production of immunosuppressive cytokines, and alterations in HLA molecules (Kalaora et al., 2022; Méndez et al., 2008; Teixido et al., 2021). These mechanisms are known to contribute to the high mortality in cutaneous melanoma. The following gene types are involved in melanoma development: HLA genes, immune checkpoint genes, and tumor antigen genes (Qin et al., 2021).

Significant advancements have been made in melanoma and HLA immunogenetics, focusing on improving personalized treatment approaches and understanding the immune response to melanoma antigens. HLA genes are responsible for stimulating immune cells to provide protection and defense against cancer (Mosaad, 2015). In addition to this, the HLA alleles affect the overall survival of cancer patients because of their capacity to recognize cancer-associated molecules (Hazini et al., 2021). HLA genes are polymorphic and are involved in MHCs, responsible for over 200 immune-related genes associated with white blood cell development (Monos and Winchester, 2019; Navarrete, 2000).

Melanoma cells evade immune checkpoints and proliferate rapidly; they are known to downregulate HLA expression (Attrill et al., 2021). Advances in immunogenetics have led to the development of personalized cancer vaccines and therapies targeting specific HLA types (Blass and Ott, 2021). The integration of HLA typing with genomic data has facilitated the advancement of precision medicine approaches. By considering HLA diversity, clinicians can tailor treatments to individual patients based on their genetic predispositions and immune profiles (Pagliuca et al., 2022). Moreover, advances in genomic and transcriptomic sequencing technologies have enabled the identification of tumor-specific antigens, including mutated peptides and overexpressed peptides on melanoma cells (Li et al., 2023; Smith et al., 2019). This has paved the way for developing personalized cancer vaccines that target these specific antigens. Sahin et al. (2017) conducted a groundbreaking study on personalized RNA mutanome vaccines for melanoma, showcasing their potential to mobilize immune responses against cancer mutations. By identifying individual mutations and predicting neo-epitopes, the researchers designed unique vaccines for each patient. All patients developed T-cell responses to multiple neo-epitopes, and a significant reduction in metastatic events was observed, resulting in sustained progression-free survival. Additionally, vaccine-induced T-cell infiltration and tumor cell killing were confirmed in post-vaccination samples (Sahin et al., 2017).

Techniques, such as the XPRESIDENT™ platform (Tübingen approach), have been developed to analyze the HLA ligandome of tumor tissues (Freudenmann et al., 2018). This approach involves extracting tumor samples, isolating HLA-bound peptides, and using mass spectrometry to identify mutated peptides unique to the patient's tumor. These peptides are then used to formulate personalized cancer vaccines, aiming to induce robust immune responses against melanoma (Freudenmann et al., 2018). Overall, these advancements in melanoma and HLA immunogenetics represent a paradigm shift toward precision medicine, where treatment strategies are increasingly tailored to individual genetic profiles and tumor characteristics. These developments hold promise for improving outcomes in melanoma patients and are shaping the future of cancer immunotherapy.

Synthetic biology also offers promising avenues for advancing melanoma research and treatment through innovative approaches. This is conducted through the engineering of T-cell therapies (Caliendo et al., 2019). Another advancement is through the use of gene editing tools, tools like clustered regularly interspaced palindromic repeats (CRISPR)—CRISPR-associated (Cas) 9, which enable precise genetic modifications in melanoma cells. A recent study by Christodoulou et al. (2021) focused on targeting the MAPK signaling pathway in metastatic melanoma utilizing CRISPR-Cas9 genetic screens to uncover novel genetic dependencies that could serve as therapeutic targets. The study reported significantly reduced melanoma cell fitness upon inactivation, including both known and novel melanoma fitness genes, suggesting that its loss further activates MAPK signaling, which is deleterious to melanoma cells (Christodoulou et al., 2021). Overall, synthetic biology holds immense potential for transforming melanoma treatment by providing innovative solutions that enhance specificity, efficacy, and personalized therapies. Continued research and technological advancements in this field are essential for realizing these therapeutic opportunities and improving patient outcomes. Bioinformatics and computational modeling also benefit from advanced computational tools and bioinformatics algorithms that facilitate the design and optimization of synthetic biological systems for melanoma therapy (Rahman et al., 2022).

IMMUNOCOMPUTING AND BIOINFORMATICS

Researchers are currently leveraging computational models and artificial intelligence (AI) to develop sophisticated tools for analyzing and predicting immune system behavior. This research holds the potential for tailoring treatment strategies to an individual's unique immune profile and for identifying new targets and approaches for therapy. The field of melanoma treatment has seen remarkable progress due to the emergence of immunotherapy. Through the integration of immunocomputing and bioinformatics, a novel approach to utilizing the immune system for more effective melanoma treatment has arisen. These advanced technologies have the potential to enhance the precision and effectiveness of immunotherapy through personalized treatment strategies and the discovery of new therapeutics (Zakariya et al., 2024).

LEVERAGING IMMUNOCOMPUTING AND ARTIFICIAL INTELLIGENCE

Computational approaches are utilized to advance and optimize immunotherapy (immunocomputing). These technologies enable researchers to create advanced tools for analyzing and predicting immune system behavior with unparalleled accuracy. These models replicate various elements of the immune response, such as the interactions between cancer cells and immune cells, the impacts of different therapeutic agents, and the dynamics of the tumor microenvironment. This facilitates a more precise comprehension of how various treatments can influence melanoma progression and immune responses (Ricker et al., 2024).

In recent years, immunotherapy has revolutionized cancer treatment. However, one of the major challenges has been identifying the most suitable candidates for this form of treatment. To address this challenge, AI has been integrated into clinical practices to handle tasks that traditionally rely on human intelligence, such as language interpretation, visual perception, and decision-making (Sebastian and Peter, 2022). AI technologies have significantly improved the precision and effectiveness of diagnosing and predicting responses to cancer treatments. With AI, clinicians can accurately categorize patients who are likely to respond favorably to cancer immunotherapy, ensuring that only appropriate candidates receive the treatment (Esteva et al., 2017).

PERSONALIZED TREATMENT STRATEGIES

One of the most promising applications of immunocomputing and bioinformatics lies in the development of personalized treatment strategies. Understanding the uniqueness of each individual's immune system is crucial for effective immunotherapy. By analyzing an individual's immune profile, encompassing genetic, proteomic, and cellular data, computational models can forecast how a patient is likely to respond to different immunotherapeutic agents. This personalized approach empowers clinicians to customize treatments tailored to the patient's immune system, potentially enhancing the therapy's efficacy and reducing adverse effects (Kourou et al., 2015).

Personalized neoantigen vaccines represent a rapidly advancing area where bioinformatics plays a critical role. These vaccines are customized based on the unique set of neoantigens (mutated proteins expressed by tumor cells) found in an individual's melanoma. Computational tools are utilized to identify these neoantigens from sequencing data, enabling the development of vaccines that can effectively train the immune system to target melanoma cells. Studies have illustrated that patients who have received personalized neoantigen vaccines exhibited robust immune responses and prolonged disease-free survival (Ott et al., 2017). Tumor neoantigens are essential for the success of immunotherapy, as they serve as targets for the immune system's attacks. One of the primary challenges is the rapid and accurate prediction of immunogenic tumor antigens. AI, particularly machine learning (ML) techniques, holds the potential to streamline this process by identifying the factors that determine tumor immunogenicity and the peptides presented by MHC-I. These capabilities can be leveraged to assess neoantigen binding and predict treatment responses in cancer immunotherapy (Tabari et al., 2023).

For instance, artificial neural networks have enabled the identification of tumor antigen T-cell epitopes in melanoma patients, thereby facilitating personalized cancer immunotherapy (Nielsen et al., 2010). AI, especially through neural-based models, has significantly advanced the understanding of the tumor immune microenvironment, which is crucial for comprehending patients' responses to cancer immunotherapy. Integrating RNA sequencing with imaging data in clinical settings has allowed for a more precise characterization of these environments for solid tumors like colorectal, breast, lung, and pancreatic cancers (Lin et al., 2023; Xie et al., 2023). These advancements have paved the way for more accurate patient stratification and personalized treatment plans.

DISCOVERY OF NEW DRUG TARGETS AND THERAPEUTIC APPROACHES

AI and bioinformatics play a crucial role in discovering new drug targets and therapeutic approaches. These technologies analyze large datasets from genomic and proteomic studies to identify potential targets for immunotherapy that were previously unknown. ML algorithms can sift through complex biological data to find patterns and correlations that suggest new mechanisms of tumor immune evasion or resistance. For example, computational approaches have helped in the identification of novel immune checkpoints beyond PD-1/PD-L1 and CTLA-4. These discoveries have led to the development of next-generation ICIs that are currently being evaluated in clinical trials (Topalian et al., 2016). Furthermore, AI has been used to identify biomarkers that predict which patients are most likely to benefit from specific immunotherapies, thereby optimizing patient selection and treatment outcomes (Prelaj et al., 2023).

Numerous research groups and companies are dedicated to developing AI programs that aim to enhance the efficiency, precision, and affordability of cancer screening. AI acts as a supplementary visual aid, empowering medical professionals to identify and diagnose cancer with greater precision than traditional methods, leading to improved diagnostic accuracy and better patient insights (Jha and Topol, 2016). In particular, deep learning (DL) methods enable the precise and automated identification of changes in tumor size and gene status, which are critical for monitoring the efficacy of immunotherapy (Litjens et al., 2017). AI is also instrumental in predicting responses to immunotherapy by evaluating immune signatures, medical imaging, and histologic analysis. As the knowledge of molecular mechanisms of tumors expands, AI helps refine immunotherapy strategies, ensuring that treatments are tailored to enhance the immune system's ability to recognize and target cancer cells (Topol, 2019). AI tools have been used to identify biomarkers and immune signatures that predict how well a patient will respond to specific immunotherapies, thereby optimizing treatment protocols (Kather et al., 2018).

CASE STUDIES AND EXAMPLES

Several studies illustrate the impact of using immunocomputing and bioinformatics in melanoma treatment. For example, Gibney et al. (2016) conducted a study using ML models to predict patient responses to anti-PD-1 therapy based on pre-treatment tumor biopsies. These models incorporated features such as gene expression profiles and patterns of immune cell infiltration, achieving high predictive accuracy and enabling more informed treatment decisions. Furthermore, bioinformatics tools have been employed to analyze the tumor microenvironment and identify biomarkers associated with response or resistance to immunotherapy (Gibney et al., 2016). A study by Hegde et al. (2016) demonstrated how bioinformatics analysis of tumor samples from melanoma patients treated with ICIs revealed distinct immune signatures correlated with clinical outcomes. This valuable information helps in refining treatment strategies and improving patient management.

Radiomics, an advanced AI technique, is transforming cancer management by analyzing detailed patterns from medical images obtained through computed tomography (CT), magnetic resonance imaging (MRI), and positron emission tomography (PET) (Gillies et al., 2016). These patterns play a crucial role in various clinical applications, including monitoring response rates, customizing therapy, stratifying risks, analyzing survival, predicting metastatic potential, and patient monitoring (Lambin et al., 2012). Radiomics is particularly effective in customizing therapy by identifying subtle differences in medical images that can significantly impact treatment decisions. For example, the predictive signatures obtained from radiomic analysis have been associated with immune markers, such as CD8+ expression in melanoma (Lambin et al., 2012). This expression is inversely related to the mean of positive pixel (MPP) and standard deviation (SD), which in turn correlates with patient prognostic outcomes (Trebeschi et al., 2019). This application is not limited to melanoma; it has also been effectively used in non-small-cell lung cancer and renal cancers, providing valuable insights into patient survival outcomes, especially in those treated with pembrolizumab (Sun et al., 2018).

The integration of immunocomputing and bioinformatics into melanoma immunotherapy marks a groundbreaking advancement in cancer treatment. These technologies enable the development of personalized treatment strategies, enhancing the precision and efficacy of immunotherapy and facilitating the discovery of new drug targets and therapeutic approaches. As computational models and AI continue to evolve, their application in melanoma treatment promises to improve patient outcomes and revolutionize the field of oncology. The integration of AI in cancer immunotherapy represents a significant advancement, enhancing the precision, efficacy, and personalization of cancer treatments. By leveraging AI for patient stratification, tumor characterization, and treatment monitoring, clinicians can offer more targeted and effective therapies. As AI and biotechnology continue to evolve, their combined application promises to revolutionize cancer treatment and improve patient outcomes.

CHALLENGES AND LIMITATIONS

Immunomodulation devices hold significant potential for treating various conditions but are confronted with substantial challenges and limitations that must be overcome to enable effective clinical application. A primary challenge lies in achieving precise control over immune modulation. The complex nature of the immune system implies that imprecise modulation may lead to unintended consequences such as off-target effects, over-activation, or suppression, resulting in undesirable immune responses. While researchers are actively pursuing the development of advanced algorithms and feedback systems to enhance the precision of these devices, attaining the requisite control level remains a major obstacle (Hancock et al., 2016).

Ensuring the biocompatibility of immunomodulation devices is imperative to prevent adverse immune reactions. Key considerations encompass material rejection, cytotoxicity, and chronic inflammation. Current advancements in biomaterials science concentrate on creating materials that are not only biocompatible but also capable of seamless integration with biological tissues (Ratner et al., 2013). Safeguarding the long-term stability and functionality of devices intended for chronic conditions is of utmost importance. These devices encounter challenges related to degradation, power supply, and maintenance. Continuous research efforts aim to enhance the durability and reliability of these devices, thereby ensuring effective performance over extended periods (Schmalz et al., 2018). Navigating the regulatory landscape is essential to ensure the safety and efficacy of immunomodulation devices for clinical adoption. Challenges in this realm include intricate regulations, extensive clinical trials, and post-market surveillance. As highlighted by Wilkinson & Boxtel (2019), successfully navigating these regulatory requirements is vital for the introduction of new immunomodulation devices to the market (Wilkinson and Van Boxtel, 2020).

While immunomodulation devices present the potential to revolutionize the treatment of various immune-related conditions, they confront significant challenges that warrant attention. Overcoming these challenges will necessitate persistent research and innovation in materials science, bioengineering, and regulatory science.

FUTURE PERSPECTIVES

Developing new materials that improve the efficacy and safety of these devices, combining immunomodulation devices with digital health technologies for real-time monitoring and adjustment of immune responses is crucial (Mahara et al., 2023). The future of immunomodulation devices lies in their ability to provide personalized treatment, and advances in nanotechnology will likely lead to the development of more sophisticated nanoparticle devices capable of real-time monitoring and adjustment of immune responses (Chehelgerdi et al., 2023). Integration with AI could further enhance the precision and efficacy of these devices, allowing for continuous optimization based on patient-specific data (Alowais et al., 2023).

Advancements in synthetic biology could lead to the engineering of immune cells with enhanced functionalities. This includes improved antigen recognition, resistance to immunosuppression, and the ability to target melanoma cells more effectively. Techniques like CRISPR-Cas9 could be used to modify genetic components of immune cells, making them more robust against cancer evasion mechanisms (Roybal and Lim, 2017). Insights from immunogenetics will inform the development of personalized therapies targeting specific genetic variations affecting immune function. Personalized cancer vaccines, developed by analyzing tumor-specific antigens and HLA ligandome, will become more prevalent, offering robust immune responses against melanoma (Gubin et al., 2015). AI and computational models are transforming cancer therapy by enabling precise analysis and prediction of immune system behavior (Xu et al., 2021). These technologies will continue to evolve, providing more sophisticated tools for understanding interactions between cancer cells and immune cells, the effects of different therapeutic agents, and the dynamics of the tumor microenvironment. AI can identify candidates for immunotherapy, predict responses, and optimize treatment plans based on individual immune profiles. By using bioinformatics to identify unique neoantigens from tumor sequencing data, vaccines can be tailored to train the immune system to target melanoma cells effectively (Biswas et al., 2023). The integration of immunogenetics, synthetic biology, and AI will drive the field toward precision medicine. Treatments will be increasingly tailored to individual patients, considering their genetic makeup, immune profiles, and tumor characteristics. This approach promises to improve patient outcomes, reduce treatment-related toxicity, and provide more effective long-term management of melanomas (Villani et al., 2021). Advancements in technologies such as 3D printing, nanorobotics, and electromagnetic devices will further revolutionize melanoma treatment. 3D-printed scaffolds customized to patient-specific needs will deliver precise immunomodulatory treatments (Facklam et al., 2020).

CONCLUSION

In conclusion, the rapid advancements in immunotherapy, driven by innovations in immunomodulation devices, synthetic biology, and bioinformatics, offer exciting prospects for the future of melanoma treatment. Personalized and precision medicine approaches, supported by cutting-edge technology, will significantly enhance therapeutic outcomes and improve the quality of life for melanoma patients. The integration of technology with the immune system holds tremendous potential to revolutionize healthcare and address some of the most challenging medical conditions of our time.

REFERENCES

Abbott, M. and Ustoyev, Y. 2019. Cancer and the immune system: The history and background of immunotherapy, *Seminars in Oncology Nursing*, 35, p. 150923.

Abdelaziz, A. G., Nageh, H., Abdo, S. M., Abdalla, M. S., Amer, A. A., Abdal-Hay, A. and Barhoum, A. 2023. A review of 3D polymeric scaffolds for bone tissue engineering: Principles, fabrication techniques, immunomodulatory roles, and challenges, *Bioengineering*, 10, p. 204.

Ahmadian, Z., Gheybi, H. and Adeli, M. 2022. Efficient wound healing by antibacterial property: Advances and trends of hydrogels, hydrogel-metal NP composites and photothermal therapy platforms, *Journal of Drug Delivery Science and Technology*, 73, p. 103458.

Alowais, S. A., Alghamdi, S. S., Alsuhebany, N., Alqahtani, T., Alshaya, A. I., Almohareb, S. N., Aldairem, A., Alrashed, M., Bin Saleh, K., Badreldin, H. A., Al Yami, M. S., Al Harbi, S. and Albekairy, A. M. 2023. Revolutionizing healthcare: The role of artificial intelligence in clinical practice, *BMC Medical Education*, 23, p. 689.

Amreddy, N., Babu, A., Muralidharan, R., Panneerselvam, J., Srivastava, A., Ahmed, R., Mehta, M., Munshi, A. and Ramesh, R. 2018. Recent advances in nanoparticle-based cancer drug and gene delivery, *Advances in Cancer Research*, 137, pp. 115–170.

Anu Mary Ealia, S. and Saravanakumar, M. P. 2017. A review on the classification, characterisation, synthesis of nanoparticles and their application, *IOP Conference Series: Materials Science and Engineering*, 263, p. 032019.

Attrill, G. H., Ferguson, P. M., Palendira, U., Long, G. V., Wilmott, J. S. and Scolyer, R. A. 2021. The tumour immune landscape and its implications in cutaneous melanoma, *Pigment Cell & Melanoma Research*, 34, pp. 529–549.

Bear, A. S., Kennedy, L. C., Young, J. K., Perna, S. K., Mattos Almeida, J. P., Lin, A. Y., Eckels, P. C., Drezek, R. A. and Foster, A. E. 2013. Elimination of metastatic melanoma using gold nanoshell-enabled photothermal therapy and adoptive T cell transfer, *PLOS ONE*, 8, p. e69073.

Biswas, N., Chakrabarti, S., Padul, V., Jones, L. D. and Ashili, S. 2023. Designing neoantigen cancer vaccines, trials, and outcomes, *Frontiers in Immunology*, 14, p. 1105420.

Blanco, E., Shen, H. and Ferrari, M. 2015. Principles of nanoparticle design for overcoming biological barriers to drug delivery, *Nature Biotechnology*, 33, pp. 941–951.

Blass, E. and Ott, P. A. 2021. Advances in the development of personalized neoantigen-based therapeutic cancer vaccines, *Nature Reviews Clinical Oncology*, 18, pp. 215–229.

Boateng, F. and Ngwa, W. 2019. Delivery of nanoparticle-based radiosensitizers for radiotherapy applications, *International Journal of Molecular Science*, 21, p. 273.

Brenner, J., Cho, J. H., Wong, N. M. and Wong, W. W. 2018. Synthetic biology: Immunotherapy by design, *Annual Review of Biomedical Engineering*, 20, pp. 95–118.

Caliendo, F., Dukhinova, M. and Siciliano, V. 2019. Engineered cell-based therapeutics: Synthetic biology meets immunology, *Front Bioeng Biotechnol*, 7, p. 43.

Carnevale, L., Perrotta, M. and Lembo, G. 2021. A focused review of neural recording and stimulation techniques with immune-modulatory targets, *Frontiers in Immunology*, 12, p. 689344.

Chatterjee, D. K., Diagaradjane, P. and Krishnan, S. 2011. Nanoparticle-mediated hyperthermia in cancer therapy, *Therapeutic Delivery*, 2, pp. 1001–1014.

Chehelgerdi, M., Chehelgerdi, M., Allela, O. Q. B., Pecho, R. D. C., Jayasankar, N., Rao, D. P., Thamaraikani, T., Vasanthan, M., Viktor, P., Lakshmaiya, N., Saadh, M. J., Amajd, A., Abo-Zaid, M. A., Castillo-Acobo, R. Y., Ismail, A. H., Amin, A. H. and Akhavan-Sigari, R. 2023. Progressing nanotechnology to improve targeted cancer treatment: Overcoming hurdles in its clinical implementation, *Molecular Cancer*, 22, p. 169.

Chen, D. S. and Mellman, I. 2013. Oncology meets immunology: The cancer-immunity cycle, *Immunity*, 39, pp. 1–10.

Christodoulou, E., Rashid, M., Pacini, C., Droop, A., Robertson, H., Groningen, T. V., Teunisse, A. F. A. S., Iorio, F., Jochemsen, A. G., Adams, D. J. and Doorn, R. V. 2021. Analysis of CRISPR-Cas9 screens identifies genetic dependencies in melanoma, *Pigment Cell & Melanoma Research*, 34, pp. 122–131.

Cracchiolo, M., Ottaviani, M. M., Panarese, A., Strauss, I., Vallone, F., Mazzoni, A. and Micera, S. 2021. Bioelectronic medicine for the autonomic nervous system: Clinical applications and perspectives, *Journal of Neural Engineering*, 18, p. 041002.

Dai, H., Fan, Q. and Wang, C. 2022. Recent applications of immunomodulatory biomaterials for disease immunotherapy, *Exploration (Beijing)*, 2, p. 20210157.

Davis, L. E., Shalin, S. C. and Tackett, A. J. 2019. Current state of melanoma diagnosis and treatment, *Cancer Biology & Therapy*, 20, pp. 1366–1379.

Demir, G., Klein, H. O. and Tuzuner, N. 2003. Low dose daily rhGM-CSF application activates monocytes and dendritic cells in vivo, *Leukemia Research*, 27, pp. 1105–1108.

Deweese, T. L., Van Der Poel, H., Li, S., Mikhak, B., Drew, R., Goemann, M., Hamper, U., Dejong, R., Detorie, N., Rodriguez, R., Haulk, T., Demarzo, A. M., Piantadosi, S., Yu, D. C., Chen, Y., Henderson, D. R., Carducci, M. A., Nelson, W. G. and Simons, J. W. 2001. A phase I trial of CV706, a replication-competent, PSA selective oncolytic adenovirus, for the treatment of locally recurrent prostate cancer following radiation therapy, *Cancer Research*, 61, pp. 7464–7472.

Diaz, M. J., Natarelli, N., Aflatooni, S., Aleman, S. J., Neelam, S., Tran, J. T., Taneja, K., Lucke-Wold, B. and Forouzandeh, M. 2023. Nanoparticle-based treatment approaches for skin cancer: A systematic review, *Current Oncology*, 30, pp. 7112–7131.

Ding, F., Zhang, L., Chen, X., Yin, W., Ni, L. and Wang, M. 2022. Photothermal nanohybrid hydrogels for biomedical applications, *Frontiers in Bioengineering and Biotechnology*, 10, p. 1066617.

Doughty, A. C. V., Hoover, A. R., Layton, E., Murray, C. K., Howard, E. W. and Chen, W. R. 2019. Nanomaterial applications in photothermal therapy for cancer, *Materials (Basel)*, 12, p. 779.

Eddy, K., Shah, R. and Chen, S. 2021. Decoding melanoma development and progression: Identification of therapeutic vulnerabilities, *Frontiers in Oncology*, 10, p. 626129.

Esteva, A., Kuprel, B., Novoa, R. A., Ko, J., Swetter, S. M., Blau, H. M. and Thrun, S. 2017. Dermatologist-level classification of skin cancer with deep neural networks, *Nature*, 542, pp. 115–118.

Facklam, A. L., Volpatti, L. R. and Anderson, D. G. 2020. Biomaterials for personalized cell therapy, *Advanced Materials*, 32, p. 1902005.

Fang, R. H. and Zhang, L. 2016. Nanoparticle-based modulation of the immune system, *Annual Review of Chemical and Biomolecular Engineering*, 7, pp. 305–326.

Farhana, A. 2023. Enhancing skin cancer immunotheranostics and precision medicine through functionalized nanomodulators and nanosensors: Recent development and prospects, *International Journal of Molecular Sciences*, 24, p. 3493.

Farhoudi, L., Fobian, S.-F., Oei, A. L., Amin, M., Jaafari, M. R. and Ten Hagen, T. L. M. 2023. Applications of biomimetic nanoparticles in breast cancer as a blueprint for improved next-generation cervical cancer therapy, *Nano Today*, 53, p. 102032.

Ferrucci, P. F., Pala, L., Conforti, F. and Cocorocchio, E. 2021. Talimogene laherparepvec (T-VEC): An intralesional cancer immunotherapy for advanced melanoma, *Cancers*, 13, p. 1383.

Freudenmann, L. K., Marcu, A. and Stevanović, S. 2018. Mapping the tumour human leukocyte antigen (HLA) ligandome by mass spectrometry, *Immunology*, 154, pp. 331–345.

Garnock-Jones, K. P. 2016. Talimogene laherparepvec: A review in unresectable metastatic melanoma, *BioDrugs*, 30, pp. 461–468.

Gibney, G. T., Weiner, L. M. and Atkins, M. B. 2016. Predictive biomarkers for checkpoint inhibitor-based immunotherapy, *Lancet Oncology*, 17, pp. e542–e551.

Gillies, R. J., Kinahan, P. E. and Hricak, H. 2016. Radiomics: Images are more than pictures, they are data, *Radiology*, 278, pp. 563–577.

Giri, G., Maddahi, Y. and Zareinia, K. 2021. A brief review on challenges in design and development of nanorobots for medical applications, *Applied Sciences*, 11, p. 10385.

Gubin, M. M., Artyomov, M. N., Mardis, E. R. and Schreiber, R. D. 2015. Tumor neoantigens: Building a framework for personalized cancer immunotherapy, *Journal of Clinical Investigation*, 125, pp. 3413–3421.

Gunter, N. V., Yap, B. J. M., Chua, C. L. L. and Yap, W. H. 2019. Combining understanding of immunological mechanisms and genetic variants toward development of personalized medicine for psoriasis patients, *Frontiers in Genetics*, 10, p. 440505.

Haleem, A., Javaid, M., Singh, R. P., Rab, S. and Suman, R. 2023. Applications of nanotechnology in medical field: A brief review, *Global Health Journal*, 7, pp. 70–77.

Hancock, R. E., Haney, E. F. and Gill, E. E. 2016. The immunology of host defence peptides: Beyond antimicrobial activity, *Nature Reviews Immunology*, 16, pp. 321–334.

Hazini, A., Fisher, K. and Seymour, L. 2021. Deregulation of HLA-I in cancer and its central importance for immunotherapy. *Journal for ImmunoTherapy of Cancer*, 9, p. e002899.

Hegde, P. S., Karanikas, V. and Evers, S. 2016. The where, the when, and the how of immune monitoring for cancer immunotherapies in the era of checkpoint inhibition, *Clinical Cancer Research*, 22, pp. 1865–1874.

Hoffner, B., Iodice, G. M. and Gasal, E. 2016. Administration and handling of talimogene laherparepvec: An intralesional oncolytic immunotherapy for melanoma, *Oncology Nursing Forum*, 43, pp. 219–226.

Jain, K. K. and Jain, K. K. 2021. Personalized Immuno-Oncology. In: *Textbook of Personalized Medicine*, Cham: Springer, 479–508.

Jha, S. and Topol, E. J. 2016. Adapting to artificial intelligence: Radiologists and pathologists as information specialists, *JAMA*, 316, pp. 2353–2354.

Kalaora, S., Nagler, A., Wargo, J. A. and Samuels, Y. 2022. Mechanisms of immune activation and regulation: Lessons from melanoma, *Nature Reviews Cancer*, 22, pp. 195–207.

Kather, J. N., Halama, N. and Jaeger, D. 2018. Genomics and emerging biomarkers for immunotherapy of colorectal cancer, *Seminars in Cancer Biology*, 52, pp. 189–197.

Khatun, S., Putta, C. L., Hak, A. and Rengan, A. K. 2023. Immunomodulatory nanosystems: An emerging strategy to combat viral infections, *Biomater Biosyst*, 9, p. 100073.

Knight, A., Karapetyan, L. and Kirkwood, J. M. 2023. Immunotherapy in melanoma: Recent advances and future directions, *Cancers*, 15, p. 1106.

Kong, X., Gao, P., Wang, J., Fang, Y. and Hwang, K. C. 2023. Advances of medical nanorobots for future cancer treatments, *Journal of Hematology & Oncology*, 16, p. 74.

Kourou, K., Exarchos, T. P., Exarchos, K. P., Karamouzis, M. V. and Fotiadis, D. I. 2015. Machine learning applications in cancer prognosis and prediction, *Computational and Structural Biotechnology Journal*, 13, pp. 8–17.

Krishna, K. S., Li, Y., Li, S. and Kumar, C. S. 2013. Lab-on-a-chip synthesis of inorganic nanomaterials and quantum dots for biomedical applications, *Adv Drug Deliv Rev*, 65, pp. 1470–1495.

Kunert, A., Straetemans, T., Govers, C., Lamers, C., Mathijssen, R., Sleijfer, S. and Debets, R. 2013. TCR-engineered T cells meet new challenges to treat solid tumors: Choice of antigen, T cell fitness, and sensitization of tumor milieu, *Frontiers in Immunology*, 4, p. 363.

Lambin, P., Rios-Velazquez, E., Leijenaar, R., Carvalho, S., Van Stiphout, R. G., Granton, P., Zegers, C. M., Gillies, R., Boellard, R. and Dekker, A. 2012. Radiomics: Extracting more information from medical images using advanced feature analysis, *European Journal of Cancer*, 48, pp. 441–446.

Li, D., Li, X., Zhou, W.-L., Huang, Y., Liang, X., Jiang, L., Yang, X., Sun, J., Li, Z., Han, W.-D. and Wang, W. 2019. Genetically engineered T cells for cancer immunotherapy, *Signal Transduction and Targeted Therapy*, 4, p. 35.

Li, J., Xiao, Z., Wang, D., Jia, L., Nie, S., Zeng, X. and Hu, W. 2023. The screening, identification, design and clinical application of tumor-specific neoantigens for TCR-T cells, *Molecular Cancer*, 22, p. 141.

Lin, L., Zhang, W., Chen, Y., Ren, W., Zhao, J., Ouyang, W., He, Z., Su, W., Yao, H. and Yu, Y. 2023. Immune gene patterns and characterization of the tumor immune microenvironment associated with cancer immunotherapy efficacy, *Heliyon*, 9, p. e14450.

Litjens, G., Kooi, T., Bejnordi, B. E., Setio, A. A. A., Ciompi, F., Ghafoorian, M., Van Der Laak, J. A., Van Ginneken, B. and Sánchez, C. I. 2017. A survey on deep learning in medical image analysis, *Medical Image Analysis*, 42, pp. 60–88.

Liu, W. S., Chen, Z., Lu, Z. M., Dong, J. H., Wu, J. H., Gao, J., Deng, D. and Li, M. 2024. Multifunctional hydrogels based on photothermal therapy: A prospective platform for the postoperative management of melanoma, *J Control Release*, 371, pp. 406–428.

Mahara, G., Tian, C., Xu, X. and Wang, W. 2023. Revolutionising health care: Exploring the latest advances in medical sciences, *Journal of Global Health*, 13, p. 03042.

Malachowski, T. and Hassel, A. 2020. Engineering nanoparticles to overcome immunological barriers for enhanced drug delivery, *Engineered Regeneration*, 1, pp. 35–50.

Mariani, E., Lisignoli, G., Borzì, R. M. and Pulsatelli, L. 2019. Biomaterials: Foreign bodies or tuners for the immune response? *International Journal of Molecular Sciences*, 20, p. 636.

Mellman, I., Chen, D. S., Powles, T. and Turley, S. J. 2023. The cancer-immunity cycle: Indication, genotype, and immunotype, *Immunity*, 56, pp. 2188–2205.

Méndez, R., Rodríguez, T., Del Campo, A., Monge, E., Maleno, I., Aptsiauri, N., Jiménez, P., Pedrinaci, S., Pawelec, G. and Ruiz-Cabello, F. 2008. Characterization of HLA class I altered phenotypes in a panel of human melanoma cell lines, *Cancer Immunology, Immunotherapy*, 57, pp. 719–729.

Mitchell, M. J., Billingsley, M. M., Haley, R. M., Wechsler, M. E., Peppas, N. A. and Langer, R. 2021. Engineering precision nanoparticles for drug delivery, *Nature Reviews Drug Discovery*, 20, pp. 101–124.

Monos, D. S. and Winchester, R. J. 2019. The Major Histocompatibility Complex. *Clinical Immunology*. Elsevier.

Mosaad, Y. 2015. Clinical role of human leukocyte antigen in health and disease, *Scandinavian Journal of Immunology*, 82, pp. 283–306.

Navarrete, C. V. 2000. The HLA system in blood transfusion, *Best Practice & Research Clinical Haematology*, 13, pp. 511–532.

Nielsen, M., Lund, O., Buus, S. and Lundegaard, C. 2010. MHC class II epitope predictive algorithms, *Immunology*, 130, pp. 319–328.

Ott, P. A., Hu, Z., Keskin, D. B., Shukla, S. A., Sun, J., Bozym, D. J., Zhang, W., Luoma, A., Giobbie-Hurder, A. and Peter, L. 2017. An immunogenic personal neoantigen vaccine for patients with melanoma, *Nature*, 547, pp. 217–221.

Pagliuca, S., Gurnari, C., Rubio, M. T., Visconte, V. and Lenz, T. L. 2022. Individual HLA heterogeneity and its implications for cellular immune evasion in cancer and beyond, *Frontiers in Immunology*, 13, p. 944872.

Piszczek, P., wójcik-piotrowicz, K., Gil, K. and kaszuba-zwoińska, J. 2021. Immunity and electromagnetic fields, *Environmental Research*, 200, p. 111505.

Prelaj, A., Miskovic, V., Zanitti, M., Trovo, F., Genova, C., Viscardi, G., Rebuzzi, S., Mazzeo, L., Provenzano, L. and Kosta, S. 2023. Artificial intelligence for predictive biomarker discovery in immuno-oncology: A systematic review, *Annals of Oncology*, 35, pp. 29–65.

Qin, R., Peng, W., Wang, X., Li, C., Xi, Y., Zhong, Z. and Sun, C. 2021. Identification of genes related to immune infiltration in the tumor microenvironment of cutaneous melanoma, *Frontiers in Oncology*, 11, p. 615963.

Queirolo, P., Boutros, A., Tanda, E., Spagnolo, F. and Quaglino, P. 2019. Immune-checkpoint inhibitors for the treatment of metastatic melanoma: A model of cancer immunotherapy, *Seminars in Cancer Biology*, 59, pp. 290–297.

Rahman, M. M., Islam, M. R., Rahman, F., Rahaman, M. S., Khan, M. S., Abrar, S., Ray, T. K., Uddin, M. B., Kali, M. S. K. and Dua, K. 2022. Emerging promise of computational techniques in anti-cancer research: At a glance, *Bioengineering*, 9, p. 335.

Rahmati, M. and Mozafari, M. 2019. Biological response to carbon-family nanomaterials: Interactions at the nano-bio interface, *Frontiers in Bioengineering and Biotechnology*, 7, p. 4.

Ratner, B. D., Hoffman, A. S., Schoen, F. J. and Lemons, J. E. 2013. *Biomaterials Science: An Introduction to Materials in Medicine*. Academic Press.

Ricker, C. A., Meli, K. and Van Allen, E. M. 2024. Historical perspective and future directions: Computational science in immuno-oncology, *Journal for Immunotherapy of Cancer*, 12, p. e008306.

Robbins, P. F., Kassim, S. H., Tran, T. L., Crystal, J. S., Morgan, R. A., Feldman, S. A., Yang, J. C., Dudley, M. E., Wunderlich, J. R., Sherry, R. M., Kammula, U. S., Hughes, M. S., Restifo, N. P., Raffeld, M., Lee, C. C., Li, Y. F., El-Gamil, M. and Rosenberg, S. A. 2015. A pilot trial using lymphocytes genetically engineered with an NY-ESO-1-reactive T-cell receptor: Long-term follow-up and correlates with response, *Clinical Cancer Research*, 21, pp. 1019–1027.

Robbins, P. F., Morgan, R. A., Feldman, S. A., Yang, J. C., Sherry, R. M., Dudley, M. E., Wunderlich, J. R., Nahvi, A. V., Helman, L. J., Mackall, C. L., Kammula, U. S., Hughes, M. S., Restifo, N. P., Raffeld, M., Lee, C. C., Levy, C. L., Li, Y. F., El-Gamil, M., Schwarz, S. L., Laurencot, C. and Rosenberg, S. A. 2011. Tumor regression in patients with metastatic synovial cell sarcoma and melanoma using genetically engineered lymphocytes reactive with NY-ESO-1, *Journal of Clinical Oncology*, 29, pp. 917–924.

Rodrigues, D., Barbosa, A. I., Rebelo, R., Kwon, I. K., Reis, R. L. and Correlo, V. M. 2020. Skin-integrated wearable systems and implantable biosensors: A comprehensive review, *Biosensors*, 10, p. 79.

Rohaan, M. W., Wilgenhof, S. and Haanen, J. 2019. Adoptive cellular therapies: The current landscape, *Virchows Archiv*, 474, pp. 449–461.

Ross, C. L., Teli, T. and Harrison, B. S. 2016. Electromagnetic field devices and their effects on nociception and peripheral inflammatory pain mechanisms, *Alternative Therapies in Health & Medicine*, 22, pp. 52–64.

Roybal, K. T. and Lim, W. A. 2017. Synthetic immunology: Hacking immune cells to expand their therapeutic capabilities, *Annual Review of Immunology*, 35, pp. 229–253.

Sabit, H., Abdel-Hakeem, M., Shoala, T., Abdel-Ghany, S., Abdel-Latif, M. M., Almulhim, J. and Mansy, M. 2022. Nanocarriers: A reliable tool for the delivery of anticancer drugs, *Pharmaceutics*, 14, p. 1566.

Sahin, U., Derhovanessian, E., Miller, M., Kloke, B. P., Simon, P., Löwer, M., Bukur, V., Tadmor, A. D., Luxemburger, U., Schrörs, B., et al. 2017. Personalized RNA mutanome vaccines mobilize poly-specific therapeutic immunity against cancer, *Nature*, 547, pp. 222–226.

Sarnaik, A. A., Hamid, O., Khushalani, N. I., Lewis, K. D., Medina, T., Kluger, H. M., Thomas, S. S., Domingo-Musibay, E., Pavlick, A. C., Whitman, E. D., Martin-Algarra, S., Corrie, P., Curti, B. D., Oláh, J., Lutzky, J., Weber, J. S., Larkin, J. M. G., Shi, W., Takamura, T., Jagasia, M., Qin, H., Wu, X., Chartier, C., Graf Finckenstein, F., Fardis, M., Kirkwood, J. M. and Chesney, J. A. 2021. Lifileucel, a tumor-infiltrating lymphocyte therapy, in metastatic melanoma, *Journal of Clinical Oncology*, 39, pp. 2656–2666.

Schmalz, G., Hickel, R., van Landuyt, K.L. and Reichl, F.-X. (2018). Scientific update on nanoparticles in dentistry†, *Int Dent J*, 68, pp. 299–305. https://doi.org/10.1111/idj.12394

Sebastian, A. M. and Peter, D. 2022. Artificial intelligence in cancer research: Trends, challenges and future directions, *Life*, 12, p. 1991.

Shafi, N., Costantine, J., Kanj, R., Tawk, Y., Ramadan, A. H., Kurban, M., Rahal, J. A. and Eid, A. A. 2023. A portable non-invasive electromagnetic lesion-optimized sensing device for the diagnosis of skin cancer (SkanMD), *IEEE Transactions on Biomedical Circuits and Systems*, 17, pp. 558–573.

Smith, C. C., Selitsky, S. R., Chai, S., Armistead, P. M., Vincent, B. G. and Serody, J. S. 2019. Alternative tumour-specific antigens, *Nature Reviews Cancer*, 19, pp. 465–478.

Sobhani, Z., Behnam, M. A., Emami, F., Dehghanian, A. and Jamhiri, I. 2017. Photothermal therapy of melanoma tumor using multiwalled carbon nanotubes, *International Journal of Nanomedicine*, 12, pp. 4509–4517.

Souiade, L., Domingo-Diez, J., Alcaide, C., Gámez, B., Gámez, L., Ramos, M. and Serrano Olmedo, J. J. 2023. Improving the efficacy of magnetic nanoparticle-mediated hyperthermia using trapezoidal pulsed electromagnetic fields as an in vitro anticancer treatment in melanoma and glioblastoma multiforme cell lines, *International Journal of Molecular Sciences*, 24, p. 15933.

Stabler, C., Li, Y., Stewart, J. and Keselowsky, B. 2019. Engineering immunomodulatory biomaterials for type 1 diabetes, *Nature Reviews Materials*, 4, pp. 429–450.

Sun, R., Limkin, E. J., Vakalopoulou, M., Dercle, L., Champiat, S., Han, S. R., Verlingue, L., Brandao, D., Lancia, A. and Ammari, S. 2018. A radiomics approach to assess tumour-infiltrating CD8 cells and response to anti-PD-1 or anti-PD-L1 immunotherapy: An imaging biomarker, retrospective multicohort study, *Lancet Oncology*, 19, pp. 1180–1191.

Szeto, G. L. and Finley, S. D. 2019. Integrative approaches to cancer immunotherapy, *Trends in Cancer*, 5, pp. 400–410.

Tabari, A., Cox, M., D'amore, B., Mansur, A., Dabbara, H., Boland, G., Gee, M. S. and Daye, D. 2023. Machine learning improves the prediction of responses to immune checkpoint inhibitors in metastatic melanoma, *Cancers*, 15, p. 2700.

Teixido, C., Castillo, P., Martinez-Vila, C., Arance, A. and Alos, L. 2021. Molecular markers and targets in melanoma, *Cells*, 10, p. 2320.

Toda, M., Martuza, R. L. and Rabkin, S. D. 2000. Tumor growth inhibition by intratumoral inoculation of defective herpes simplex virus vectors expressing granulocyte-macrophage colony-stimulating factor, *Mol Ther*, 2, pp. 324–329.

Topalian, S. L., Taube, J. M., Anders, R. A. and Pardoll, D. M. 2016. Mechanism-driven biomarkers to guide immune checkpoint blockade in cancer therapy, *Nature Reviews Cancer*, 16, pp. 275–287.

Topol, E. J. 2019. High-performance medicine: The convergence of human and artificial intelligence, *Nature Medicine*, 25, pp. 44–56.

Toy, R. and Roy, K. 2016. Engineering nanoparticles to overcome barriers to immunotherapy, *Bioeng Transl Med*, 1, pp. 47–62.

Trebeschi, S., Drago, S., Birkbak, N., Kurilova, I., Călin, A., Pizzi, A. D., Lalezari, F., Lambregts, D., Rohaan, M. and Parmar, C. 2019. Predicting response to cancer immunotherapy using noninvasive radiomic biomarkers, *Annals of Oncology*, 30, pp. 998–1004.

Valcourt, D. M., Dang, M. N., Scully, M. A. and Day, E. S. 2020. Nanoparticle-mediated co-delivery of notch-1 antibodies and ABT-737 as a potent treatment strategy for triple-negative breast cancer, *ACS Nano*, 14, pp. 3378–3388.

Villani, A., Scalvenzi, M., Fabbrocini, G., Ocampo-Candiani, J. and Ocampo-Garza, S. S. 2021. Looking into a better future: Novel therapies for metastatic melanoma, *Dermatology and Therapy*, 11, pp. 751–767.

Wang, Y., Qiao, S. L., Wang, J., Yu, M. Z., Wang, N. N., Mamuti, M., An, H. W., Lin, Y. X. and Wang, H. 2023. Engineered CpG-loaded nanorobots drive autophagy-mediated immunity for TLR9-positive cancer therapy, *Advanced Materials*, 36, p. e2306248.

Wilkinson, B. and Van Boxtel, R. 2020. The medical device regulation of the European Union intensifies focus on clinical benefits of devices, *Therapeutic Innovation & Regulatory Science*, 54, pp. 613–617.

Wojtukiewicz, M. Z., Rek, M. M., Karpowicz, K., Górska, M., Polityńska, B., Wojtukiewicz, A. M., Moniuszko, M., Radziwon, P., Tucker, S. C. and Honn, K. V. 2021. Inhibitors of immune checkpoints—PD-1, PD-L1, CTLA-4—New opportunities for cancer patients and a new challenge for internists and general practitioners, *Cancer and Metastasis Reviews*, 40, pp. 949–982.

Won, S. M., Song, E., Reeder, J. T. and Rogers, J. A. 2020. Emerging modalities and implantable technologies for neuromodulation, *Cell*, 181, pp. 115–135.

Xie, J., Luo, X., Deng, X., Tang, Y., Tian, W., Cheng, H., Zhang, J., Zou, Y., Guo, Z. and Xie, X. 2023. Advances in artificial intelligence to predict cancer immunotherapy efficacy, *Frontiers in Immunology*, 13, p. 1076883.

Xu, Y., Su, G.-H., Ma, D., Xiao, Y., Shao, Z.-M. and Jiang, Y.-Z. 2021. Technological advances in cancer immunity: From immunogenomics to single-cell analysis and artificial intelligence, *Signal Transduction and Targeted Therapy*, 6, p. 312.

Yang, S., Wu, J., Wang, Z., Cheng, Y., Zhang, R., Yao, C. and Yang, D. 2024. A smart DNA hydrogel enables synergistic immunotherapy and photodynamic therapy of melanoma, *Angewandte Chemie*, 63, p. e202319073.

Yang, Y. 2015. Cancer immunotherapy: Harnessing the immune system to battle cancer, *Journal of Clinical Investigation*, 125, pp. 3335–3337.

Zakariya, F., Salem, F. K., Alamrain, A. A., Sanker, V., Abdelazeem, Z. G., Hosameldin, M., Tan, J. K., Howard, R., Huang, H. and Awuah, W. A. 2024. Refining mutanome-based individualised immunotherapy of melanoma using artificial intelligence, *European Journal of Medical Research*, 29, p. 25.

Zhang, Y., Zhan, X., Xiong, J., Peng, S., Huang, W., Joshi, R., Cai, Y., Liu, Y., Li, R., Yuan, K., Zhou, N. and Min, W. 2018. Temperature-dependent cell death patterns induced by functionalized gold nanoparticle photothermal therapy in melanoma cells, *Scientific Reports*, 8, p. 8720.

Zhu, Z., Liu, W. and Gotlieb, V. 2016. The rapidly evolving therapies for advanced melanoma—Towards immunotherapy, molecular targeted therapy, and beyond, *Critical Reviews in Oncology/Hematology*, 99, pp. 91–99.

5 Targeted Therapies and Nanomedicine

Precision at the Molecular Level

Rahaba Marima, Olalekan Fadebi, and Zodwa Dlamini
SAMRC Precision Oncology Research Unit (PORU), DSTI/NRF SARChI Chair in Precision Oncology and Cancer Prevention (POCP), Pan African Cancer Research Institute (PACRI), University of Pretoria, Pretoria, South Africa

Olalekan Fadebi
Faculty of Health Sciences, Steve Biko Academic Hospital, University of Pretoria, Pretoria, South Africa

Onyemaechi O. Azu
University of the Western Cape, Bellville, Cape Town, South Africa

Innocent Edagha
School of Medicine, Moi University, Eldoret, Kenya

Philemon Ubanako
School of Clinical Medicine, Faculty of Health Sciences, University of the Witwatersrand, Parktown, South Africa

Jyotsna Batra
Centre for Genomics and Personalized Health, Queensland University of Technology
Translational Research Institute, Queensland University of Technology
School of Biomedical Sciences, Faculty of Health, Queensland University of Technology, Brisbane, Australia

INTRODUCTION

Melanoma is the most aggressive and lethal skin cancer, which results from an oncogenic transformation of melanocytes and is usually associated with poor prognosis following metastasis (Guo et al., 2021). Conventional treatment for localized primary invasive melanoma is performed by surgical excision with an overall 5-year survival rate of up to 92% (Joyce, 2017). However, in the case of advanced metastasized melanoma, only a 10% survival rate may be achievable following surgical resection of

 DOI: 10.1201/9781003511625-5

the primary tumor, and radiotherapy is also highly unsuccessful following metastasis (Bhatia et al., 2022). The poor therapeutic responses associated with surgery, radiotherapy, and chemotherapy in advanced metastatic melanoma have necessitated the search for novel, innovative therapies for the disease (Wagstaff et al., 2022). Advanced metastatic melanoma, which is associated with high mortality, requires additional therapeutic strategies such as targeted therapy and immunotherapy (Menzer and Hassel, 2022). Nanomedicine in melanoma precision medicine is also an emerging area of research.

The FDA has approved a few targeted therapies, showing improved therapeutic response and patient survival in metastatic melanoma. Targeted therapeutic strategies comprised of BRAF and MEK inhibition are effective in individuals with metastatic melanoma harboring BRAFV600 mutations. For metastatic melanoma patients with non-BRAFV600 mutations, immunotherapy with checkpoint inhibition is the primary first-line therapy option (Menzer and Hassel, 2022). Unfortunately, about 50% of patients do not improve with immunotherapy, necessitating efficient second-line treatments (Menzer and Hassel, 2022). Although there are pitfalls, nanomedicine is a potential approach to enhancing the overall melanoma treatment. This chapter discusses molecular mechanisms involved in melanoma-targeted therapies, current nanomedicine trends in advancing melanoma treatments, the convergence of nanomedicine, targeted therapies, and other modalities as enhanced melanoma therapeutic approaches.

CURRENT TRENDS IN MELANOMA-TARGETED THERAPIES: MOLECULAR MECHANISMS AND IMPLICATIONS

MAPK Signaling

Improved understanding of the molecular pathogenesis of advanced metastatic melanoma has led to effective targeted therapies, which have improved patient survival. The most reported deregulated pathway in melanoma is the mitogen-activated protein kinase (MAPK) signal transduction pathway. The MAPK pathway is a conserved cell signaling pathway that is vital in regulating cell proliferation, viability, differentiation, and cell death in eukaryotic cells (Fernandez et al., 2023). The therapeutic relevance of this pathway is seen in the approval of several small molecule inhibitors for targeted therapy. The MAPK pathway contains three sequentially activated protein kinases: RAS, MEK, and MAPK (ERK), whose activation is required for MAPK signaling, thereby regulating diverse cellular programs (Guo et al., 2020; Li et al., 2016). MAPK signaling cascade is usually triggered by the binding of mitogens, hormones, or neurotransmitters to transmembrane receptor tyrosine kinases. This leads to the dimerization of RTK, activating oncogenic RAS and increasing cellular RAS-GDP levels. The sequential phosphorylation of RAF, MEK, and ERK subsequently regulates the expression of genes that control vital cellular processes such as cell viability, proliferation, differentiation, and apoptosis (Grimaldi et al., 2017; Y.-J. Guo et al., 2020; Li et al., 2016). Deregulation of this pathway, as seen in mutations of BRAF and NRAS, leads to their constitutive activation without the need for mitogenic signals, thereby inducing uncontrolled proliferation and metastasis.

Targeting BRAF

The RAF protein has three isoforms: ARAF, BRAF, and CRAF. BRAF (v-RAF murine sarcoma viral oncogene homolog B1) is a serine/threonine kinase that activates the MAP kinase/ERK-signaling pathway (Riegel and Rajalingam, 2020; Zhao and Luo, 2022). The most common genetic lesion in melanoma is mutations in the *BRAF* oncogene, which is shown to be mutated in 40–60% of melanoma cases (Castellani et al., 2023; Tatjana and Sergejs, 2022). About 90% of BRAF mutations are a result of point mutations in which valine (V) is substituted by glutamic acid (E) on position 600 of the BRAF protein (V600E mutation), which also represents about half of all metastatic melanomas (Czarnecka et al., 2020; Palmieri et al., 2021; Sanchez et al., 2021). The second most common BRAF mutation in malignant melanoma is the V600K mutation, which also occurs in 68%

of benign nevi. The fact that V600K mutations are present in both benign and malignant melanoma raises the question of the involvement of BRAF in melanoma carcinogenesis. Early-stage melanoma shows a mutation rate of 10% BRAF, shown to stimulate proliferation and viability as its key strategy in promoting tumor growth. $BRAF^{V600E}$ exerts constitutive activity, which is implicated in tumor cell proliferation, survival, invasion, and metastasis (Montico et al., 2020). BRAF is a critical target for small-molecule or RNAi-based therapeutics as gain-of-function, and its mutations are strongly linked with tumorigenicity (Roa et al., 2024).

BRAF has proven to be an attractive target as it is mutated and constitutively activated in many melanoma cases and can induce cell proliferation, invasion, and metastasis. Vemurafenib is a small-molecule drug developed to inhibit mutant BRAF in melanoma, specifically (Han et al., 2020). The $BRAF^{V600E}$ mutations are sensitive to small molecules that inhibit the hyperactive $BRAF^{V600E}$ activity. The most clinically effective BRAF inhibitors are vemurafenib and dabrafenib.

Targeting NRAS

NRAS is a small GTPase mutated in approximately 20% of melanomas harboring wild-type BRAF. Glutamine-leucine point mutations at position 61 (Q61L) account for 80% of NRAS mutations (Muñoz-Couselo et al., 2017; Muñoz-Maldonado et al., 2019). Mutant NRAS leads to the aberrant accumulation of GTP due to impaired GTPase activity, thereby leading to the deregulation of GTP by GTPase-activating proteins (GAPs) and guanine nucleotide exchange factors (GEFs) (Wagstaff et al., 2022). NRAS-mutant melanomas are usually diagnosed in patients above 55 years of age and are associated with higher EMT and lymph node metastasis. NRAS tumors generally display a more aggressive phenotype and usually show adverse prognosis (Wagstaff et al., 2022).

Although NRAS and BRAF are found in the same RAS-RAF mitogen-activating kinase pathway, mutations in both genes rarely occur in the same patient. Nevertheless, NRAS mutations have been observed in some BRAF-mutant melanoma patients with aggressive melanoma who failed to respond to targeted BRAF therapy (Castellani et al., 2023). This evidence highlights the importance of NRAS in advanced malignant melanoma and suggests some redundancy in the molecular mechanisms of melanoma progression in the context of NRAS and BRAF. Benign nevi harbor high rates of NRAS and BRAF mutations, thereby limiting the possibility of both mutations being involved in the initiation phase of melanoma. Nevertheless, studies have shown that higher rates of NRAS and BRAF mutations are observed in metastatic melanoma compared with primary melanoma lesions, thereby implicating these mutations in the oncogenic transformation from primary to metastatic melanoma (Houben et al., 2004; Vanni et al., 2020a).

Since NRAS mutations are associated with deregulated tumor cell proliferation and metastasis, targeting NRAS represents a viable therapeutic strategy in melanoma. Although RAS was the first oncogene discovered in melanoma, treating NRAS mutant melanoma has been challenging. Farnesyl transferase inhibitors (FTIs) are small-molecule drugs that have been developed to target RAS localization by inhibiting post-translational RAS modifications, thereby preventing its insertion into the phospholipid bilayer of the plasma membrane (Appels et al., 2005; Nair and Saha, 2023).

NRAS-mutant tumors are challenging to target with FTIs due to their nonspecificity. FTIs are nonspecific because numerous membrane-bound proteins are also prone to farnesylation following FTI treatment. Salirasib is a small molecule FTI that induces apoptosis in RAS-transformed cells by interfering with the localization of RAS at the plasma membrane, thereby preventing galactin 1 on the plasma membrane from being bound by RAS-GTP (Korzeniecki and Priefer, 2021). Salirasib has shown some promise in preclinical studies, but further research is essential. Targeting NRAS mutant melanomas can also be accomplished using interfering RNAs (siRNAs) (Wagstaff et al., 2022). Nevertheless, challenges associated with nucleic acid delivery in preclinical models and other biological systems have slowed the delayed progress of siRNA therapeutics.

Targeting MEK

Despite a relatively low occurrence of MEK mutations in human tumors, the activity of MEK is observed in more than 85% of tumors, partly as a result of mutations of upstream RAS or RAF proteins (Song et al., 2022). MEK inhibitors inhibit cell proliferation and induce cell death in melanoma cells harboring NRAS and BRAF mutations. Patients with BRAF- and NRAS-mutated metastatic melanoma treated with MEK inhibitors have a high response rate, progression-free survival, and overall survival (Priantti et al., 2023). Standard therapy in patients with BRAF-mutant melanoma combines MEK and BRAF inhibitors, which show higher efficacy and less systemic toxicity than BRAF inhibitors alone (Menzer and Hassel, 2022). Furthermore, combination therapies using MEK inhibitors and non-BRAF inhibitor regimens, immune checkpoint inhibitors such as anti-PD-1/anti-PD-L1 and CDK 4/6 inhibitors have also yielded improved therapeutic responses in metastatic melanoma (Cancer Genome Atlas Network, 2015; De Meza et al., 2023; Schuler et al., 2022).

Several FDA-approved combinations of therapeutic strategies involving BRAF and MEK inhibitors have been used to effectively inhibit the growth of tumors in patients with RAS or RAF mutations (Song et al., 2023). Trametinib is a non-ATP-competitive inhibitor of MEK1 and MEK2 approved in 2013 to treat $BRAF^{V600E/K}$-mutant metastatic melanoma (Pan and Mader, 2022). Cobimetinib is a very selective and highly effective allosteric MEK1/2 inhibitor, which is effective in targeting cell lines harboring KRAS and BRAF mutations and $BRAF^{V600E/K}$-mutant patients (Pan and Mader, 2022; Patel et al., 2020). In 2015, the European Medicines Agency and the FDA authorized vemurafenib and carbometinib for the treatment of $BRAF^{V600E/K}$ mutant and unresectable melanoma (Schummer et al., 2020).

Targeting CDK4/CDKN2A

Genetic susceptibility to familial melanoma occurs in 5–10% of melanoma patients (Zocchi et al., 2021). Cyclin-dependent kinase 4 (*CDK4*) oncogene and cyclin-dependent kinase inhibitor 2A (*CDKN2A*) are associated with familial melanoma genesis (Sargen et al., 2020). Cell cycle progression from the G1 to S phase is regulated partly by CDK4 and p16INK4a (Crozier et al., 2022). While p16INK4a suppresses CDK4 activity, inhibiting cell division, cyclin D1-activated CDK4 functions as a proto-oncogene that stimulates the transition from G1 to S phase, permitting cell proliferation (Crozier et al., 2022). Research has shown that although CDK4 mutations are relatively rare, inactivated p16INK4A mutations on 9p21 account for 25–60% of familial melanoma patients (Hedberg et al., 2022; Ribeiro Moura Brasil Arnaut et al., 2021). To curb melanoma progression with such a molecular phenotype, it seems plausible to inhibit CDK4, thereby arresting cell cycle progression and inhibiting uncontrolled proliferation. CDK4/6 inhibitors have been used as monotherapy or combined with other immunotherapies, such as PD-L1 or BRAF/MEK inhibitors (Garutti et al., 2021).

Targeting MC1R

Melanocortin 1 receptor (MC1R) is a G-protein-coupled receptor in melanocytes that plays a significant role in regulating skin pigmentation (Guida et al., 2022). Studies have reported that Caucasian populations display an increased risk of melanoma development attributable to some MC1R mutations (Manganelli et al., 2021). Mutations in the BRAF, NRAS, or CDKN2A genes can occur in people with MC1R mutations, which result in reduced melanin synthesis because they are prone to UV-induced DNA mutagenesis (Li et al., 2022; Zaidi et al., 2020).

Patients with constitutively activated BRAF melanoma and no history of chronic sun exposure have been discovered to carry these variations (Colombino et al., 2024; Loras et al., 2022; Patel et al., 2020). In BRAF mutant melanomas, wild-type MC1R alleles are sporadically detected (Vanni et al., 2020b). Interestingly, BRAF mutations are six times more common in American adults with non-chronic sun-damaged melanomas and are frequently detected in younger patients who harbored the MC1R polymorphism (Castellani et al., 2023; Neville et al., 2024). Recent studies suggest that FDA-approved BRAF and HDAC inhibitors, such as vorinostat, could enhance the efficacy of MC1R-targeted therapies by improving drug delivery through upregulated MC1R expression (Lara-Vega et al., 2023).

Targeting PI3K-AKT Pathway

Another molecular pathway involved in cell survival and proliferation is the PI3K-AKT pathway (Peng et al., 2022). When constitutively activated, PI3K-AKT promotes melanoma cells' proliferation and metastasis, similar to the RAS-RAF-MEK-ERK pathway (Fresno Vara et al., 2004; Peng et al., 2022). Molecular aberrations such as gain-of-function mutations or chromosomal copy number variations in PIK3CA and AKT1 genes are responsible for a hyperactive PI3K/AKT pathway (Ma et al., 2024). Moreover, up to 3% PI3K missense mutation rate has been found in examining melanoma tumor samples (Vanni et al., 2020b). The low mutation rate of PI3K-AKT pathway-associated genes suggests that this pathway may be insignificant in melanoma initiation or progression. However, the PI3K-AKT pathway can also be hyperactivated through (i) the inactivation or loss of PTEN and (ii) the influence of NRAS mutations (Cuesta et al., 2021). An NRAS mutation stimulating PI3K-AKT pathway hyperactivation means that the RAS/RAF/MEK/ERK and PI3K-AKT pathways are defective. Furthermore, in RAS- and RAF-mutant melanomas, PTEN loss or inactivation leads to PI3K/AKT pathway activation, which drives the metastasis of melanomas.

ERK Signaling

The protein extracellular signal-regulated kinase (ERK) is a downstream component of the MAPK pathway. When activated, it catalyzes the phosphorylation of nuclear transcription factors, thereby conveying growth and mitogenic signals from RAS GTPases and other proteins (Dillon et al., 2021). In melanoma, mutations in BRAF and NRAS can abrogate ERK signaling, rendering it independent of upstream feedback mechanisms (Al Mahi and Ablain, 2022). Resistance to targeted therapy such as MEK and RAS inhibitors poses a considerable challenge in melanoma therapy. Tsamis and colleagues (2023) showed that ERK signaling could be restored in patients who acquired resistance to MEK and RAF inhibitors, thereby addressing drug resistance in melanoma. **Figure 5.1** illustrates various dysregulated pathways in melanoma.

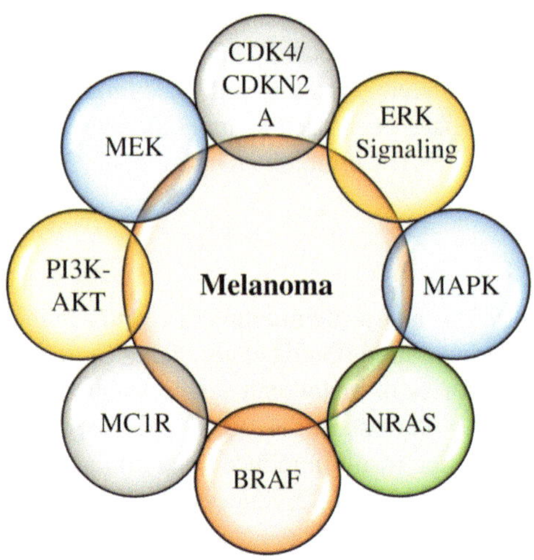

FIGURE 5.1 **A representation of dysregulated pathways in melanoma.** Mutations in these pathways may influence other pathways and may be targeted for treatment.

NANOMEDICINE IN ADVANCING MELANOMA TREATMENT

In the context of the sophisticated and complex emergence of nanotechnology as applied to disease therapy, it is essential to highlight that recent advances in nanomedicine can play critical roles in the clinical treatment of advanced melanoma. This is because nanomaterials can target drug delivery at the cellular level by overcoming biological barriers in the body. Briefly, nanomedicine refers to the use of nanotechnology and nanoscience in preventing, diagnosing, and treating human diseases (Soares et al., 2018; Zhang et al., 2020). Due to their small size (10–100 nm), high specific surface area, and flexible surface functionalization, nanotherapeutics commonly show higher therapeutic efficacy than traditional small molecule medicines because of reduced toxicity, better bioavailability, and improved pharmacokinetics, and this overall contributes to their improved therapeutic outcome. As a result, nanotherapeutics overcome barriers that traditional medications cannot, and they may be able to satisfy market needs for illness treatments in the future (Zhang et al., 2020). To deliver anticancer drugs to tumors, nanoparticles can be used in three different ways: (i) passively, by focusing on the tumor microenvironment and the Enhanced Permeation and Retention (EPR) effect of leaky tumor blood vessels; (ii) triggered by responding to changes in temperature, pH, light, ultrasound, or magnetic fields; and (iii) actively, by using ligands attached to the nanoparticles to target particular receptors or markers on tumor cells (De la Puente and Azab, 2017). Nanotherapeutics have a critical role in oncology since they provide a controlled release of active components of drugs, ensuring maximum activity in the body. Thus, it allows targeted and guided therapy by improving therapeutic efficacy and minimizing off-target toxicities (Bhatia et al., 2022). Various nanomedicine drugs for melanoma are discussed in **Table 5.1**.

NANOMEDICINE AS A ROLE PLAYER IN COMBINED MELANOMA THERAPEUTICS

Combination therapy regarding nanomedicine is an upcoming and promising therapeutic approach to melanoma. It exhibits benefits such as enhanced sensitivity to tumor cells, reactive oxygen species (ROS), heat, and radiation therapy, and improved therapeutic efficacy synergistically (Guan et al., 2021). Examples of combination nanotherapies for melanoma are synergistic radio/photothermal/photodynamic therapy, synergistic sono/chemo/photothermal therapy, synergistic chemo/immuno/photothermal therapy, and synergistic immuno/photodynamic therapy (Guan et al., 2021). The efficacy of radiotherapy (RT) was improved by combining it with photothermal therapy (PTT). In addition, using gold nanocages modified with polyethylene glycol (PEG) and coupled with the CD44 antibody, PTT and RT had a synergistic effect against the destruction of four T1 cells. The combination of hyperthermia and RT of hollow spike-like gold nanostructures minimized tumor growth more than when RT was used alone (Daneshvar et al., 2020). A combination of immunotherapy and PDT showed that nanoparticles effectively eradicated melanoma cells and prevented the recurrence and metastasis of tumor cells by improving immune markers such as cytokine levels, immune cell proportions, and serum antibodies (Zhu et al., 2020). Nanomedicine-based combination therapy can minimize long-term toxicity and high resistance to drugs and improve the efficacy of monotherapies and conventional treatments, resulting in an increased survival rate of melanoma patients (Guan et al., 2021).

A study demonstrated that the delivery of gold nanoparticles into the bloodstream acted like bacteria and was taken up by immune cells *in vivo* (Gao et al., 2022). Activation of these nanoparticle immune complexes that are naturally attracted to melanoma cells by PTT-induced destruction of melanoma cells led to recruitment and aggregation of immune cells,

TABLE 5.1
Nanomedicine Drugs for Melanoma

Nanoparticle	Drug	Mechanism of Action	Effect	References
Polymeric nanoparticles	Poly (lactic-co-glycolic acid) (PLGA) [e.g., Leuprolide acetate (Lupron Depot)] 43 (PLGA) polylactic acid (PLA) [e.g., Goserelin acetate (Zoladex implant)] and polycaprolactone (PCL) combined with polyethylene glycol (PEG) [e.g., PEGylated granulocyte colony-stimulating factor (Neulasta)]	• PLGA acts as a biodegradable drug delivery system. In formulations like Lupron Depot, PLGA encapsulates the drug (e.g., Leuprolide acetate), protecting it and controlling its release. • As PLGA undergoes hydrolysis in the body, it gradually breaks down into lactic and glycolic acids, releasing the encapsulated drug over an extended period. • This mechanism allows for sustained drug delivery, reducing dosing frequency and improving patient compliance.	Enhanced amphipathic, biocompatibility, and better delivery of hydrophilic drugs	El-Kenawy et al. (2017) Arasi et al. (2020)
Liposomes	Phosphatidylethanolamine liposomal cisplatin	• Phosphatidylethanolamine liposomal cisplatin encapsulates cisplatin in pH-sensitive liposomes, enhancing tumor targeting and reducing systemic toxicity. • The liposomes accumulate in tumors via the Enhanced Permeability and Retention (EPR) effect and release cisplatin in acidic tumor environments. • This formulation improves cellular uptake through endocytosis or membrane fusion. • Once inside cancer cells, cisplatin forms DNA crosslinks, inhibiting replication and transcription, ultimately inducing apoptosis.	Improved cytotoxicity and delivery of the drug by 3.6-fold due to high drug concentration	El-Kenawy et al. (2017)
	Cabazitaxel conjugated with lipoprodug	• Cabazitaxel conjugated with lipoprodrug combines the microtubule-stabilizing action of cabazitaxel with enhanced drug delivery. • The lipid conjugation improves tumor targeting through the EPR effect and increases cellular uptake. • Upon internalization, the pH-sensitive bond releases cabazitaxel in acidic tumor environments, allowing it to bind tubulin, disrupting the process of mitosis, and triggering apoptosis in cancer cells.	Expressed improved safety profile and tolerability in animal studies compared to free cabazitaxel	Shi et al. (2020)
	Glutathione disulfide loaded with liposomes	• Glutathione disulfide (GSSG) liposomes effectively deliver GSSG into cells, overcoming its poor membrane permeability. • This increases intracellular GSSG levels, promoting protein S-glutathionylation, a regulatory mechanism during oxidative stress. • The liposomes enhance GSSG's ability to modulate cellular redox state, potentially affecting various physiological and pathological processes associated with oxidative stress and protein function regulation.	The improved survival rate of melanoma-bearing mice because of the deceleration of the growth of tumor cells by 85–90%	Arasi et al. (2020)

(Continued)

TABLE 5.1 *(Continued)*
Nanomedicine Drugs for Melanoma

Nanoparticle	Drug	Mechanism of Action	Effect	References
Niosomes	Artemisinin encapsulated in noisome	• Artemisinin encapsulated in niosomes enhances drug delivery and efficacy against malaria parasites. • The noisome protects and transports artemisinin to infected cells. • Upon release, artemisinin's endoperoxide bridge is cleaved by iron, generating free radicals. • These radicals alkylate heme and parasite proteins, disrupting vital processes and killing the parasite. • This formulation improves artemisinin's bioavailability and antimalarial activity.	Selectively targeted melanoma cells sparing normal cells	El-Kenawy et al. (2017)
Nanohydrogels	Doxorubicin (DOX) loaded into polymersomes	• DOX-loaded polymersomes enhance drug delivery and efficacy against cancer cells. • The polymersomes protect and transport DOX, accumulating in tumors via the EPR effect. • The polymersomes release DOX upon cellular uptake in response to specific stimuli (e.g., pH, redox conditions). • Once released, DOX intercalates with DNA, inhibits topoisomerase II, and generates free radicals, leading to DNA damage and cancer cell apoptosis.	Selective uptake of DOX by melanoma cells	Kumar et al. (2023)
Solid Lipid Nanoparticles (SLN)	Temozolomide (TMZ) encapsulated in SLN	• TMZ encapsulated in Solid Lipid Nanoparticles (SLNs) enhances drug stability and delivery. • SLNs protect TMZ from premature degradation and improve its pharmacokinetics. • The nanoparticles accumulate in tumors via the EPR effect, releasing TMZ in a sustained manner. • Once released, TMZ undergoes pH-dependent activation, forming the active metabolite MTIC, which methylates DNA, causing cell cycle arrest and apoptosis in cancer cells.	Improved therapeutic efficacy via inhibition of vascularization and growth of B16-F10 melanoma in C57/BL6 mice with minimal toxicity	Cassano et al. (2021)

(Continued)

TABLE 5.1 *(Continued)*
Nanomedicine Drugs for Melanoma

Nanoparticle	Drug	Mechanism of Action	Effect	References
Dendrimers	Encapsulation of DOX and immunoadjuvant cytosine-phosphate-guanine oligonucleotides (CpG ODNs) in amino-terminated polyamidoamine (PAMAM) dendrimer	• Encapsulation of doxorubicincytosine-phosphate-guanine oligonucleotides (CpG ODNs) in PAMAM dendrimer enhances drug delivery and immunostimulation. • The dendrimer protects and transports both agents, accumulating in tumors via the EPR effect. • Upon cellular uptake, DOX intercalates DNA and inhibits topoisomerase II, while CpG ODNs activate Toll-like receptor 9, stimulating innate immunity. • This dual-action approach combines direct cytotoxicity with immune system activation against cancer cells.	Improved therapeutic efficacy	Cassano et al. (2021)
Carbon nanotubes (CNT)	Prodrug of DOX encapsulated in CNT (CNT-DOX)	• Carbon nanotubes encapsulating DOX prodrug (CNT-DOX) enhance drug delivery and reduce toxicity. • CNTs protect and transport DOX, accumulating in tumors via the EPR effect. • The prodrug design allows controlled release in the tumor microenvironment. • Once released, DOX intercalates DNA, inhibits topoisomerase II, and generates free radicals, leading to DNA damage and cancer cell apoptosis. • CNTs may also synergistically enhance DOX's cytotoxicity.	*In vitro* induction of cell death in B16-F10 melanoma *In vivo* inhibition of growth of tumor with minimal side effects compared to free DOX	Cassano et al. (2021)
	Polypyrrole-coated multi-walled carbon nanotubes composite (PPy@MWCNTs)	• PPy@MWCNTs combine the conductivity of MWCNTs with the electroactive properties of polypyrrole. • The composite enhances electron transfer and increases surface area. • PPy provides additional active sites, while MWCNTs improve mechanical strength and electrical conductivity. • This synergistic effect results in improved electrochemical performance, making PPy@MWCNTs suitable for applications in supercapacitors, sensors, and electrochemical catalysis.	Better access to deeper tumors with selective uptake and minimal side effects and histologically 50% tumor reduction and 75% necrosis 10 days after therapy	Cassano et al. (2021)

(Continued)

TABLE 5.1 *(Continued)*
Nanomedicine Drugs for Melanoma

Nanoparticle	Drug	Mechanism of Action	Effect	References
Metal nanoparticles	DOX encapsulated in gold nanoparticles (AgNP@CMC-DOX)	• AuNP@CMC-DOX enhances drug delivery and efficacy against cancer cells. • The nanoparticles protect and transport DOX, accumulating in tumors via the EPR effect. • Upon cellular uptake, the acidic environment triggers DOX release. • Once freed, DOX intercalates DNA, inhibits topoisomerase II, and generates free radicals, leading to DNA damage and cancer cell apoptosis. • The gold nanoparticles may also synergistically enhance DOX's cytotoxicity.	Synergistic cytotoxicity against melanoma cells and antimicrobial activity against Gram-negative and Gram-positive bacteria	Cassano et al. (2021)
	Conjugation of type I topoisomerase inhibitor and miRNA with gold nanoparticles [miRNA-34a with traditional chemotherapeutic agents (like the topoisomerase inhibitor SN-38)]	• The conjugation of a type I topoisomerase inhibitor (like SN-38) and miRNA-34a with gold nanoparticles creates a synergistic therapeutic system. • Gold nanoparticles protect and deliver both agents to cancer cells via the EPR effect. • The topoisomerase inhibitor induces DNA damage, while miRNA-34a suppresses oncogenes and enhances apoptosis. • This combination overcomes drug resistance, increases cellular uptake, and improves the overall anticancer efficacy compared to individual treatments.	Enhanced cytotoxic effect against human uveal melanoma synergistically with miRNA exhibiting improved solubility in water	Synoradzki et al. (2024)
	Platinum nanoparticles combined with DOX	• Platinum nanoparticles combined with DOX enhance drug delivery and efficacy against cancer cells. • The nanoparticles protect and transport DOX, accumulating in tumors via the EPR effect. • Upon cellular uptake, DOX intercalates DNA and inhibits topoisomerase II, while platinum nanoparticles deplete intracellular glutathione and generate reactive oxygen species. • This dual mechanism induces DNA damage, triggers apoptosis, and overcomes drug resistance in cancer cells.	Induction of apoptosis and remarkable reduction in the growth of tumor in a model of subcutaneous murine melanoma tumor	Cassano et al. (2021)

(Continued)

TABLE 5.1 *(Continued)*
Nanomedicine Drugs for Melanoma

Nanoparticle	Drug	Mechanism of Action	Effect	References
Chitosan	Conjugation of chitosan/alginate nanoparticles with DOX	• Chitosan/alginate nanoparticles conjugated with DOX enhance drug delivery and efficacy against cancer cells. • The nanoparticles protect and transport DOX, accumulating in tumors via the EPR effect. • The pH-sensitive nature of the nanoparticles allows controlled release in acidic tumor environments. • Once released, DOX intercalates DNA, inhibits topoisomerase II, and generates free radicals, leading to DNA damage and cancer cell apoptosis. • This formulation improves DOX's bioavailability and reduces systemic toxicity (Li et al., 2022).	Inhibition of growth and viability of melanoma cells in a mouse model through production of cytotoxic effect that lasts longer	Arasi et al. (2020)
	Encapsulation of specific siRNAs into alginate-conjugated trimethyl chitosan (ATMC) nanoparticles	• Encapsulation of specific siRNAs in ATMC nanoparticles enhances siRNA delivery and stability. • The nanoparticles protect siRNA from degradation and facilitate cellular uptake. • Upon internalization, the nanoparticles release siRNA in the cytoplasm, where it binds to target mRNA, leading to its degradation and subsequent gene silencing. • This approach allows for targeted inhibition of specific genes involved in cancer progression, potentially improving therapeutic outcomes.	Silences the GP130 and S1PR1 genes in melanoma B16-F10 potentially producing an anticancer effect	Arasi et al. (2020)
Albumin-based nanoparticles	Albumin-based nanostructures containing AZD8055 (ABN-AZD)	• ABN-AZD enhances drug delivery and efficacy against uveal melanoma. • The nanostructures protect and transport AZD8055, accumulating in tumors via the EPR effect. • A disulfide linker allows selective drug release in the glutathione-rich tumor environment. • Once released, AZD8055 inhibits mTOR kinase, disrupting cell growth and proliferation pathways. • This formulation improves AZD8055's bioavailability, selectivity, and antitumor activity while reducing systemic toxicity.	Selective toxicity against uveal melanoma cells significantly minimizes the size of the tumor in comparison to free AZD8055 in mouse models	Synoradzki et al. (2024)

thus targeting melanoma cells more effectively. Nanotechnology can improve various targeted melanoma therapies, including cancer immunotherapy, molecularly targeted therapy, cytotoxic chemotherapy, gene therapy, PTT, radiation therapy, and photodynamic therapy (Beiu et al., 2020). To improve the target delivery of chemotherapeutics into tumor cells, nanoparticles were combined with target ligands. PPC@HA was manufactured by encapsulating amphiphilic platinum (IV)-polyethylenimine-chlorin e6 (Pt (IV)-PEI-Ce6) NPs in an aqueous solution after the polymer was developed, which was then synthesized and self-assembled into NPs (PPC). The already formed PPC@HA, when injected into mice with melanoma cells, demonstrated a synergistic photodynamic and chemotherapy antitumor effect (Huang et al., 2022).

Theranostic nanomedicine, the combination of diagnostics and therapy, is a steadily rising medical field aimed at making personalized medicine successful. Gold nanoparticles (AGuIX) have effectively been used in experimental animal models of melanoma metastases as an MRI contrast agent and treatment (El-Kenawy et al., 2017). In addition, photoluminescent polymer—poly (lactic acid) (BPLP-PLA), which is a biodegradable nanoparticle when loaded with anti-$BRAF^{V600E}$-specific drug (PLX4032) and muramyl peptide, can be used for imaging and treatment of melanoma (El-Kenawy et al., 2017). Delivery of drugs to the target site through the magnetic field with the help of Superparamagnetic Iron Oxide Nanoparticles (SPION) helps increase the concentration of drugs at the target site overall, minimizing side effects (Jin et al., 2020). More research is aimed at engineering fluorescent dyes that are more stable and can be used to access areas situated deep into the body to aid in diagnosing and treating melanoma through shifting wavelengths. Additionally, studies are underway on ultrasound microbubbles that can be used to deliver drugs more effectively and using nanoparticles combined with ultrasound to kill cancer cells (Jin et al., 2020). **Figure 5.2** illustrates the role of nanomedicine in melanoma treatment.

Multifunctionally designed nanomedicine significantly enhances the susceptibility of malignant cells to medications, heat, X-ray radiation, and ROS. This improves the therapeutic benefits of many therapies in a synergistic way. This section emphasizes combination therapy and discusses many common multimodal synergistic treatments to determine the optimum therapeutic outcome for melanoma. A new age in melanoma treatment has been brought about by combination therapy, which has the potential to increase therapeutic benefits to an improved level of efficacy (Zhu et al., 2020).

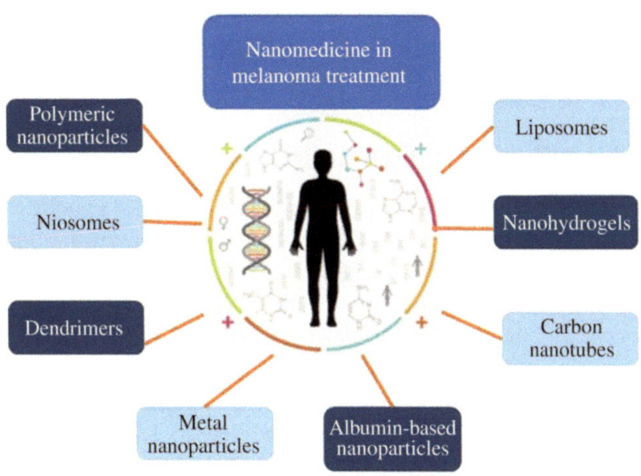

FIGURE 5.2 **Nanomedicine as a frontier in melanoma treatment.** Various nanoparticles may be used in melanoma-enhanced treatment.

SYNERGISTIC RADIO/PHOTOTHERMAL/PHOTODYNAMIC THERAPY

Platinum nanoparticles (PtNPs) may convert energy by acting as absorbers for X-rays and laser light (Daneshvar et al., 2020). Furthermore, they could function as radiosensitizers in cancer treatment. Due to the modest radiation dosages administered for safety and the limited absorption of radiation beams by soft tissue tumors, conventional radiotherapy could be more effective. In light of this, the scientists showed that PtNPs treated the B16/F10 cells more deeply and produced more ROS when combined with laser light radiation than when they used X-rays or only laser radiation (Daneshvar et al., 2020; Guan et al., 2021). Using platinum mesoporous as a unique NIR photosensitizer for PTT and an X-ray absorption agent for X-ray-induced photodynamic therapy (X-PDT) for melanoma cancer cells was another comparable strategy. Comparing PTT and X-PDT combined exposure to that of PTT or X-PDT alone, the latter resulted in increased efficacy and cooperativity, more profound treatment, and a meager survival rate of melanoma cells (Salehi et al., 2019).

SYNERGISTIC SONO/CHEMO/PHOTOTHERMAL THERAPY

To treat skin cancer, a sono/chemo/photothermal approach combined the mechanical wounding, cytotoxic, and photothermal effects of melanin, chemotherapeutic medications, and ultrasonic contrast agents. For the treatment of melanoma, self-assembling perfluoropentane nanodroplets with outstanding biocompatibility were created (Chiang et al., 2018). The Ouzo effect spontaneously manufactured polyvinyl alcohol (PVA)-shelled and melanin-cored nanodroplets. The anti-cancer medication DOX was then injected into the PVA shells of the nanodroplets. Optoacoustic irradiation was applied after the loading procedure to create the nanocavity structure by vaporizing the nanodroplets. In both *in vitro* and *in vivo* experiments, the nanodroplets effectively eliminated melanoma tumors when combined with optoacoustic synergistic irradiation treatment and laser irradiation after the tumor structures were mechanically disrupted in the *in vivo* animal experiments.

SYNERGISTIC CHEMO/IMMUNO/PHOTOTHERMAL-THERAPY

An adjuvant molecule called CpG that can cause DC mutations, indocyanine green (ICG), a photothermal agent, and DOX were coupled in a combination treatment based on an α-cyclodextrin (CD)-based gel system (Qin et al., 2020). The original tumor growth may be successfully inhibited by the chemo/immuno/photothermal treatment approach. PD-L1 inhibition unexpectedly prevented tumor development in both primary and metastatic melanoma, decreased tumor size, and prevented tumor recurrence (Guan et al., 2021; Qin et al., 2020). Tumor-specific antigens are sustainably released, which makes combinatorial treatment an enhanced therapeutic approach. Additionally, this unique therapy produced a robust tumor-specific immunity that may cover a wide variety of solid tumors, in contrast to conventional immunotherapy.

SYNERGISTIC IMMUNO/PHOTODYNAMIC THERAPY

Using aluminum hydroxide as an immunoadjuvant and chlorin e6 as a photosensitizer, this innovative nanosystem [Al-bovine serum albumin (BSA)-Ce6 NPs] combines immunotherapy with PDT (Guan et al., 2021; Zhu et al., 2020). By inducing a potent antitumor immune response, which in turn enhances immune response indicators like serum antibody levels, cytokine levels, and immune cell proportions, they showed that the nanoparticles effectively killed melanoma cells and prevented tumor relapse or metastasis. Combination therapy based on nanomedicines for melanoma may decrease high drug resistance, boost the efficacy of monotherapies and conventional treatments, and decrease long-term toxicity. Consequently, combination therapy based on nanomedicine may offer the advantages of monotherapy while lowering the risk of metastasis and recurrence and improving the survival rate.

CHALLENGES AND LIMITATIONS IMPEDING NANOMEDICINE AND TARGETED THERAPIES IN MELANOMA TREATMENT

One major challenge encountered in nanomedicine is the presence of undesired effects due to the interaction of nanoparticles and the hosts' immune system forming biocorona. El-Kenawy et al. (2017) shed light on using macrophages to directly deliver active pharmacological agents to tumor cells, minimizing such interactions. Notable progress in nanomedicine clinical trials has been witnessed. However, this comes with limitations that must be overcome. Following their entry into the biological system, the nanodrug's complex interaction with the immune system leads to premature clearance of the drugs, toxicity, and side effect activation. In addition to the complex immunological interactions, the intended biological targets and biological barriers hindering the availability of nanodrugs are significant limitations that should be overcome. Targeted therapies also focused on signaling pathways and molecular mechanisms may be limited by the interactions, activations, and deactivations in the inter-pathways signaling, impeding with small molecule inhibitor drugs' mode of action.

CONCLUSIONS AND PERSPECTIVES

Nanomedicine forms an essential part of a combined melanoma therapeutic approach. This, however, comes with complex host immunological interactions. The continued evaluation of nanomaterials' physicochemical properties *in vitro* and *in vivo* models will provide invaluable insights into nanomedicine therapeutic use in melanoma. Furthermore, while human systems may react differently to animal models, current and future research efforts should focus on the translational use of nanodrugs from preclinical to clinical applications in melanoma nanomedicine treatment.

Nanotechnology drug-driven platforms represent a promising tool in melanoma precision medicine. The complex nanodrug-host immune system interaction may be invertedly used to trigger immunogenicity. This may be favored by immunotherapy and targeted and combinatorial therapies. Understanding the molecular mechanisms underlying melanoma will enhance melanoma-targeted therapies and hold the key to melanoma nanomedicine and precision medicine through a combinatorial and convergence therapeutic approach (**Figure 5.3**).

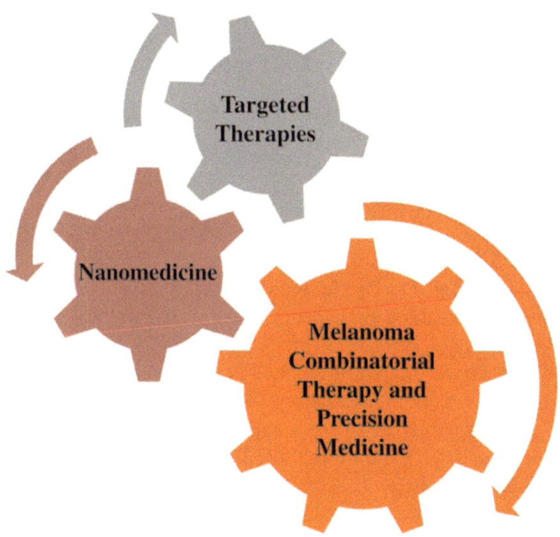

FIGURE 5.3 **The combinatorial therapy approach.** This approach includes nanomedicine and targeted therapies, which collaboratively hold enhanced melanoma treatment options.

REFERENCES

Al Mahi, A. and Ablain, J. 2022. RAS pathway regulation in melanoma, *Disease Models & Mechanisms*, 15, p. dmm049229.

Appels, N. M. G. M., Beijnen, J. H. and Schellens, J. H. M. 2005. Development of farnesyl transferase inhibitors: A review, *The Oncologist*, 10(8), pp. 565–578. https://doi.org/10.1634/theoncologist.10-8-565

Arasi, M. B., Pedini, F., Valentini, S., Felli, N. and Felicetti, F. 2020. Advances in natural or synthetic nanoparticles for metastatic melanoma therapy and diagnosis, *Cancers*, 12(10), p. 2893.

Beiu, C., Giurcaneanu, C., Grumezescu, A. M., Holban, A. M., Popa, L. G. and Mihai, M. M. 2020. Nanosystems for improved targeted therapies in melanoma, *Journal of Clinical Medicine*, 9(2), p. 318.

Bhatia, S. N., Chen, X., Dobrovolskaia, M. A. and Lammers, T. 2022. Cancer nanomedicine, *Nature Reviews Cancer*, 22, pp. 550–556.

Cancer Genome Atlas Network. 2015. Genomic classification of cutaneous melanoma, *Cell*, 161(7), pp. 1681–1696. https://doi.org/10.1016/j.cell.2015.05.044

Cassano, R., Cuconato, M., Calviello, G., Serini, S. and Trombino, S. 2021. Recent advances in nanotechnology for the treatment of melanoma, *Molecules*, 26(4), p. 785.

Castellani, G., Buccarelli, M., Arasi, M. B., Rossi, S., Pisanu, M. E., Bellenghi, M., Lintas, C. and Tabolacci, C. 2023. BRAF mutations in melanoma: Biological aspects, therapeutic implications, and circulating biomarkers, *Cancers (Basel)*, 15, p. 4026.

Chiang, C.-S., Lin, Y.-J., Lee, R., Lai, Y.-H., Cheng, H.-W., Hsieh, C.-H., Shyu, W.-C. and Chen, S.-Y. 2018. Combination of fucoidan-based magnetic nanoparticles and immunomodulators enhances tumour-localized immunotherapy, *Nature Nanotechnology*, 13, pp. 746–754.

Colombino, M., Casula, M., Paliogiannis, P., Manca, A., Sini, M. C., Pisano, M., Santeufemia, D. A., Cossu, A. and Palmieri, G. 2024. Heterogeneous pathogenesis of melanoma: BRAF mutations and beyond, *Critical Reviews in Oncology/Hematology*, 201, p. 104435.

Crozier, L., Foy, R., Mouery, B. L., Whitaker, R. H., Corno, A., Spanos, C., Ly, T., Gowen Cook, J. and Saurin, A. T. 2022. CDK4/6 inhibitors induce replication stress to cause long-term cell cycle withdrawal, *The EMBO Journal*, 41(6), p. e108599. https://doi.org/10.15252/embj.2021108599

Cuesta, C., Arévalo-Alameda, C. and Castellano, E. 2021. The importance of being PI3K in the RAS signaling network, *Genes*, 12, p. 1094.

Czarnecka, A. M., Bartnik, E., Fiedorowicz, M. and Rutkowski, P. 2020. Targeted therapy in melanoma and mechanisms of resistance, *International Journal of Molecular Sciences*, 21, p. 4576.

Daneshvar, F., Salehi, F., Karimi, M., Vais, R. D., Mosleh-Shirazi, M. and Sattarahmady, N. 2020. Combined X-ray radiotherapy and laser photothermal therapy of melanoma cancer cells using dual-sensitization of platinum nanoparticles, *Journal of Photochemistry and Photobiology B: Biology*, 203, p. 111737.

De la Puente, P. and Azab, A. K. 2017. Nanoparticle delivery systems, general approaches, and their implementation in multiple myeloma, *European Journal of Haematology*, 98(6), pp. 529–541. https://doi.org/10.1111/ejh.12870

De Meza, M. M., Blokx, W. A. M., Bonenkamp, J. J., Blank, C. U., Aarts, M. J. B., van den Berkmortel, F. W. P. J., Boers-Sonderen, M. J., De Groot, J. W. B., Haanen, J. B. A. G., Hospers, G. A. P., Kapiteijn, E., Van Not, O. J., Piersma, D., Van Rijn, R. S., Stevense-den Boer, M., Van der Veldt, A. A. M., Vreugdenhil, G., Van den Eertwegh, A. J. M., Suijkerbuijk, K. P. M. and Wouters, M. W. J. M. 2023. Adjuvant BRAF-MEK inhibitors versus anti PD-1 therapy in stage III melanoma: A propensity-matched outcome analysis, *Cancers*, 15(2), p. 409. https://doi.org/10.3390/cancers15020409

Dillon, M., Lopez, A., Lin, E., Sales, D., Perets, R. and Jain, P. 2021. Progress on Ras/MAPK signaling research and targeting in blood and solid cancers, *Cancers (Basel)*, 13.

El-Kenawy, A. E. M., Constantin, C., Hassan, S. M. A., et al. 2017. Nanomedicine in Melanoma: Current Trends and Future Perspectives. *In*: Ward, W.H., Farma, J.M. (eds.) *Cutaneous Melanoma: Etiology and Therapy*. Brisbane (AU): Codon Publications. doi: 10.15586/codon.cutaneousmelanoma.2017.ch10

Fernandez, M. F., Choi, J. and Sosman, J. 2023. New approaches to targeted therapy in melanoma, *Cancers*, 15(12), 3224. https://doi.org/10.3390/cancers15123224

Fresno Vara, J. A., Casado, E., de Castro, J., Cejas, P., Belda-Iniesta, C. and González-Barón, M. 2004. PI3K/Akt signalling pathway and cancer, *Cancer Treatment Reviews*, 30(2), pp. 193–204. https://doi.org/10.1016/j.ctrv.2003.07.007

Gao, C., Wang, Q., Li, J., Kwong, C. H. T., Wei, J., Xie, B., Lu, S., Lee, S. M. Y. and Wang, R. 2022. In vivo hitchhiking of immune cells by intracellular self-assembly of bacteria-mimetic nanomedicine for targeted therapy of melanoma, *Science Advances*, 8, p. eabn1805.

Garutti, M., Targato, G., Buriolla, S., Palmero, L., Minisini, A. M. and Puglisi, F. 2021. CDK4/6 inhibitors in melanoma: A comprehensive review, *Cells*, 10(6), p. 1334. https://doi.org/10.3390/cells10061334

Grimaldi, A. M., Simeone, E., Festino, L., Vanella, V., Strudel, M. and Ascierto, P. A. 2017. MEK inhibitors in the treatment of metastatic melanoma and solid tumors, *American Journal of Clinical Dermatology*, 18(6), 745–754. https://doi.org/10.1007/s40257-017-0292-y

Guan, M., Zhu, S. and Li, S. 2021. Recent progress in nanomedicine for melanoma theranostics with emphasis on combination therapy, *Frontiers in Bioengineering and Biotechnology*, 9, p. 661214.

Guida, S., Guida, G. and Goding, C. R. 2022. MC1R functions, expression, and implications for targeted therapy, *Journal of Investigative Dermatology*, 142, pp. 293–302.e1.

Guo, W., Wang, H. and Li, C. 2021. Signal pathways of melanoma and targeted therapy, *Signal Transduction and Targeted Therapy*, 6(1), p. 424. https://doi.org/10.1038/s41392-021-00827-6

Guo, Y.-J., Pan, W.-W., Liu, S.-B., Shen, Z.-F., Xu, Y. and Hu, L.-L. 2020. ERK/MAPK signalling pathway and tumorigenesis, *Experimental and Therapeutic Medicine*, 19(3), pp. 1997–2007. https://doi.org/10.3892/etm.2020.8454

Han, X.-R., Chen, L., Wei, Y., Yu, W., Chen, Y., Zhang, C., Jiao, B., Shi, T., Sun, L. and Zhang, C. 2020. Discovery of selective small molecule degraders of BRAF-V600E, *Journal of Medicinal Chemistry*, 63, pp. 4069–4080.

Hedberg, M. L., Berry, C. T., Moshiri, A. S., Xiang, Y., Yeh, C. J., Attilasoy, C., Capell, B. C. and Seykora, J. T. 2022. Molecular mechanisms of cutaneous squamous cell carcinoma, *International Journal of Molecular Sciences*, 23, p. 3478.

Houben, R., Becker, J. C., Kappel, A., Terheyden, P., Bröcker, E.-B., Goetz, R. and Rapp, U. R. 2004. Constitutive activation of the Ras-Raf signaling pathway in metastatic melanoma is associated with poor prognosis, *Journal of Carcinogenesis*, 3, p. 6. https://doi.org/10.1186/1477-3163-3-6

Huang, X., Mu, N., Ding, Y., Lam, H. W., Yue, L., Gao, C., Chen, T., Yuan, Z. and Wang, R. 2022. Targeted delivery and enhanced uptake of chemo-photodynamic nanomedicine for melanoma treatment, *Acta Biomaterialia*, 147, pp. 356–365.

Jin, G., Cheah, P., Qu, J., Liu, L. and Zhao, Y. 2020. Applications of nanomaterials for theranostics of melanoma, *Journal of Nanotheranostics*, 1(1), pp. 39–55.

Joyce, K. M. 2017. Surgical Management of Melanoma. *In*: Ward, W. H. and Farma, J. M. (eds.) *Cutaneous Melanoma: Etiology and Therapy [Internet]*. Brisbane (AU): Codon Publications; Available from: https://www.ncbi.nlm.nih.gov/books/NBK481850/ doi: 10.15586/codon.cutaneousmelanoma.2017.ch7

Korzeniecki, C. and Priefer, R. 2021. Targeting KRAS mutant cancers by preventing signaling transduction in the MAPK pathway, *European Journal of Medicinal Chemistry*, 211, p. 113006.

Kumar, G., Virmani, T., Sharma, A. and Pathak, K. 2023. Codelivery of phytochemicals with conventional anticancer drugs in form of nanocarriers. *Pharmaceutics*, 15(3), p. 889.

Lara-Vega, I., Correa-Lara, M. V. M. and Vega-López, A. 2023. Effectiveness of radiotherapy and targeted radionuclide therapy for melanoma in preclinical mouse models: A combination treatments overview, *Bulletin du Cancer*, 110, pp. 912–936.

Li, C., Kuai, L., Cui, R. and Miao, X. 2022. Melanogenesis and the targeted therapy of melanoma, *Biomolecules*, 12, p. 1874.

Li, L., Zhao, G.-D., Shi, Z., Qi, L.-L., Zhou, L.-Y. and Fu, Z.-X. 2016. The Ras/Raf/MEK/ERK signaling pathway and its role in the occurrence and development of HCC, *Oncology Letters*, 12(5), pp. 3045–3050. https://doi.org/10.3892/ol.2016.5110

Loras, A., Gil-Barrachina, M., Marqués-Torrejón, M. Á., Perez-Pastor, G. and Martinez-Cadenas, C. 2022. UV-induced somatic mutations driving clonal evolution in healthy skin, nevus, and cutaneous melanoma, *Life*, 12, p. 1339.

Ma, Q., Chen, G., Li, Y., Guo, Z. and Zhang, X. 2024. The molecular genetics of PI3K/PTEN/AKT/mTOR pathway in the malformations of cortical development, *Genes & Diseases*, 11, p. 101021.

Manganelli, M., Guida, S., Ferretta, A., Pellacani, G., Porcelli, L., Azzariti, A. and Guida, G. 2021. Behind the scene: Exploiting MC1R in skin cancer risk and prevention, *Genes*, 12, p. 1093.

Menzer, C. and Hassel, J. C. 2022. Targeted therapy for melanomas without BRAF V600 mutations, *Current Treatment Options in Oncology*, 23(6), pp. 831–842. https://doi.org/10.1007/s11864-022-00946-4

Montico, B., Colizzi, F., Giurato, G., Rizzo, A., Salvati, A., Baboci, L., Benedetti, D., Pivetta, E., Covre, A. and Bo, M. D. 2020. Loss of Spry1 reduces growth of BRAFV600-mutant cutaneous melanoma and improves response to targeted therapy, *Cell Death & Disease*, 11, p. 392.

Muñoz-Couselo, E., Adelantado, E. Z., Ortiz, C., García, J. S. and Perez-Garcia, J. 2017. NRAS-mutant melanoma: Current challenges and future prospect, *OncoTargets and Therapy*, 10, pp. 3941–3947.

Muñoz-Maldonado, C., Zimmer, Y. and Medová, M. 2019. A comparative analysis of individual RAS mutations in cancer biology, *Frontiers in Oncology*, 9, p. 1088.

Nair, A. and Saha, B. 2023. Regulation of Ras-GTPase signaling and localization by post-translational modifications, *Kinases and Phosphatases*, 1, pp. 97–116.

Neville, G., Marzario, B., Shilling, D., Hand, C. and Heffron, C. 2024. Low incidence of BRAF and NRAS mutations in a population with a high incidence of melanoma, *Virchows Archiv*, 484, pp. 1–5.

Palmieri, G., Colombino, M., Casula, M., Sini, M. C., Manca, A., Pisano, M., Paliogiannis, P. and Cossu, A. 2021. Molecular Landscape Profile of Melanoma. In: *New Therapies in Advanced Cutaneous Malignancies*, 31–55. Springer.

Pan, Y. and Mader, M. M. 2022. Principles of kinase allosteric inhibition and pocket validation, *Journal of Medicinal Chemistry*, 65, pp. 5288–5299.

Patel, H., Yacoub, N., Mishra, R., White, A., Yuan, L., Alanazi, S. and Garrett, J. T. 2020. Current advances in the treatment of BRAF-mutant melanoma, *Cancers*, 12, p. 482.

Peng, Y., Wang, Y., Zhou, C., Mei, W. and Zeng, C. 2022. PI3K/Akt/mTOR pathway and its role in cancer therapeutics: Are we making headway? *Frontiers in Oncology*, 12. https://doi.org/10.3389/fonc.2022.819128

Priantti, J. N., Vilbert, M., Madeira, T., Moraes, F. C. A., Hein, E. C. K., Saeed, A. and Cavalcante, L. 2023. Efficacy and safety of rechallenge with BRAF/MEK inhibitors in advanced melanoma patients: A systematic review and meta-analysis, *Cancers*, 15(15), p. 3754. https://doi.org/10.3390/cancers15153754

Qin, L., Cao, J., Shao, K., Tong, F., Yang, Z., Lei, T., Wang, Y., Hu, C., Umeshappa, C. S. and Gao, H. 2020. A tumor-to-lymph procedure navigated versatile gel system for combinatorial therapy against tumor recurrence and metastasis, *Science Advances*, 6, p. eabb3116.

Ribeiro Moura Brasil Arnaut, J., Dos Santos Guimarães, I., Evangelista Dos Santos, A. C., De Moraes Lino Da Silva, F., Machado, J. R. and De Melo, A. C. 2021. Molecular landscape of hereditary melanoma, *Critical Reviews in Oncology/Hematology*, 164, p. 103425.

Riegel, K. and Rajalingam, K. 2020. The non-linearity of RAF-MEK signaling in dendritic cells, *Cell Cycle*, 19, pp. 2249–2259.

Roa, P., Bremer, N. V., Foglizzo, V. and Cocco, E. 2024. Mutations in the Serine/Threonine kinase BRAF: Oncogenic drivers in solid tumors, *Cancers*, 16, p. 1215.

Salehi, F., Daneshvar, F., Karimi, M., Vais, R. D., Mosleh-Shirazi, M. and Sattarahmady, N. 2019. Enhanced melanoma cell-killing by combined phototherapy/radiotherapy using a mesoporous platinum nanostructure, *Photodiagnosis and Photodynamic Therapy*, 28, pp. 300–307.

Sanchez, J. N., Subramanian, C., Chanda, M., Shanguan, G., Zhang, N., Wang, T., Timmermann, B. N., Blagg, B. S. J. and Cohen, M. S. 2021. A novel C-terminal Hsp90 inhibitor KU758 synergizes efficacy in combination with BRAF or MEK inhibitors and targets drug-resistant pathways in BRAF-mutant melanomas, *Melanoma Research*, 31(3), pp. 197–207. doi: 10.1097/CMR.0000000000000734

Sargen, M. R., Pfeiffer, R. M., Yang, X. R., Tucker, M. A. and Goldstein, A. M. 2020. Variation in cutaneous patterns of melanomagenesis according to germline CDKN2A/CDK4 status in melanoma-prone families, *Journal of Investigative Dermatology*, 140, pp. 174–181.e3.

Schuler, M., Zimmer, L., Kim, K. B., Sosman, J. A., Ascierto, P. A., Postow, M. A., De Vos, F. Y. F. L., van Herpen, C. M. L., Carlino, M. S., Johnson, D. B., Berking, C., Reddy, M. B., Harney, A. S., Berlin, J. D. and Amaria, R. N. 2022. Phase Ib/II trial of ribociclib in combination with binimetinib in patients with NRAS-mutant melanoma, *Clinical Cancer Research*, 28(14), pp. 3002–3010. https://doi.org/10.1158/1078-0432.CCR-21-3872

Schummer, P., Schilling, B. and Gesierich, A. 2020. Long-term outcomes in BRAF-mutated melanoma treated with combined targeted therapy or immune checkpoint blockade: Are we approaching a true cure? *American Journal of Clinical Dermatology*, 21, pp. 493–504.

Shi, L., Wang, Y., Wang, Q., Jiang, Z., Ren, L., Yan, Y., Liu, Z., Wan, J., Huang, L., Cen, B. and Han, W. 2020. Transforming a toxic drug into an efficacious nanomedicine using a lipoprodrug strategy to treat patient-derived melanoma xenografts, *Journal of Controlled Release*, 324, pp. 289–302.

Soares, S., Sousa, J., Pais, A. and Vitorino, C. 2018. Nanomedicine: Principles, properties, and regulatory issues, *Frontiers in Chemistry*, 6, p. 356901.

Song, Y., Bi, Z., Liu, Y., Qin, F., Wei, Y. and Wei, X. 2022. Targeting RAS–RAF–MEK–ERK signaling pathway in human cancer: Current status in clinical trials, *Genes & Diseases*, 10(1), 76–88. https://doi.org/10.1016/j.gendis.2022.05.006

Song, Y., Bi, Z., Liu, Y., Qin, F., Wei, Y. and Wei, X. 2023. Targeting RAS–RAF–MEK–ERK signaling pathway in human cancer: Current status in clinical trials, *Genes & Diseases*, 10, pp. 76–88.

Synoradzki, K. J., Paduszyńska, N., Solnik, M., Toro, M. D., Bilmin, K., Bylina, E., Rutkowski, P., Yousef, Y. A., Bucolo, C., Zweifel, S. A. and Reibaldi, M. 2024. From molecular biology to novel immunotherapies and nanomedicine in uveal melanoma, *Current Oncology*, 31(2), pp. 778–800.

Tatjana, Z. and Sergejs, I. 2022. The Value of Histopathological Characteristics and BRAF and NRAS Mutations for the Diagnosis, Risk Stratification, and Prognosis of Malignant Invasive Melanoma. *In*: Sonia, M. and Eduardo, C. (eds.) *Melanoma*. Rijeka: IntechOpen.

Tsamis, I., Gomatou, G., Chachali, S. P., Trontzas, I. P., Patriarcheas, V., Panagiotou, E. and Kotteas, E. 2023. BRAF/MEK inhibition in NSCLC: Mechanisms of resistance and how to overcome it, *Clinical and Translational Oncology*, 25, pp. 10–20.

Vanni, I., Tanda, E. T., Dalmasso, B., Pastorino, L., Andreotti, V., Bruno, W., Boutros, A., Spagnolo, F. and Ghiorzo, P. 2020a. Non-BRAF mutant melanoma: Molecular features and therapeutical implications, *Frontiers in Molecular Biosciences*, 7, p. 172.

Vanni, I., Tanda, E. T., Spagnolo, F., Andreotti, V., Bruno, W. and Ghiorzo, P. 2020b. The current state of molecular testing in the BRAF-mutated melanoma landscape, *Frontiers in Molecular Biosciences*, 7, p. 113.

Wagstaff, W., Mwamba, R. N., Grullon, K., Armstrong, M., Zhao, P., Hendren-Santiago, B., Qin, K. H., Li, A. J., Hu, D. A., Youssef, A., Reid, R. R., Luu, H. H., Shen, L., He, T.-C. and Haydon, R. C. 2022. Melanoma: Molecular genetics, metastasis, targeted therapies, immunotherapies, and therapeutic resistance, *Genes & Diseases*, 9, pp. 1608–1623. https://doi.org/10.1016/j.gendis.2022.04.004

Zaidi, M. R., Fisher, D. E. and Rizos, H. 2020. Biology of Melanocytes and Primary Melanoma. *In*: Balch, C. M., Atkins, M. B., Garbe, C., Gershenwald, J. E., Halpern, A. C., Kirkwood, J. M., Mcarthur, G. A., Thompson, J. F. and Sober, A. J. (eds.) *Cutaneous Melanoma*. Cham: Springer International Publishing.

Zhang, C., Yan, L., Wang, X., Zhu, S., Chen, C., Gu, Z. and Zhao, Y. 2020. Progress, challenges, and future of nanomedicine, *Nano Today*, 35, p. 101008.

Zhao, J. and Luo, Z. 2022. Discovery of Raf family is a milestone in deciphering the Ras-mediated intracellular signaling pathway, *International Journal of Molecular Sciences*, 23, p. 5158.

Zhu, Y., Xue, J., Chen, W., Bai, S., Zheng, T., He, C., Guo, Z., Jiang, M., Du, G. and Sun, X. 2020. Albumin-biomineralized nanoparticles to synergize phototherapy and immunotherapy against melanoma, *Journal of Controlled Release*, 322, pp. 300–311.

Zocchi, L., Lontano, A., Merli, M., Dika, E., Nagore, E., Quaglino, P., Puig, S. and Ribero, S. 2021. Familial melanoma and susceptibility genes: A review of the most common clinical and dermoscopic phenotypic aspect, associated malignancies and practical tips for management. *Journal of Clinical Medicine*, 10, p. 3760.

6 Overcoming Resistance
Molecular Insights and Therapeutic Options

Benny Mosoane and Lesedi Nevondo
Department of Anatomical Pathology, National Health Laboratory Services, Tshwane Academic Division, Faculty of Health Sciences, University of Pretoria, Pretoria, South Africa

Thabiso Victor Miya and Zodwa Dlamini
SAMRC Precision Oncology Research Unit (PORU), DSTI/NRF SARChI Chair in Precision Oncology and Cancer Prevention (POCP), Pan African Cancer Research Institute (PACRI), University of Pretoria, Pretoria, South Africa

Paulina Czajka-Francuz and Paulo Nunes
Fortrea Inc., Durham, North Carolina, USA

Kamal S. Saini
Fortrea Inc., Durham, North Carolina, USA
Addenbrooke's Hospital, Cambridge University Hospitals NHS Foundation Trust, Cambridge, UK

INTRODUCTION

Melanoma is a malignant neoplasm of the skin that originates from the transformation of the melanocytes. Melanoma accounts for 1% of cutaneous malignancy, but it is a leading cause of skin cancer-related mortality (Society, 2024). According to the 2019 National Cancer Registry of South Africa, the overall incidence of melanoma was recorded at 2.7 per 100,000 and ranked fifth most prevalent cancer among men and sixth most prevalent cancer among women (CANSA, 2024; Tod et al., 2019). In South Africa, the incidence of melanoma among White Africans is nearly 20 times greater than that observed in Black Africans (Norval and Wright, 2017).

The risk factors for melanoma are multifaceted, often interrelated, and may vary across different anatomical sites and population groups. Melanoma growth and progression are associated with the accumulation of genetic mutations that result in the hyperactivation of cell survival pathways. The most prevalent mutation in melanoma is in the V-Raf Murine Sarcoma Viral Oncogene Homolog B (BRAF) oncogene (Castellani et al., 2023). Other complex ranges of genes involved include cyclin dependent kinase inhibitor 2A (CDKN2A) but also CDK4 and BAP1 genes, as well as murine double minute 2 (MDM2), amongst others (Tod et al., 2019).

Surgical excision is regarded as an effective measure in the treatment of early-stage melanoma. In recent years, the treatment has undergone significant changes, particularly in the landscape of

DOI: 10.1201/9781003511625-6

metastatic disease. The combination of BRAF inhibitors (vemurafenib, encorafenib, and dabrafenib) and mitogen-activated protein kinase (MEK) inhibitors (cobimetinib, binimetinib, and trametinib) has resulted in a substantial reduction in melanoma-related mortality (Yu et al., 2019). The occurrence of drug resistance toward these combinations poses a challenge that continues to drive the efforts of research community in identifying new therapeutic targets.

Employment of immunotherapy-based strategies and disruption of metabolic pathways, which confer survival advantage, are among other avenues that may prove beneficial in overcoming melanoma resistance. Gaining better insight into the compensatory pathways activated by melanoma cells in response to treatment with clinically available agents, we anticipate further improvement in the cure of melanoma patients. This chapter addresses the formidable issues of treatment resistance, and the readers are guided through the latest molecular insights and therapeutic strategies aimed at overcoming resistance mechanisms. Furthermore, the chapter explores how cutting-edge technologies are unraveling the complexities of resistance mechanisms and guiding the development of innovative solutions.

CHALLENGES OF TREATMENT RESISTANCE

Genetic mutations in BRAF, members of the Ras family (HRAS, KRAS, and NRAS), MEK, receptor tyrosine kinase (c-KIT), mesenchymal-epithelial transition factor (c-Met), vascular endothelial growth factor receptor (VEGFR), and phosphatidylinositol-3-kinase (PI3K) are principal targets for molecularly targeted therapies in melanoma (Patel et al., 2021). These genetic alterations induce the activation of downstream pathways that promote oncogenesis by facilitating cell survival and proliferation, including the RAS/MAPK, AKT/PI3K, and Janus kinase/signal transducers and activators of transcription (JAK/STAT) pathways (**Figure 6.1**).

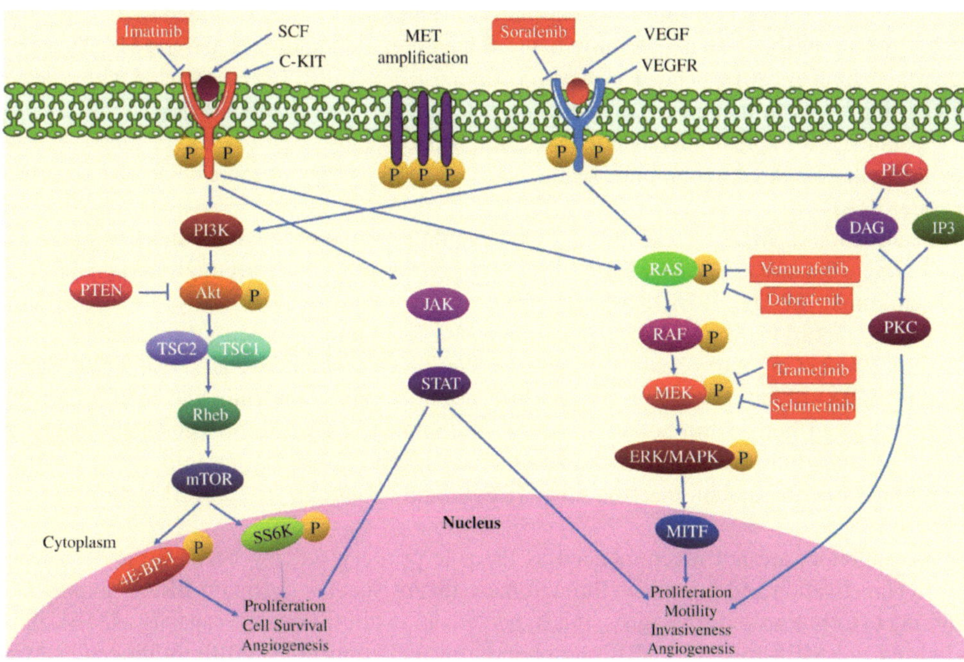

FIGURE 6.1 The main signaling pathways that contribute to the development of melanoma and its progression. Phosphorylation of mesenchymal epithelial transition factor (c-MET), receptor-tyrosine kinase Kit (c-KIT), and vascular endothelial growth factor receptor (VEGFR) initiates signaling pathways that drive angiogenesis, motility, proliferation, and survival. Activating mutations in downstream pathway components—such as MEK, rapidly accelerated fibrosarcoma (RAF), and Rat sarcoma virus GTPases (RAS)—can lead to constitutive pathway activation. This activation occurs even in the absence of external growth signals, contributing to persistent tumor growth and progression. (From Montor et al., 2018; Patel et al., 2021.)

BRAF, a serine/threonine protein kinase, plays a crucial role in regulating cell survival, division, and proliferation via the RAS/RAF/MAPK signaling pathway. Mutations in BRAF are present in over 60% of cutaneous melanoma cases (Hawryluk and Tsao, 2014). The V600E substitution accounts for approximately 80% of these mutations, while V600K and V600D mutations represent most of the remaining 20% (Pollock et al., 2003). Vemurafenib, a highly selective inhibitor targeting the V600E and V600K BRAF mutations, competes with ATP at the kinase domain, thereby inhibiting BRAF kinase activity. This disruption leads to reduced tumor progression and increased tumor cell death (Kim and Cohen, 2016). In addition, all three of the V600 BRAF mutations are targeted by dabrafenib, another ATP-competitive BRAF inhibitor (Ryu et al., 2017).

Melanoma often develops resistance to BRAF inhibitors, potentially due to reactivation or bypass mechanisms within the MAPK pathway. These mechanisms may involve the overexpression of PI3K, insulin-like growth factor receptor I (IGF-1R), and platelet-derived growth factor receptor beta (PDGFR-β), as well as the presence of MEK mutations (Nazarian et al., 2010; Poulikakos et al., 2011; Shi, 2017). Additional resistance pathways associated with BRAF-targeted treatments include the loss of *neurofibromin* (NF1) activity, amplification of mutant BRAF signaling, the presence of BRAF variants that are independent of RAS signaling, and the amplification of the microphthalmia-associated transcription factor (MITF) (Luebker and Koepsell, 2019; Nissan et al., 2014; Zhong et al., 2022).

It has been proposed that miR-211-5p, miR-204-5p, and miR-1246 play crucial roles in the mechanism of acquired resistance to BRAF inhibitors (Díaz-Martínez et al., 2018; Kim et al., 2017). It has been established that the response to vemurafenib is affected by the increased expression of miR-204-5p and miR-211-5p in vemurafenib-resistant cells (Patel et al., 2021). Vemurafenib treatment led to rapid RNA stabilization, thereby influencing the expression of these miRNAs. Díaz-Martínez and colleagues observed that following exposure to vemurafenib, the combined overexpression of miR-204-5p and miR-211-5p consistently induced the upregulation of Ras and the MAPK pathway (Díaz-Martínez et al., 2018). The identification of microRNAs (miRNAs) associated with resistance to BRAF inhibitors in melanoma suggests the potential for a mechanism-based strategy to mitigate resistance and improve therapeutic outcomes. Monotherapy targeting BRAF may not achieve optimal results compared to combination therapies that address one or more co-activated pathways alongside BRAF.

The activation of MEK/extracellular signal-regulated kinases (ERK) 1 and 2 regulates secondary targets that are critical for cell proliferation, survival, and differentiation (Dhanasekaran and Premkumar Reddy, 1998; Roskoski, 2012). Given that approximately 5% of melanoma cases harbor mutations in the MEK1/2 pathway, MEK1/2 are promising therapeutic targets in melanoma (Lian et al., 2019; Savoia et al., 2019; Wellbrock and Hurlstone, 2010). For melanoma treatment, MEK inhibitors, such as binimetinib, cobimetinib, trametinib, and selumetinib, have been investigated both as monotherapies and in combination with anti-BRAF therapies. The FDA has approved the combination therapies of encorafenib plus binimetinib and vemurafenib plus cobimetinib for melanoma treatment (Davis and Wayman, 2022; Sarkisian and Davar, 2018).

MEK inhibitors are not recommended as the sole primary therapy because they can lead to MEK hyperactivation and resistance through mechanisms such as upstream BRAF amplification. According to Corcoran and colleagues, this hyperactivation diminishes the capacity of MEK inhibitors to influence MEK-mediated ERK phosphorylation (Corcoran et al., 2010). Additionally, MEK1 mutations, including P124L and Q56P, are associated with resistance to both vemurafenib (a BRAF inhibitor) and selumetinib (a MEK inhibitor). These mutations can either directly interfere with the binding of the drug or cause conformational alterations that change the drug-binding site's position (Emery et al., 2009).

Resistance to MEK inhibitors is also attributed to the disruption of Bcl-2-like protein 11 (BIM), a critical protein for apoptosis, through the activation of the STAT-3 pathway (Dai et al., 2011). Moreover, the development of acquired resistance to MEK inhibitors has been associated with the overexpression of the immunoglobulin transcription factor 2 (ITF-2) gene. Elevated ITF-2 levels have been observed in melanoma cell lines resistant to MEK inhibitors, and ITF-2 knockdown has been shown to enhance the responsiveness of these resistant cells to selumetinib (Hur et al., 2017).

The treatment of melanoma may be optimized by the synergistic combination of immune checkpoint inhibitors (ICIs), BRAF inhibitors, and MEK inhibitors. The combination of pembrolizumab, a programmed death-1 (PD-1) inhibitor, with dabrafenib (a BRAF inhibitor) and trametinib (a MEK inhibitor) has been shown to reduce the incidence of treatment-resistant melanoma (Sarkisian and Davar, 2018). In the IMspire150 study, progression-free survival (PFS) for patients with BRAFV600 mutation-positive advanced melanoma significantly increased from 10.6 months to 15.1 months when treated with atezolizumab (a checkpoint inhibitor), vemurafenib, and cobimetinib (Ascierto et al., 2023; Czarnecka et al., 2020).

In the RAS subfamily of proteins, NRAS has been associated with melanoma in predominantly patients that are older than 55 years (Fedorenko et al., 2013). Tumors harboring NRAS mutations turn out to be thicker and carry poor clinical outcomes compared to BRAF-mutant tumors (Heppt et al., 2017; Vanni et al., 2020; Yan et al., 2018). RAS phosphorylated MEK1 and MEK2 to affect the MAPK pathway leading to the cell cycle progression and interacting with PI3K subunit of PI3K/AKT pathway to contribute directly to anti-apoptotic activity (**Figure 6.2**) (Downward, 2003; Zou et al., 2019).

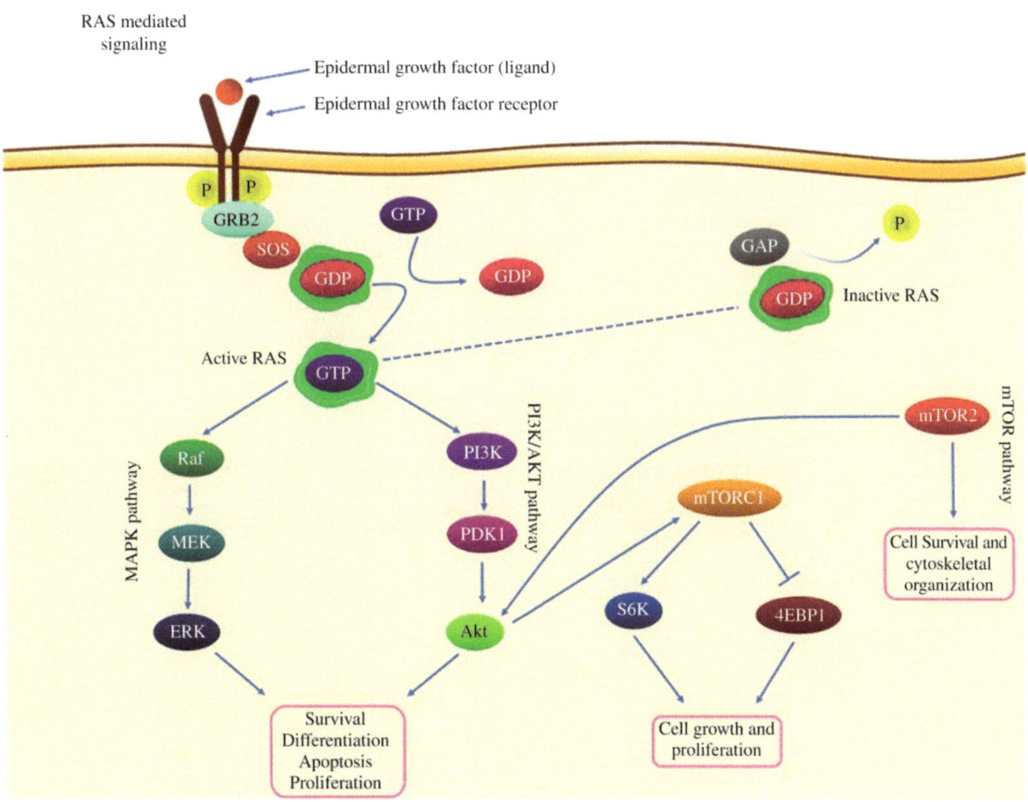

FIGURE 6.2 **RAS-mediated signaling pathway.** RAS can affect the mitogen-activated pathway kinase (MAPK) pathway through phosphorylation of MEK1 and MEK2, which activate extracellular-signal regulated kinase 1 and 2 (ERK1 and ERK2), leading to cell cycle progression. RAS can affect the phosphatidylinositol-3-kinase (PI3K)/Ak strain transforming (AKT)/mammalian target of rapamycin (mTOR) pathway through interaction with the PI3K subunit and directly contribute to anti-apoptotic activity.

Despite the extensively studied involvement of RAS in multiple signaling pathways, the direct inhibitors of NRAS are yet to be found. Current targeted therapies interrupt downstream signaling pathways of mutant RAS proteins, such as the PI3K and MAPK pathways. In a Phase II clinical trial, the MEK inhibitor MEK 162 achieved a 21% response rate in melanomas with NRAS mutations (Petit et al., 2019; Van Herpen et al., 2019). In a multicenter study, MEK inhibitor monotherapy has been demonstrated to be a viable treatment option in advanced NRAS-mutated melanoma in patients who failed treatment with ICIs (Salzmann et al., 2022).

The increased activity of parallel growth factor receptors, such as EGFR, PDGFR-β, and IGF1R, which can activate RAS, complicates the direct inhibition of RAS mutations (Ji et al., 2012; Takashima and Faller, 2013). Additionally, the mitogen-activated protein kinase 8 (MAP3K8) gene, encoding a serine-threonine kinase (STK) known as cancer Osaka thyroid (COT), has been identified as an agonist of the MAPK pathway that contributes to resistance to RAF inhibition (Ji et al., 2012; Johannessen et al., 2010). By activating ERK through MEK-dependent pathways, COT evades RAF signaling. Moreover, the frequent co-occurrence of NF1 deletion and RAS mutation in melanoma, which leads to a lack of negative feedback on RAS activation, poses another challenge (Nissan et al., 2014). As a result, there is an increase in RAS activity and resistance to RAF inhibition downstream.

A type III transmembrane receptor tyrosine kinase, c-KIT is composed of five distinct domains: a glycosylated extracellular ligand-binding domain encoded by exons 1–9, a hydrophobic transmembrane domain encoded by exon 10, an intracellular juxtamembrane domain encoded by exon 11, and two tyrosine kinase domains encoded by exons 12–21 (**Figure 6.3**) (Ma et al., 2017; Pham et al., 2020). The stem cell factor (SCF) is a glycoprotein ligand that exerts its biological functions by binding to and activating c-KIT receptor (Lennartsson and Rönnstrand, 2012). Mutations

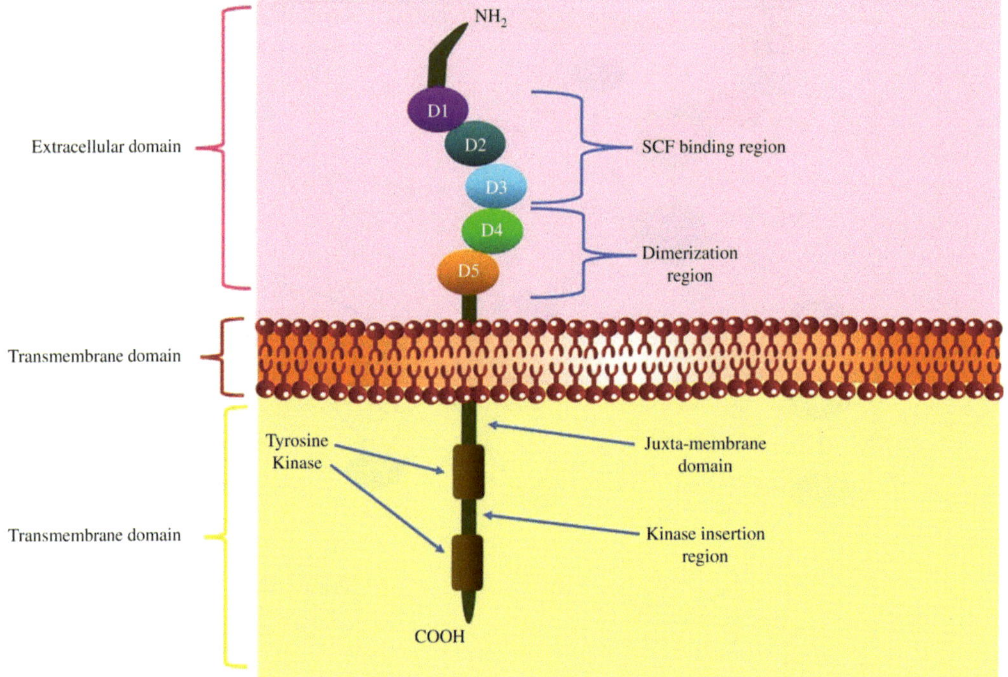

FIGURE 6.3 **The structure of c-kIT.** Five different domains make up the c-KIT protein: two tyrosine kinase domains, an intracellular juxtamembrane domain, a hydrophobic transmembrane domain, and a glycosylated extracellular ligand-binding region.

in c-KIT show varying downstream functional consequences in melanoma. Activated c-KIT in uveal melanoma triggers downstream intracellular signaling through the JAK-STAT, PI3K-Akt, and MAPK pathways, which leads to specific responses that promote cell survival and proliferation (Curtin et al., 2006). Through the PI3K/AKT pathway, c-KIT controls apoptosis in metastatic melanoma (Abbaspour Babaei et al., 2016; Ma et al., 2017).

In melanoma, c-KIT mutations predominantly occur in exons 9 and 11, with exons 13 and 17 being less frequently affected (Doma et al., 2020). In patients with c-KIT mutations in exons 11 and 13 treated with the c-KIT inhibitor imatinib, the disease control rate (DCR) is 66.7%, while the objective response rate (ORR) is 24.4% (Pham et al., 2020). Imatinib has demonstrated a DCR of 90% and an ORR of 80% in gastrointestinal stromal tumors (GIST) (Blanke et al., 2008; Din and Woll, 2008). Imatinib's comparatively lower clinical efficacy in melanoma with c-KIT mutations is thought to be caused by secondary acquired resistance mechanisms, which include higher genetic mutation loads, cytokines from the tumor microenvironment (TME), reactivation of redundant downstream survival signaling pathways, and/or activating or secondary c-KIT mutations (Bello et al., 2014; Todd et al., 2014; Wei et al., 2019). For patients with c-KIT-mutant melanoma who are resistant to imatinib, newer c-KIT inhibitors—such as dasatinib, masitinib, nilotinib, and sunitinib—show moderate efficacy when combined with immunotherapy (Pham et al., 2020; Rager et al., 2022). Additionally, regorafenib has recently demonstrated notable activity in patients with metastatic melanoma harboring c-KIT mutations, particularly in second- or later-line settings (Kim et al., 2023).

Melanoma, along with various other malignancies, stimulates angiogenesis through the overexpression of vascular endothelial growth factor (VEGF). Cancer cells produce VEGF in significantly higher concentrations than normal cells (Strizzi et al., 2001). Therapeutic strategies targeting angiogenesis in melanoma can focus on VEGF ligands and/or their receptors. Axitinib, a selective VEGFR inhibitor, exerts its effects by competitively binding to the ATP-binding sites of VEGFR-1, VEGFR-2, and VEGFR-3. Treatment outcomes have been shown to improve when anti-PD-1 monoclonal antibodies, such as toripalimab, are combined with selective VEGFR inhibitors (Sheng et al., 2019; Zhang et al., 2014). Bevacizumab, a monoclonal antibody targeting VEGF-A, has shown potential against various malignancies, including melanoma. It can be administered as a monotherapy or in combination with chemotherapeutic agents like carboplatin and paclitaxel. In a phase II clinical trial, the combination of bevacizumab and ipilimumab—an anti-CTLA-4 monoclonal antibody—showed enhanced therapeutic efficacy (Hodi et al., 2014).

The FGF2 signaling pathway, crucial for sustaining the tumor vasculature by mediating interactions between endothelial cells and pericytes, has been connected to the emergence of VEGFR inhibitor-acquired resistance (Ichikawa et al., 2020). A nonselective multi-kinase inhibitor, sorafenib targets BRAF, c-KIT, VEGFR-1, VEGFR-2, and VEGFR-3. It has been demonstrated to impede tumor formation and angiogenesis in a range of cancer cell lines (Liu et al., 2006; Zanotto-Filho et al., 2018). In BRAF-mutant melanoma, sorafenib has not been successful in selectively targeting mutant BRAF; however, it led to intolerable off-target side effects by inhibiting wild-type BRAF (Eisen et al., 2006; Finn et al., 2012; Hauschild et al., 2009; Liu et al., 2006).

THE ROLE OF TUMOR MICROENVIRONMENT ON THERAPY RESISTANCE OF CANCER CELLS

The TME is composed of the extracellular matrix (ECM), soluble factors, immune cells, fibroblasts, tumor stroma, and microvasculature (**Figure 6.4**) (Zhou et al., 2023). Tumor cell proliferation, invasion, and metastasis are all contingent upon the dynamic interaction between the TME and the tumor cells. The TME induces a localized inflammatory response within the tumor, which hinders the immune system's ability to eradicate tumor cells and ultimately leads to the development of drug resistance (Li and Tian, 2023; Wu et al., 2022; Zhou et al., 2023).

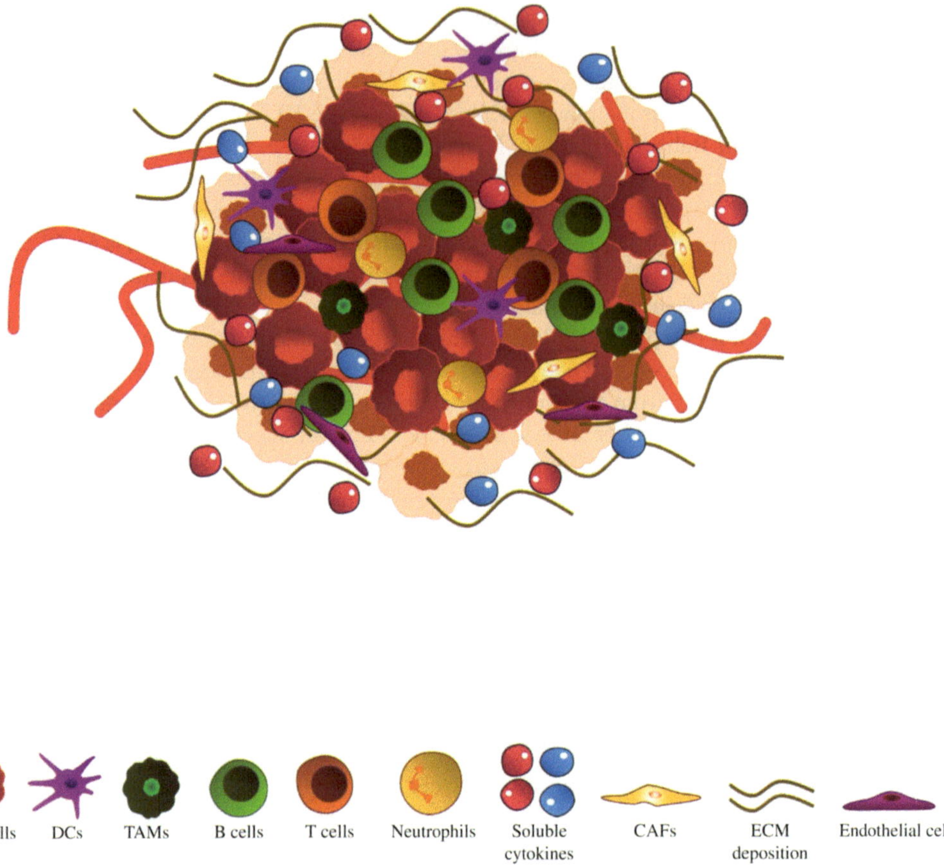

FIGURE 6.4 Composition of tumor microenvironment (TME). The TME micro-ecosystem comprises extracellular matrix (ECM), cancer-associated fibroblasts (CAFs), soluble factors, endothelial cells, tumor-associated macrophages (TAMs), lymphocytes, and dendritic cells (DCs).

The efficacy of immunotherapies seems to be influenced by the presence of preexisting immunity, characterized by the infiltration of immune cells into the tumor. TME has been classified into three groups, namely the immunologically excluded TME (intermediate stage); the inflammatory (hot) TME, which indicates preexisting immunity; and the noninflammatory TME, also referred to as immunologically ignorant or cold. The classification is based on the microscopic location of CD8 cytotoxic T lymphocytes (CTLs) within the tumor (Tian and Quek, 2024).

Tumor-infiltrating lymphocytes (TILs) are generally regarded as a favorable prognostic marker in melanoma, as they indicate a more robust antitumor immune response from the host (Azimi et al., 2012; Clemente et al., 1996; Fu et al., 2019). In contrast, the exclusion of immune cells from the TME has been identified as a significant resistance mechanism to ICIs (Tian and Quek, 2024). However, some studies have not demonstrated a clear correlation between the presence of TILs and improved prognosis in melanoma (Antohe et al., 2019; Gooden et al., 2011; Maibach et al., 2020). Although the presence of Forkhead box P3+ (FOXP3) regulatory cells has not been consistently associated with overall patient survival, the presence of CD3+ and CD8+ T lymphocytes has been linked to positive effects on patient survival (Giavina-Bianchi et al., 2017; Gooden et al., 2011).

The immune cells of the TME play a role in the complex process of immunoediting. This process results in the production of numerous cytokines, chemokines, and growth factors, which are essential for controlling cell differentiation, regulating cell-to-cell interactions, and activating many cell types (Shurin et al., 2006). Tumor-immune system interactions may result in the eradication of cancerous cells, an equilibrium condition, or the release of cancerous cells (Mittal et al., 2014). In some instances where not all tumor cells are eradicated, tumor cells may proliferate to an equilibrium state and remain latent for varying periods (Bhatia and Kumar, 2011; Koebel et al., 2007).

Melanoma cells can employ multiple tactics to evade and suppress the immune system. One such strategy involves the manipulation of tumor-specific antigens (TSAs), which can lead melanoma cells to downregulate tumor-associated antigens (TAAs) and cause T-cell depletion following prolonged exposure (Durrant and Ramage, 2005; Lee et al., 2016). TSAs, also referred to as "neoantigens," are newly formed antigens absent from normal human DNA (Xie et al., 2023). Additionally, cancer cells often exhibit low levels of major histocompatibility complex (MHC) expression, express immune checkpoint proteins to protect themselves from attacks by macrophages and T cells, recruit tolerogenic T-regulatory cells (T-regs), and avoid being recognized by natural killer (NK) cells (Hirano et al., 2005; Jandus et al., 2008; Schatton et al., 2010; Solana et al., 2007).

The Role of Immune Checkpoint Inhibitors

Ipilimumab is a monoclonal antibody that acts against the cytotoxic T-lymphocyte-associated protein 4 (CTLA-4) receptor, and it was approved by the FDA in 2011 for metastatic melanoma (Cohen et al., 1987). Activated CTLA-4 blocks the activation of helper T lymphocytes and increases the regulatory action of regulatory T lymphocytes. Therefore, ipilimumab inhibits lymphocyte blockade to allow the immune system to fight the tumor.

Pembrolizumab was the first PD-1 inhibitor to receive approval in 2014 for the treatment of unresectable or metastatic melanoma that had not responded to prior therapies (Raedler, 2015). In advanced melanoma, the combination of CTLA-4 inhibitors and PD-1 inhibitors, such as pembrolizumab, has been associated with increased chances of achieving long-lasting, durable remissions, with overall survival rates extending up to five years (Hassel et al., 2023). Tumor cells, hematopoietic cells, and non-hematopoietic cells produce two ligands for PD-1, namely PD-L1 and PD-L2 (Zodwa et al., 2016). The binding of PD-1 to these ligands delivers inhibitory signals to T cells, which can lead to T-cell anergy and impair the antitumor immune response (Dong et al., 2017; Zou and Chen, 2008). The expression of PD-1 ligands by tumor cells is a mechanism through which they evade immune detection within the TME (Ishida et al., 1992).

Nivolumab monotherapy has proven to be more effective than ipilimumab alone and is now considered the standard treatment for patients with metastatic melanoma, either as a standalone therapy or in combination with ipilimumab (Hirano et al., 2005). An additional promising approach to reprogramming the melanoma microenvironment was the approval of nivolumab in combination with relatlimab, an inhibitor of the lymphocyte activation gene-3 (LAG-3) receptor, for first-line treatment of advanced melanoma in 2022, following the encouraging results from the phase II/III trial (RELATIVITY-047) (Tawbi, 2023). Relatlimab targets LAG-3 expressed on NK cells and TILs, potentially enhancing antigen-specific T-cell responses and cytotoxic T-cell-mediated tumor cell lysis, thereby inhibiting tumor growth (Tawbi et al., 2022).

Targeting Cancer-Associated Fibroblasts

The cancer stroma is predominantly composed of CAFs, which are essential for tumor growth, metastasis, and resistance to treatment (Kharouf et al., 2023). CAFs are instrumental in tumor formation and ECM remodeling, processes essential for both local invasion and distant metastasis. Moreover, CAFs enhance the inflammatory response in melanoma by secreting a range of immunosuppressive and pro-tumor chemokines and cytokines, including IL-1β, IL-6, IL-8, IFN-γ, TNF-α, and various C-X-C motif chemokine ligands (Papaccio et al., 2021).

Fibroblasts associated with melanoma have also been demonstrated to promote immunological suppression through their interactions with melanoma-stroma cells (Guido et al., 2012). Hugo and colleagues demonstrated that, in advanced melanoma, the abundance of

CAFs is associated with resistance to both checkpoint inhibitors and targeted therapies (Hugo et al., 2016). Therefore, CAFs are potential targets for cancer treatment, including melanoma. Fibroblast activation protein (FAP), PDGFR, and vitamin D are identified targets for CAFs (De Smedt et al., 2024; Fujimura, 2022; Shariev et al., 2022; Zhou et al., 2015). FAP is a type II transmembrane serine protease overexpressed by CAFs and chiefly associated with unfavorable prognosis in melanoma (Hutchenreuther et al., 2018; Zhang and Ertl, 2016; Zhou et al., 2024). Novel approaches are being investigated to investigate the reduction of CAFs by focusing on markers specific to CAFs, such as FAP (Glabman et al., 2022; Wang et al., 2022; Xu et al., 2023). At the moment there is one phase I trial assessing FAP-IL-2v in humans (NCT03875079) (ClinicalTrials.gov, 2021).

Targeting Tumor-Associated Macrophages

The TME is predominantly composed of TAMs (Bied et al., 2023). TAMs within the TME can exhibit two distinct phenotypes: the pro-tumor, immunosuppressive M2 phenotype, and the antitumor M1 phenotype. These phenotypes differ in their functions and the cytokines they produce. Repolarization of immunosuppressive M2 TAMs into the M1 phenotype under certain conditions can enhance their antitumor activity. This repolarization can be achieved through genetic reprogramming, converting M2 TAMs into M1 macrophages to stimulate an antitumor response (Andreesen et al., 1990). The presence of TAMs has been associated with adverse clinical outcomes (Allison et al., 2023; Habib et al., 2024). Targeting colony-stimulating factor 1 receptor (CSF1R) signaling is a strategy to inhibit TAM proliferation, differentiation, and function. Both preclinical and clinical studies are ongoing for direct inhibitors of CSF1R signaling, such as edicotinib, pexidartinib, ARRY-382, as well as CSF1 neutralizing antibodies (Adams et al., 2022; Habib et al., 2024; Johnson et al., 2022; Siddiqui et al., 2023; Wesolowski et al., 2019).

Targeting Tumor-Associated Neutrophils (TANs)

TANs with a pro-tumor N2 phenotype (N2 TANs) are actively involved in tumor progression and metastatic spread within the TME. To promote tumor invasion, N2 TANs alter the TME by releasing granules that contain several proteases, for example, neutrophil elastase and matrix metalloproteinase 9 (MMP-9) (Augoff et al., 2022; Xiao and Yu, 2021). Additionally, TANs produce transforming growth factor-β (TGF-β) and arginase 1, both of which contribute to the suppression of adaptive immunity (Batlle and Massagué, 2019; Grzywa et al., 2020). The release of hepatocyte growth factor (HGF), also called scatter factor, promotes tumor progression (Mizuno et al., 2019). The chemokine receptor 2 (CXCR2) regulates and mobilizes neutrophils, thus making it a potential target for controlling TANs (Wang et al., 2019). Small molecules such as SX-682, which prevent the interaction between CXCR2 and CXCL8 (its ligand), are the novel approaches to improve the treatment efficacy of chemotherapy (Han et al., 2021; Horn et al., 2020; Singh et al., 2023).

THE ROLE OF PHF8 IN RESISTANCE TO MELANOMA-TARGETED THERAPIES

Plant homeodomain finger protein 8 (PHF8) is a member of the Jumonji C protein finger histone demethylase family (Qi et al., 2010). PFH8 is known to have an established role in neuronal differentiation as well as in the development of the brain and craniofacial structures. Mutations in PHF8 have led to outcomes such as cleft lip palate and X-linked mental retardation (Laumonnier et al., 2005). PHF8 not only plays a role in neuronal development but also its overexpression has been identified in malignant cells of carcinomas of the breast, colorectum, prostate, stomach, and liver, as well as in lymphoblastic leukemias (Audia and Campbell, 2016; Franci et al., 2014; Ma et al., 2015; Mccann et al., 2019). In most of these tumors, PHF8 plays a role in the regulation of cell cycle progression, which is not the case in melanoma. The study, conducted by Moubarak and colleagues in the United States, found that PHF8 was upregulated in cases of metastatic melanoma versus in the primary melanoma (Moubarak et al., 2022). PHF8 immunohistochemistry revealed not only an increased positivity in a host of metastatic melanoma cells but also a strong intensity of staining versus that seen in a primary melanoma (Liu et al., 2023; Moubarak et al., 2022; Siegel and Massagué, 2003). Moubarak et al. (2022) continued to show that when PHF8 was knocked out, there was reduced invasive capacity of the tumor cells of the primary melanoma. This inhibition of invasion was noted in both melanoma cells with BRAF and NRAS mutations. However, PHF8 gene knockout was shown to have no effect on the growth of the primary tumor (Moubarak et al., 2022).

In recent years, no studies have been able to adequately explain the genetic mutations responsible for tumor development and metastasis in individuals with melanoma. However, it has been proposed that epigenetic mechanisms regulate the transcriptional changes necessary for melanoma tumor cells to acquire metastatic capabilities. PHF8 has been implicated in controlling the transcription of various invasive and metastatic genes, with the TGF-β signaling pathway being the most significantly regulated pathway (Moubarak et al., 2022). PHF8 controls the transcription of several ligands and receptors of the TGF-β pathway (Liu et al., 2019). Data shows that PHF8 is a direct transcriptional activator of pro-metastatic genes (Franci et al., 2014; Shao et al., 2017). Thus, silencing of PFH8 suppresses the downstream TGF-β signaling cascade. This has given birth to exciting exploration of the potential targeted therapies.

Currently, TGF-β targeting drugs have undergone clinical trials and have shown promising results (Gómez-Muñoz et al., 2023; Shao et al., 2017; Teixeira et al., 2020). Another role that PHF8 modulation or TGF-β inhibition may play is in the prevention of BRAF and MAPK inhibitors (Sun et al., 2014). As TGF-β signaling cross-talks with MAPK pathway, which may contribute to drug resistance, the combination of PHF8 modulators and MAPK inhibitors may prove useful in preventing MAPK inhibitors drug resistance. PHF8 modulation and its effect of inhibiting the TGF-β pathway may also play a role in improved responses to ICIs (Liu et al., 2023). TGF-β produced by tumor cells is known to decrease the cytolytic and pro-apoptotic factors of CD8, resulting in decreased immune surveillance. Thus, inhibition of TGF-β by PHF8 may result in better outcomes for patients with tumors that are refractory to PD-1 inhibition (Moubarak et al., 2022; Siewe and Friedman, 2021). PHF8 epigenetic regulation of the TGF-β pathway opens up a whole new world of possibilities for therapeutic interventions in patients with metastatic melanoma.

THE GUT MICROBIOTA AND TREATMENT RESISTANCE IN MELANOMA

The emergence of new treatments and a deeper understanding of the underlying molecular pathways have facilitated improvements in the care and quality of life for melanoma patients. Still, there is much to gain because treatment resistance is a significant issue that has not yet been resolved. Currently, precision medicine research is concentrating on gut microbiota (GM) (Guardamagna et al., 2022; Makaranka et al., 2022). GM has been said to be important for both oncogenesis and immunological homeostasis in connection to immunotherapy (Grochowska et al., 2022; Laborda-Illanes et al., 2020; Wu and Wu, 2012; Xu et al., 2021). Certain gut bacteria may influence ICIs response, resistance development, and susceptibility to immune-related adverse events (irAE) (Usyk et al., 2021). This influence is primarily being studied to gain a deeper understanding of the intricate relationship between what appear to be important pathways in molecular oncology (Guardamagna et al., 2022).

IMMUNOTHERAPY

Exciting advancements in cancer immunotherapy, such as the development of ICIs and a deeper understanding of cancer immune checkpoints, have revolutionized the treatment landscape for melanoma (Ascierto et al., 2019; Larkin et al., 2019; Miller and Sadelain, 2015). One of the first drugs introduced into clinical practice was ipilimumab, a monoclonal antibody that targets cytotoxic CTLA-4. More recently, two inhibitors of PD-1 were introduced into the market: nivolumab and pembrolizumab (Larkin et al., 2015). However, because response rates vary, it is important to find biomarkers so that we can comprehend the mechanisms underlying ICIs resistance (Elkrief et al., 2019; Larkin et al., 2019). The relationship between the immune system and cancer cells is intricate and dynamic. The efficacy of ICIs is modulated by tumor-associated cellular markers, the extent of tumor immune infiltration, and various environmental factors (Cristescu et al., 2018; Elkrief et al., 2019; Sharma et al., 2017). The importance of the microbiota has come to light more recently, and numerous investigations comparing the intestinal microbiota of patients who responded to ICIs treatment with nonresponders have shown notable variations in the variety and composition of flora (Chaput et al., 2017; Gopalakrishnan et al., 2018; Limeta et al., 2020; Matson et al., 2018; Routy et al., 2018a, 2018b; Sivan et al., 2015; Vétizou et al., 2015). Beneficial microorganisms in the context of ICIs have been identified using preclinical animal models. Several species of bacteria, including *Akkermansia muciniphila*, *Bifidobacterium* species, *Faecalibacterium* species, and *Bacteroides fragilis*, have been identified as potentially beneficial (Routy et al., 2018a, b; Sivan et al., 2015; Vétizou et al., 2015).

Other studies have investigated fecal samples from patients receiving ICIs therapy using methods like 16S rRNA gene sequencing (Chaput et al., 2017; Gopalakrishnan et al., 2018; Matson et al., 2018; Routy et al., 2018a, b). *Akkermansia muciniphila* was identified by Routy and colleagues as a crucial player in their discovery that a poor response to PD-1/PD-L1 inhibitors is related to an altered microbial environment (Routy et al., 2018b). Metagenomic analysis of fecal samples revealed that treatment responders had significantly higher levels of this bacterium. Furthermore, the efficacy of immunotherapy was improved by oral supplementation with these bacteria or by performing fecal microbiota transplantation (FMT) from responder patients to germ-free mice (Routy et al., 2018b). The authors also noted greater levels of *Faecalibacterium* species, *Bifidobacterium* species, and *B. fragilis* in treatment responders in a different research (Routy et al., 2018a). *Enterococcus faecium*, *Bifidobacterium longum*, and *Collinsella aerofaciens* were found by Matson et al. (2018) through a metagenomic analysis of stool samples from patients receiving ICI therapy for melanoma. These bacteria may increase the effectiveness of PD-L1 inhibitors. Using comparable methods, Gopalakrishnan and colleagues discovered that patients undergoing anti-PD-1 therapy had better response rates when their fecal levels of the *Ruminococcaceae* family of *Clostridiales* were greater (Gopalakrishnan et al., 2018). Additionally, the researchers showed that germ-free mice responded to anti-PD-1 therapy by having a higher intra-tumoral CD8+ T lymphocyte count and slower progression of melanoma when used in conjunction with FMT (Gopalakrishnan et al., 2018).

However, results regarding the impacts of particular microorganisms vary throughout research projects. For example, although some researchers discovered that a positive reaction to ICIs is linked to a higher representation of the *Bacteroides* species, others pointed out that the same species was detrimental to efficacy (Chaput et al., 2017; Routy et al., 2018a; Vétizou et al., 2015). To investigate this further, Limeta and colleagues conducted a meta-analysis of four trials with 130 patients in total (Limeta et al., 2020). They found that the overrepresentation of the *Faecalibacterium* taxa, along with the existence of *Barnesiella intestinihominis* and *Ruminococcacea*, were advantageous. Additionally, they discovered a connection between *Bifidobacterium dentium*, *Adlercreutzia equolifaciens*, *B. thetaiotaomicron*, and an unidentified *Mogibacterium* microorganism and poor response to ICIs treatment. Subsequently, they employed these discoveries to create a classifier that accurately predicted the prognosis and ICI responses in a separate group of 27 patients (Limeta et al., 2020).

The side effects of ICI treatment are also a topic of concern since they can provide serious difficulties for patients and physicians alike. The compounds most frequently used in treating melanoma include cutaneous, gastrointestinal, renal, hepatic, and endocrine toxicities in addition to arthritis and pneumonitis. These are varied and depend on the medications and dosage (Xu et al., 2018). While supportive care combined with glucocorticoids may be sufficient for certain patients, in other cases, ICIs therapy may need to be postponed or stopped because of intolerable side effects (Larkin et al., 2015). According to Xu and colleagues, the rates of events that pose a threat to life are as follows: 28.6% for ipilimumab, 19.8% for pembrolizumab, and 14.1% for nivolumab (Xu et al., 2018). According to several researchers, GM may potentially contribute to an individual's vulnerability to ICIs toxicity. Vetizou and colleagues found that in mice injected with a mix of *Burkholderia fragilis* and *B. cepacian*, there was a decrease in colitis rates associated with CTLA-4 suppression (Vétizou et al., 2015). Meanwhile, a study by Chaput and colleagues involving 26 patients undergoing ipilimumab treatment for melanoma revealed a correlation between high concentration of *Firmicutes* phylum and onset of colitis (Chaput et al., 2017).

Some studies have correlated a high concentration of the *Bacteroides* phylum to a decreased likelihood of adverse effects (Dubin et al., 2016; Saâda-Bouzid et al., 2017; Sun et al., 2020). The overall implication of these findings is that antitumor immunity and thus, the immune checkpoint response in cancer patients may be impacted by commensal microbiota, and there is preliminary evidence suggesting that adverse events related to treatment may also be affected. Even though it is probably unduly optimistic to believe that a particular gut microbial profile can directly correlate with response, the suggestion is that treatment efficacy can be increased if microbiota can be altered (Lee et al., 2021). The majority of this research has used preclinical models, and the processes underlying these effects are not well understood. To gain further insights into these effects, large-scale clinical trials involving FMT are needed (Lee et al., 2021).

Chemotherapy

Chemotherapy drugs can still be useful in treating more severe illnesses, even though they are not the first line of treatment for melanoma (*Cancer*, 2015). Dacarbazine was once often used for advanced disease, and even though immunotherapy has generally replaced it, it is still taken into consideration for patients with metastatic melanoma (stage IV) when targeted treatments are not appropriate (*Cancer*, 2015; Wilson and Schuchter, 2016). In the locoregional, palliative context, bleomycin and cisplatin are also utilized in hyperthermic isolated limb perfusion (HILP) in conjunction with electrochemotherapy with good efficacy (Health and Excellence, 2013; Schellerer et al., 2021). Although there are few published studies examining the precise interaction between microbiota and these drugs, there is growing evidence that chemotherapeutic medicines in general, including their toxicity and efficacy, can be impacted by GM (Alexander et al., 2017). Numerous explanations have been put forth for this, such as immunomodulation, metabolism, enzymatic breakdown, translocation, decreased diversity, and ecological variety (Alexander et al., 2017; Yang et al., 2021). According to Viaud and colleagues, doxorubicin and cyclophosphamide-induced alterations in the intestinal barrier permit certain bacteria to translocate into secondary lymphoid organs in mouse models (Viaud et al., 2013). As a result, specific T helper cells (pTh17) mounted a response, increasing the effectiveness of the aforementioned chemotherapeutic drugs. Similarly, there was a correlation between tumor resistance to cyclophosphamide and broad-spectrum antibiotics (Viaud et al., 2013).

Several studies have also looked into the potential harm of the relationship between chemotherapy and gut bacteria. Mucositis, or mucosal barrier injury, is a common and occasionally crippling side effect of chemotherapy and radiation therapy. It is characterized by loss of intestinal epithelial cells and inflammation (Blijlevens et al., 2000; Sonis, 2004). The findings discussed above highlight the crucial and intricate relationship between the toxicity and efficacy of antimicrobial agents and the microbiota. However, further investigation, including clinical trials involving melanoma patients, is necessary to fully understand the specifics of this association and apply these findings to the general population.

Radiation Therapy

Radiation therapy has long been a crucial adjuvant treatment for melanoma patients, even though the cancer is usually less radiosensitive than other cutaneous and non-cutaneous cancers. It is frequently used to lower the risk of a local or nodal recurrence following the excision of primary melanoma or after therapeutic lymph node dissection (Hong, 2021; Shi, 2017). However, due to recent developments in immunotherapy and targeted therapy, radiotherapy is now primarily employed in palliative settings for conditions such as soft tissue metastases, bony metastases, and spinal cord compression. Furthermore, individuals with residual disease who are not responding fully to systemic treatment may receive radiation (Hong, 2021). Conversely, desmoplastic melanoma is another subtype for which radiation therapy is frequently used and has been demonstrated to enhance local tumor management in salvage and adjuvant settings (Oliver et al., 2016). Even with the advancement of accurate radiation treatments, a significant number of patients still experience side effects from radiation due to damage to adjacent premorbid tissue, like the intestinal epithelium (Tonneau et al., 2021). Modifications in the microbiota composition of epithelial surfaces have also been linked to radiotherapy, and these changes may be the cause of bone marrow failure, colitis, and mucositis (Ma et al., 2019).

According to research by Ciorba and colleagues, the probiotic *Lactobacillus rhamnosus* GG decreased radiation-induced epithelium damage by decreasing epithelial cell apoptosis and increasing crypt survival in mice (Ciorba et al., 2012). Delia and colleagues demonstrated that the probiotic formulation VSL#3 is an effective and safe method for preventing radiation-induced diarrhea (Delia et al., 2007). Some probiotic preparations that contain *Bifidobacterium bifidum*, *Lactobacillus casei*, and *L. acidophilus* have also been demonstrated to offer similar benefits (Ma et al., 2019). These findings underscore the significant role of gut bacteria in the healing process of radiation-induced damage and suggest the potential benefit of therapeutically modifying genetic material to mitigate or prevent adverse effects. However, despite the promising nature of these investigations, there is limited evidence supporting the hypothesis that interactions between GM and radiation therapy occur in melanoma. Radiation therapy is not a standard treatment modality for melanoma, which raises uncertainty about the applicability of research findings from non-melanoma cancers to clinical practice in this context.

COMBINING IMMUNOTHERAPY WITH RADIATION TO OVERCOME RESISTANCE

The immunomodulatory effects of radiation therapy in the era of immunotherapy are gaining renewed interest. Several preclinical models suggest that radiation therapy has the potential to improve the efficacy of ICIs, and conversely, the ICIs have been found to increase the local and systemic efficacy of radiation therapy (Bida et al., 2024; Davidson et al., 2022; Hsu et al., 2022; Park et al., 2015; Zhao and Shao, 2020). When a primary tumor is subjected to radiation therapy and/or combined with immunotherapy, the immune response observed in tumors outside the irradiated field is referred to as the "abscopal phenomenon" (Nelson et al., 2023).

From the preclinical models, it is postulated that radiation therapy increases diverse T-cell activation by modulating the local expression of MHC class 1 molecules, which improves the function of antigen-presenting cells (APCs) (Chen et al., 2021; Reits et al., 2006; Tailor et al., 2022). Blockage of CTLA-4 can suppress T-regs resulting in increased CD8/T-regs ratio and the addition of PD-1/PD-L1 inhibitors increases the overall population of effector CD8+ T cells (Ji et al., 2020; Relecom et al., 2021; Sobhani et al., 2021; Yuan et al., 2011). Immune therapy induction before radiation therapy is a preferred sequence in melanoma (Tagliaferri et al., 2022). Based on clinical experience, immunotherapy and radiation therapy can be combined either prior to or following disease progression. Prospective and retrospective clinical experiences on the combination of radiation therapy and immune therapy during the induction phase or peri-induction radiotherapy are summarized in **Table 6.1**.

TABLE 6.1
Summary of the Prospective and Retrospective Clinical Studies on Immune Therapy during the Induction Phase or Peri-Induction Phase of Radiation Therapy in Melanoma

Type of Study	Immune Therapy Used	Number of Patients	Median Induction to Peri-Induction Radiation Therapy Time	Radiation Dose and Fractionation	Principal Metastatic Irradiated Site	References
Retrospective	Ipilimumab	18	Between 0 and +16 weeks	30 Gray in 10 fractions	All other visceral metastases	Barker et al. (2013)
Prospective	Ipilimumab	22	Between 0 and +5 days	From 12 Gray in 2 fractions to 24 Gray in 3 fractions	Lung metastasis	Twyman-Saint Victor et al. (2015)
Retrospective	Ipilimumab	47	Between 0 and +28 days	30 Gray in 10 fractions	Distant skin, subcutaneous and any distant metastasis	Chandra et al. (2015)
Prospective	Ipilimumab	22	Between 0 and +5 days	From 18 Gray in 1 fraction to 50 Gray in 4 fractions	Lung metastasis and all other visceral metastases	Hiniker et al. (2016)
Retrospective	Nivolumab or pembrolizumab	27	Between −11 and +7 days	30 Gray in 10 fractions	Distant skin, subcutaneous and any distant metastasis	Liniker et al. (2016)
Retrospective	Nivolumab or pembrolizumab	4	Between −54 and 0 days	From 18 Gray in 1 fraction to 50 Gray in 25 fractions	Any distant metastasis	Kato et al. (2019)
Retrospective	Pembrolizumab	11	Between −9 and 0 days	Median 36 Gray (range 20–60) and median fraction 5 Gray (range 1.8–8)	Distant skin, subcutaneous and nodal metastases	Kim et al. (2019)

NOVEL NANOVACCINES FOR MELANOMA

Chemotherapy, radiation, immunotherapy, and targeted therapies have historically been used to treat melanoma, though these approaches often come with significant adverse side effects. Nanomedicines represent an innovative strategy in cancer treatment, with the potential not only to treat but also to prevent cancer. Nanovaccines, akin to traditional vaccines, work by introducing a foreign antigen to the immune system, which triggers immune response. This allows the body to recognize and respond more effectively to the antigen upon future exposures. Unlike conventional vaccines, nanovaccines offer several advantages: they can specifically target lymphoid tissues and APCs, co-deliver both antigens and adjuvants, facilitate efficient phagocytosis and processing by

APCs, and enhance adaptive immune responses. Furthermore, nanovaccines tend to have localized effects, resulting in fewer systemic side effects compared to traditional therapeutic modalities (Bezbaruah et al., 2022; Gurunathan et al., 2024; Priyanka et al., 2023).

In 2019, researchers at Tel Aviv University developed a melanoma nanovaccine aimed at both treating primary and metastatic melanomas and preventing the disease from occurring (Daily, 2019). Researchers created tiny particles of 170 nm in size created from a biodegradable polymer. The particle was then packed with two peptides of short amino acids found in melanoma cells. The vaccine showed promising results in the prevention of the acquisition of melanoma and in the treatment of primary tumors when in combination with immunotherapy drugs, showing delayed disease progression (Conniot et al., 2019). Currently, a photothermal nanovaccine is being used in melanomas of the skin (Pandesh et al., 2021). The efficacy of immunotherapy is dependent on the baseline level of T cells.

Nanovaccines adjuvants have been shown to regulate TME. With photothermal effect, there is increased immunogenic cell death and release of tumor-associated antigens. Nanomaterials in the vaccine mediate the delivery of tumor antigens to DCs with the resultant infiltration of cytotoxic T cells into the tumor (Yao et al., 2023). In this way, nanovaccines help to improve the efficacy of immunotherapy. Therefore, nanovaccines could have a significant role in the future of personalized immunotherapy for melanoma.

LIMITATIONS

The risk factors for melanoma development vary significantly due to the interplay of multiple complex factors across different anatomical regions and population groups. Disease progression is often associated with the mutations that lead to the hyperactivation of pathways crucial for cell survival. Given the high incidence of treatment resistance in melanoma, there is a critical need for researchers to understand the compensatory pathways that melanoma cells activate in response to therapeutic interventions. Solely targeting BRAF mutations is increasingly recognized as insufficient due to the emergence of treatment resistance. Mechanisms of resistance include the reactivation or bypass of the MAPK pathway following BRAF inhibition. Additionally, complementary mutations that may exacerbate treatment resistance involve the overexpression of PI3K, IGF-1R, PDGFR-β, or mutations in MEK.

Despite extensive research on the role of RAS signaling pathways in melanoma, effective direct inhibitors specifically targeting NRAS have yet to be identified. Current treatments primarily focus on directly disrupting the PI3K and MAPK pathways, which are downstream of mutant RAS proteins. Additionally, the challenge of directly inhibiting RAS mutations is compounded by the increased activity of parallel growth factor receptors, such as EGFR, PDGFR-β, and IGF1R, which can activate RAS signaling.

Due to the higher genetic mutation load, reactivation of redundant downstream survival signaling pathways, and complex TME components, targeting mutations such as c-KIT with direct inhibitors has not led to significant improvements in melanoma treatment. There is ongoing debate regarding the prognostic significance of TILs in melanoma. While some studies have highlighted TILs as a positive prognostic marker, suggesting that their presence indicates a more effective antitumor immune response, other research has failed to establish a clear link between TILs and improved prognosis. Moreover, melanoma cells evade and suppress the host immune response by downregulating TAAs and inducing T-cell exhaustion through prolonged exposure to TSAs.

Radiation, immunotherapy, and targeted therapies, while used to treat melanoma, often come with side effects similar to those observed in other malignancies. Recent research suggests that gut bacteria may influence the susceptibility to immune system-related adverse events, resistance development, and the response to ICIs. As new therapeutics for melanoma emerge, it is crucial to balance the development of resistance and its associated adverse effects with the potential benefits of these novel treatments.

CONCLUSION

Melanoma is still a leading cause of death amongst skin cancers. Risk factors for melanoma are complex and vary based on anatomical site and demographic characteristics. Surgical excision continues to be the gold standard for treating early-stage melanoma. For metastatic melanoma, treatment strategies target genetic alterations associated with BRAF, the RAS protein family, MEK, c-KIT, c-MET, PI3K, and VEGFR. These genetic changes are known to support the survival and progression of melanoma cells. However, acquired resistance often undermines the long-term efficacy of these targeted therapies, presenting a significant challenge to this molecularly focused approach.

Extensive research has been dedicated to addressing the limitations of current melanoma treatments. Studies suggest that combination therapy, which targets multiple pathways involved in melanoma development, could be an effective approach. Specifically, the combination of immune therapy with targeted therapies has shown promising results in treating melanoma. Additionally, recent research highlights the potential benefits of integrating immunotherapy with radiation therapy. Beyond these strategies, ongoing investigations are exploring TME reprogramming, the role of PHF8, the impact of the gut microbiome, and the development of melanoma nanovaccines. These emerging areas offer promising opportunities to enhance treatment outcomes and overcome resistance to melanoma.

REFERENCES

Abbaspour Babaei, M., Kamalidehghan, B., Saleem, M., Huri, H. Z. and Ahmadipour, F. 2016. Receptor tyrosine kinase (c-Kit) inhibitors: A potential therapeutic target in cancer cells, *Drug Design, Development and Therapy*, 10, pp. 2443–2459.

Adams, R., Osborn, G., Mukhia, B., Laddach, R., Willsmore, Z., Chenoweth, A., Geh, J. L. C., Mackenzie Ross, A. D., Healy, C., Barber, L., Tsoka, S., Sanz-Moreno, V., Lacy, K. E. and Karagiannis, S. N. 2022. Influencing tumor-associated macrophages in malignant melanoma with monoclonal antibodies, *Oncoimmunology*, 11, p. 2127284.

Alexander, J. L., Wilson, I. D., Teare, J., Marchesi, J. R., Nicholson, J. K. and Kinross, J. M. 2017. Gut microbiota modulation of chemotherapy efficacy and toxicity, *Nature Reviews Gastroenterology & Hepatology*, 14, pp. 356–365.

Allison, E., Edirimanne, S., Matthews, J. and Fuller, S. J. 2023. Breast cancer survival outcomes and tumor-associated macrophage markers: A systematic review and meta-analysis, *Oncology and Therapy*, 11, pp. 27–48.

Andreesen, R., Scheibenbogen, C., Brugger, W., Krause, S., Meerpohl, H. G., Leser, H. G., Engler, H. and Löhr, G. W. 1990. Adoptive transfer of tumor cytotoxic macrophages generated in vitro from circulating blood monocytes: A new approach to cancer immunotherapy, *Cancer Research*, 50, pp. 7450–7456.

Antohe, M., Nedelcu, R. I., Nichita, L., Popp, C. G., Cioplea, M., Brinzea, A., Hodorogea, A., Calinescu, A., Balaban, M., Ion, D. A., Diaconu, C., Bleotu, C., Pirici, D., Zurac, S. A. and Turcu, G. 2019. Tumor infiltrating lymphocytes: The regulator of melanoma evolution, *Oncology Letters*, 17, pp. 4155–4161.

Ascierto, P. A., Long, G. V., Robert, C., Brady, B., Dutriaux, C., Di Giacomo, A. M., Mortier, L., Hassel, J. C., Rutkowski, P. and Mcneil, C. 2019. Survival outcomes in patients with previously untreated BRAF wild-type advanced melanoma treated with nivolumab therapy: Three-year follow-up of a randomized phase 3 trial, *JAMA Oncology*, 5, pp. 187–194.

Ascierto, P. A., Stroyakovskiy, D., Gogas, H., Robert, C., Lewis, K., Protsenko, S., Pereira, R. P., Eigentler, T., Rutkowski, P., Demidov, L., Zhukova, N., Schachter, J., Yan, Y., Caro, I., Hertig, C., Xue, C., Kusters, L., Mcarthur, G. A. and Gutzmer, R. 2023. Overall survival with first-line atezolizumab in combination with vemurafenib and cobimetinib in BRAF(V600) mutation-positive advanced melanoma (IMspire150): Second interim analysis of a multicentre, randomised, phase 3 study, *Lancet Oncology*, 24, pp. 33–44.

Audia, J. E. and Campbell, R. M. 2016. Histone modifications and cancer, *Cold Spring Harbor Perspectives in Biology*, 8, p. a019521.

Augoff, K., Hryniewicz-Jankowska, A., Tabola, R. and Stach, K. 2022. MMP9: A tough target for targeted therapy for cancer, *Cancers (Basel)*, 14, p. 1847.

Azimi, F., Scolyer, R. A., Rumcheva, P., Moncrieff, M., Murali, R., Mccarthy, S. W., Saw, R. P. and Thompson, J. F. 2012. Tumor-infiltrating lymphocyte grade is an independent predictor of sentinel lymph node status and survival in patients with cutaneous melanoma, *Journal of Clinical Oncology*, 30, pp. 2678–2683.

Barker, C. A., Postow, M. A., Khan, S. A., Beal, K., Parhar, P. K., Yamada, Y., Lee, N. Y. and Wolchok, J. D. 2013. Concurrent radiotherapy and ipilimumab immunotherapy for patients with melanoma, *Cancer Immunology Research*, 1, pp. 92–98.

Batlle, E. and Massagué, J. 2019. Transforming growth factor-β signaling in immunity and cancer, *Immunity*, 50, pp. 924–940.

Bello, D. M., Dematteo, R. P. and Ariyan, C. E. 2014. The GIST of targeted therapy for malignant melanoma, *Annals of Surgical Oncology*, 21, pp. 2059–2067.

Bezbaruah, R., Chavda, V. P., Nongrang, L., Alom, S., Deka, K., Kalita, T., Ali, F., Bhattacharjee, B. and Vora, L. 2022. Nanoparticle-based delivery systems for vaccines, *Vaccines (Basel)*, 10, p. 1946.

Bhatia, A. and Kumar, Y. 2011. Cancer-immune equilibrium: Questions unanswered, *Cancer Microenvironment*, 4, pp. 209–217.

Bida, M., Mosoane, B., Phakathi, B., Sebitloane, M., Muallem, M. Z., Hull, R. and Dlamini, Z. 2024. Current Treatment Options and Limitations for Cervical Cancer. In: Dlamini, Z. (ed.) *Strategies for Overcoming Chemotherapy Resistance in Cervical Cancer.* Academic Press.

Bied, M., Ho, W. W., Ginhoux, F. and Blériot, C. 2023. Roles of macrophages in tumor development: A spatiotemporal perspective, *Cellular & Molecular Immunology*, 20, pp. 983–992.

Blanke, C. D., Rankin, C., Demetri, G. D., Ryan, C. W., Von Mehren, M., Benjamin, R. S., Raymond, A. K., Bramwell, V. H., Baker, L. H., Maki, R. G., Tanaka, M., Hecht, J. R., Heinrich, M. C., Fletcher, C. D., Crowley, J. J. and Borden, E. C. 2008. Phase III randomized, intergroup trial assessing imatinib mesylate at two dose levels in patients with unresectable or metastatic gastrointestinal stromal tumors expressing the kit receptor tyrosine kinase: S0033, *Journal of Clinical Oncology*, 26, pp. 626–632.

Blijlevens, N., Donnelly, J. and De Pauw, B. 2000. Mucosal barrier injury: Biology, pathology, clinical counterparts and consequences of intensive treatment for haematological malignancy: An overview, *Bone Marrow Transplantation*, 25, pp. 1269–1278.

Cancer, N. C. C. F. 2015. *Melanoma: Assessment and Management.*

CANSA. 2024. *Melanoma* [Online]. Available: https://cansa.org.za/melanoma/ [Accessed May, 19, 2024].

Castellani, G., Buccarelli, M., Arasi, M. B., Rossi, S., Pisanu, M. E., Bellenghi, M., Lintas, C. and Tabolacci, C. 2023. BRAF mutations in melanoma: Biological aspects, therapeutic implications, and circulating biomarkers. *Cancers (Basel)*, 15, p. 4026.

Chandra, R. A., Wilhite, T. J., Balboni, T. A., Alexander, B. M., Spektor, A., Ott, P. A., Ng, A. K., Hodi, F. S. and Schoenfeld, J. D. 2015. A systematic evaluation of abscopal responses following radiotherapy in patients with metastatic melanoma treated with ipilimumab, *Oncoimmunology*, 4, p. e1046028.

Chaput, N., Lepage, P., Coutzac, C., Soularue, E., Le Roux, K., Monot, C., Boselli, L., Routier, E., Cassard, L. and Collins, M. 2017. Baseline gut microbiota predicts clinical response and colitis in metastatic melanoma patients treated with ipilimumab, *Annals of Oncology*, 28, pp. 1368–1379.

Chen, C., Liu, Y. and Cui, B. 2021. Effect of radiotherapy on T cell and PD-1/PD-L1 blocking therapy in tumor microenvironment, *Hum Vaccin Immunother*, 17, pp. 1555–1567.

Ciorba, M. A., Riehl, T. E., Rao, M. S., Moon, C., Ee, X., Nava, G. M., Walker, M. R., Marinshaw, J. M., Stappenbeck, T. S. and Stenson, W. F. 2012. Lactobacillus probiotic protects intestinal epithelium from radiation injury in a TLR-2/cyclo-oxygenase-2-dependent manner, *Gut*, 61, pp. 829–838.

Clemente, C. G., Mihm, M. C., Jr., Bufalino, R., Zurrida, S., Collini, P. and Cascinelli, N. 1996. Prognostic value of tumor infiltrating lymphocytes in the vertical growth phase of primary cutaneous melanoma, *Cancer*, 77, pp. 1303–1310.

ClinicalTrials.gov. 2021. *A Study to Evaluate Safety and Therapeutic Activity of RO6874281 in Combination with Pembrolizumab, in Participants with Advanced or Metastatic Melanom* [Online]. Clinicaltrials.gov. Available: https://clinicaltrials.gov/study/NCT03875079?tab=history&a=20 [Accessed July 26, 2024].

Cohen, P. J., Lotze, M. T., Roberts, J. R., Rosenberg, S. A. and Jaffe, E. S. 1987. The immunopathology of sequential tumor biopsies in patients treated with interleukin-2. Correlation of response with T-cell infiltration and HLA-DR expression, *American Journal of Pathology*, 129, pp. 208–216.

Conniot, J., Scomparin, A., Peres, C., Yeini, E., Pozzi, S., Matos, A. I., Kleiner, R., Moura, L. I. F., Zupančič, E., Viana, A. S., Doron, H., Gois, P. M. P., Erez, N., Jung, S., Satchi-Fainaro, R. and Florindo, H. F. 2019. Immunization with mannosylated nanovaccines and inhibition of the immune-suppressing microenvironment sensitizes melanoma to immune checkpoint modulators, *Nature Nanotechnology*, 14, pp. 891–901.

Corcoran, R. B., Dias-Santagata, D., Bergethon, K., Iafrate, A. J., Settleman, J. and Engelman, J. A. 2010. BRAF gene amplification can promote acquired resistance to MEK inhibitors in cancer cells harboring the BRAF V600E mutation, *Science Signaling*, 3, p. ra84.

Cristescu, R., Mogg, R., Ayers, M., Albright, A., Murphy, E., Yearley, J., Sher, X., Liu, X. Q., Lu, H. and Nebozhyn, M. 2018. Pan-tumor genomic biomarkers for PD-1 checkpoint blockade–based immunotherapy, *Science*, 362, p. eaar3593.

Curtin, J. A., Busam, K., Pinkel, D. and Bastian, B. C. 2006. Somatic activation of KIT in distinct subtypes of melanoma, *Journal of Clinical Oncology*, 24, pp. 4340–4346.

Czarnecka, A. M., Bartnik, E., Fiedorowicz, M. and Rutkowski, P. 2020. Targeted therapy in melanoma and mechanisms of resistance, *International Journal of Molecular Sciences*, 21, p. 4576.

Dai, B., Meng, J., Peyton, M., Girard, L., Bornmann, W. G., Ji, L., Minna, J. D., Fang, B. and Roth, J. A. 2011. STAT3 mediates resistance to MEK inhibitor through microRNA miR-17, *Cancer Research*, 71, pp. 3658–3668.

Daily, S. 2019. *Novel Nano-vaccine for Melanoma* [Online]. Available: https://www.sciencedaily.com/releases/2019/08/190805134024.htm [Accessed June 3, 2024].

Davidson, T., Zhang, H., Dong, H., Grams, M. P., Park, S. S. and Yan, Y. 2022. Overcoming immunotherapy resistance with radiation therapy and dual immune checkpoint blockade, *Advances in Radiation Oncology*, 7, p. 100931.

Davis, J. and Wayman, M. 2022. Encorafenib and binimetinib combination therapy in metastatic melanoma, *Journal of the Advanced Practitioner in Oncology*, 13, pp. 450–455.

De Smedt, J., Aura, C., Van Kelst, S., Janssen, L., Marasigan, V., Boecxstaens, V., Stas, M., Bogaerts, K., Belmans, A., Cleynen, I., Vanderschueren, D., Vandenberghe, K., Bechter, O., Nikkels, A., Strobbe, T., Emri, G., Lambrechts, D. and Garmyn, M. 2024. Clinical and genetic determinants of vitamin D receptor expression in cutaneous melanoma patients, *Melanoma Research*, 34, pp. 125–133.

Delia, P., Sansotta, G., Donato, V., Frosina, P., Messina, G., De Renzis, C. and Famularo, G. 2007. Use of probiotics for prevention of radiation-induced diarrhea, *World Journal of Gastroenterology: WJG*, 13, p. 912.

Dhanasekaran, N. and Premkumar Reddy, E. 1998. Signaling by dual specificity kinases, *Oncogene*, 17, pp. 1447–1455.

Díaz-Martínez, M., Benito-Jardón, L., Alonso, L., Koetz-Ploch, L., Hernando, E. and Teixidó, J. 2018. miR-204-5p and miR-211-5p contribute to BRAF inhibitor resistance in melanoma, *Cancer Research*, 78, pp. 1017–1030.

Din, O. S. and Woll, P. J. 2008. Treatment of gastrointestinal stromal tumor: Focus on imatinib mesylate, *Therapeutics and Clinical Risk Management*, 4, pp. 149–162.

Doma, V., Barbai, T., Beleaua, M. A., Kovalszky, I., Rásó, E. and Tímár, J. 2020. KIT mutation incidence and pattern of melanoma in Central Europe, *Pathology Oncology Research*, 26, pp. 17–22.

Dong, Y., Sun, Q. and Zhang, X. 2017. PD-1 and its ligands are important immune checkpoints in cancer, *Oncotarget*, 8, pp. 2171–2186.

Downward, J. 2003. Targeting RAS signalling pathways in cancer therapy, *Nature Reviews Cancer*, 3, pp. 11–22.

Dubin, K., Callahan, M. K., Ren, B., Khanin, R., Viale, A., Ling, L., No, D., Gobourne, A., Littmann, E. and Huttenhower, C. 2016. Intestinal microbiome analyses identify melanoma patients at risk for checkpoint-blockade-induced colitis, *Nature Communications*, 7, p. 10391.

Durrant, L. G. and Ramage, J. M. 2005. Development of cancer vaccines to activate cytotoxic T lymphocytes, *Expert Opinion on Biological Therapy*, 5, pp. 555–563.

Eisen, T., Ahmad, T., Flaherty, K. T., Gore, M., Kaye, S., Marais, R., Gibbens, I., Hackett, S., James, M., Schuchter, L. M., Nathanson, K. L., Xia, C., Simantov, R., Schwartz, B., Poulin-Costello, M., O'dwyer, P. J. and Ratain, M. J. 2006. Sorafenib in advanced melanoma: A phase II randomised discontinuation trial analysis, *British Journal of Cancer*, 95, pp. 581–586.

Elkrief, A., Derosa, L., Kroemer, G., Zitvogel, L. and Routy, B. 2019. The negative impact of antibiotics on outcomes in cancer patients treated with immunotherapy: A new independent prognostic factor? *Annals of Oncology*, 30, pp. 1572–1579.

Emery, C. M., Vijayendran, K. G., Zipser, M. C., Sawyer, A. M., Niu, L., Kim, J. J., Hatton, C., Chopra, R., Oberholzer, P. A., Karpova, M. B., Macconaill, L. E., Zhang, J., Gray, N. S., Sellers, W. R., Dummer, R. and Garraway, L. A. 2009. MEK1 mutations confer resistance to MEK and B-RAF inhibition, *Proceedings of the National Academy of Sciences of the United States of America*, 106, pp. 20411–20416.

Fedorenko, I. V., Gibney, G. T. and Smalley, K. S. 2013. NRAS mutant melanoma: Biological behavior and future strategies for therapeutic management, *Oncogene*, 32, pp. 3009–3018.

Finn, L., Markovic, S. N. and Joseph, R. W. 2012. Therapy for metastatic melanoma: The past, present, and future, *BMC Medicine*, 10, p. 23.

Franci, G., Ciotta, A. and Altucci, L. 2014. The Jumonji family: Past, present and future of histone demethylases in cancer, *Biomolecular Concepts*, 5, pp. 209–224.

Fu, Q., Chen, N., Ge, C., Li, R., Li, Z., Zeng, B., Li, C., Wang, Y., Xue, Y., Song, X., Li, H. and Li, G. 2019. Prognostic value of tumor-infiltrating lymphocytes in melanoma: A systematic review and meta-analysis, *Oncoimmunology*, 8, p. 1593806.

Fujimura, T. 2022. Stromal factors as a target for immunotherapy in melanoma and non-melanoma skin cancers, *International Journal of Molecular Science*, 23, p. 4044.

Giavina-Bianchi, M. H., Giavina-Bianchi, P. F. J. and Festa, C. N. 2017. Melanoma: Tumor microenvironment and new treatments, *Anais brasileiros de dermatologia*, 92, pp. 156–166.

Glabman, R. A., Choyke, P. L. and Sato, N. 2022. Cancer-associated fibroblasts: Tumorigenicity and targeting for cancer therapy, *Cancers (Basel)*, 14, p. 3906.

Gómez-Muñoz, M. D. L. Á., Eskow, N., Delclaux, I., Moubarak, R. and Hernando-Monge, E. 2023. Role of PHF8 in resistance to melanoma targeted therapies, *Cancer Research*, 83, pp. 396–396.

Gooden, M. J., De Bock, G. H., Leffers, N., Daemen, T. and Nijman, H. W. 2011. The prognostic influence of tumour-infiltrating lymphocytes in cancer: A systematic review with meta-analysis, *British Journal of Cancer*, 105, pp. 93–103.

Gopalakrishnan, V., Spencer, C., Mcquade, J., Andrews, M., Helmink, B. and Cogdill, A. The gut microbiome of metastatic melanoma patients initiating systemic therapy is influenced by host factors including diet, probiotic and antibiotic use. Annual Meeting of the Society for Immunotherapy of Cancer SITC, 2018. 7–11.

Grochowska, M., Perlejewski, K., Laskus, T. and Radkowski, M. 2022. The role of gut microbiota in gastrointestinal tract cancers, *Archivum Immunologiae et Therapiae Experimentalis*, 70, p. 7.

Grzywa, T. M., Sosnowska, A., Matryba, P., Rydzynska, Z., Jasinski, M., Nowis, D. and Golab, J. 2020. Myeloid cell-derived arginase in cancer immune response, *Frontiers in Immunology*, 11, p. 938.

Guardamagna, M., Berciano-Guerrero, M.-A., Villaescusa-González, B., Perez-Ruiz, E., Oliver, J., Lavado-Valenzuela, R., Rueda-Dominguez, A., Barragán, I. and Queipo-Ortuño, M. I. 2022. Gut microbiota and therapy in metastatic melanoma: Focus on MAPK pathway inhibition, *International Journal of Molecular Sciences*, 23, p. 11990.

Guido, C., Whitaker-Menezes, D., Capparelli, C., Balliet, R., Lin, Z., Pestell, R. G., Howell, A., Aquila, S., Andò, S., Martinez-Outschoorn, U., Sotgia, F. and Lisanti, M. P. 2012. Metabolic reprogramming of cancer-associated fibroblasts by TGF-β drives tumor growth: Connecting TGF-β signaling with "Warburg-like" cancer metabolism and L-lactate production, *Cell Cycle*, 11, pp. 3019–3035.

Gurunathan, S., Thangaraj, P., Wang, L., Cao, Q. and Kim, J.-H. 2024. Nanovaccines: An effective therapeutic approach for cancer therapy, *Biomedicine & Pharmacotherapy*, 170, p. 115992.

Habib, S., Osborn, G., Willsmore, Z., Chew, M. W., Jakubow, S., Fitzpatrick, A., Wu, Y., Sinha, K., Lloyd-Hughes, H., Geh, J. L. C., Mackenzie-Ross, A. D., Whittaker, S., Sanz-Moreno, V., Lacy, K. E., Karagiannis, S. N. and Adams, R. 2024. Tumor associated macrophages as key contributors and targets in current and future therapies for melanoma, *Expert Review of Clinical Immunology*, 20, pp. 895–911.

Han, Z. J., Li, Y. B., Yang, L. X., Cheng, H. J., Liu, X. and Chen, H. 2021. Roles of the CXCL8-CXCR1/2 axis in the tumor microenvironment and immunotherapy, *Molecules*, 27, p. 137.

Hassel, J. C., Zimmer, L., Sickmann, T., Eigentler, T. K., Meier, F., Mohr, P., Pukrop, T., Roesch, A., Vordermark, D., Wendl, C. and Gutzmer, R. 2023. Medical needs and therapeutic options for melanoma patients resistant to anti-PD-1-directed immune checkpoint inhibition, *Cancers (Basel)*, 15, p. 3448.

Hauschild, A., Agarwala, S. S., Trefzer, U., Hogg, D., Robert, C., Hersey, P., Eggermont, A., Grabbe, S., Gonzalez, R., Gille, J., Peschel, C., Schadendorf, D., Garbe, C., O'day, S., Daud, A., White, J. M., Xia, C., Patel, K., Kirkwood, J. M. and Keilholz, U. 2009. Results of a phase III, randomized, placebo-controlled study of sorafenib in combination with carboplatin and paclitaxel as second-line treatment in patients with unresectable stage III or stage IV melanoma, *Journal of Clinical Oncology*, 27, pp. 2823–2830.

Hawryluk, E. B. and Tsao, H. 2014. Melanoma: Clinical features and genomic insights, *Cold Spring Harbor Perspectives in Medicine*, 4, p. a015388.

Health, N. I. F. and Excellence, C. 2013. *Electrochemotherapy for Metastases in the Skin from Tumours of Non-Skin Origin and Melanoma*. Interventional procedures guidance [IPG446]: NICE.

Heppt, M. V., Siepmann, T., Engel, J., Schubert-Fritschle, G., Eckel, R., Mirlach, L., Kirchner, T., Jung, A., Gesierich, A., Ruzicka, T., Flaig, M. J. and Berking, C. 2017. Prognostic significance of BRAF and NRAS mutations in melanoma: A German study from routine care, *BMC Cancer*, 17, p. 536.

Hiniker, S. M., Reddy, S. A., Maecker, H. T., Subrahmanyam, P. B., Rosenberg-Hasson, Y., Swetter, S. M., Saha, S., Shura, L. and Knox, S. J. 2016. A prospective clinical trial combining radiation therapy with systemic immunotherapy in metastatic melanoma, *International Journal of Radiation Oncology, Bioliology, Physics*, 96, pp. 578–588.

Hirano, F., Kaneko, K., Tamura, H., Dong, H., Wang, S., Ichikawa, M., Rietz, C., Flies, D. B., Lau, J. S., Zhu, G., Tamada, K. and Chen, L. 2005. Blockade of B7-H1 and PD-1 by monoclonal antibodies potentiates cancer therapeutic immunity, *Cancer Research*, 65, pp. 1089–1096.

Hodi, F. S., Lawrence, D., Lezcano, C., Wu, X., Zhou, J., Sasada, T., Zeng, W., Giobbie-Hurder, A., Atkins, M. B., Ibrahim, N., Friedlander, P., Flaherty, K. T., Murphy, G. F., Rodig, S., Velazquez, E. F., Mihm, M. C., Russell, S., Dipiro, P. J., Yap, J. T., Ramaiya, N., Van Den Abbeele, A. D., Gargano, M. and Mcdermott, D. 2014. Bevacizumab plus ipilimumab in patients with metastatic melanoma, *Cancer Immunology Research*, 2, pp. 632–642.

Hong, A. M. 2021. *Radiation Therapy in the Management of Melanoma* [Online]. UpToDate. Available: https://www.uptodate.com/contents/radiation-therapy-in-the-management-of-melanoma [Accessed June 2, 2024].

Horn, L. A., Riskin, J., Hempel, H. A., Fousek, K., Lind, H., Hamilton, D. H., Mccampbell, K. K., Maeda, D. Y., Zebala, J. A., Su, Z., Schlom, J. and Palena, C. 2020. Simultaneous inhibition of CXCR1/2, TGF-β, and PD-L1 remodels the tumor and its microenvironment to drive antitumor immunity, *Journal for Immunotherapy of Cancer*, 8, p. e000326.

Hsu, S. J., Chen, Y., Yang, P., Hu, Y., Chen, R., Zeng, Z. and Du, S. 2022. Radiotherapy enhance the immune checkpoint inhibitors efficacy in advanced liver cancer, *International Journal of Radiation Oncology, Biology, Physics*, 114, p. S105.

Hugo, W., Zaretsky, J. M., Sun, L., Song, C., Moreno, B. H., Hu-Lieskovan, S., Berent-Maoz, B., Pang, J., Chmielowski, B., Cherry, G., Seja, E., Lomeli, S., Kong, X., Kelley, M. C., Sosman, J. A., Johnson, D. B., Ribas, A. and Lo, R. S. 2016. Genomic and transcriptomic features of response to anti-PD-1 therapy in metastatic melanoma, *Cell*, 165, pp. 35–44.

Hur, E. H., Goo, B. K., Moon, J., Choi, Y., Hwang, J. J., Kim, C. S., Bae, K. S., Choi, J., Cho, S. Y., Yang, S. H., Seo, J., Lee, G. and Lee, J. H. 2017. Induction of immunoglobulin transcription factor 2 and resistance to MEK inhibitor in melanoma cells, *Oncotarget*, 8, pp. 41387–41400.

Hutchenreuther, J., Vincent, K., Norley, C., Racanelli, M., Gruber, S. B., Johnson, T. M., Fullen, D. R., Raskin, L., Perbal, B., Holdsworth, D. W., Postovit, L. M. and Leask, A. 2018. Activation of cancer-associated fibroblasts is required for tumor neovascularization in a murine model of melanoma, *Matrix Biology*, 74, pp. 52–61.

Ichikawa, K., Watanabe Miyano, S., Minoshima, Y., Matsui, J. and Funahashi, Y. 2020. Activated FGF2 signaling pathway in tumor vasculature is essential for acquired resistance to anti-VEGF therapy, *Scientific Reports*, 10, p. 2939.

Ishida, Y., Agata, Y., Shibahara, K. and Honjo, T. 1992. Induced expression of PD-1, a novel member of the immunoglobulin gene superfamily, upon programmed cell death, *EMBO Journal*, 11, pp. 3887–3895.

Jandus, C., Bioley, G., Speiser, D. E. and Romero, P. 2008. Selective accumulation of differentiated FOXP3(+) CD4 (+) T cells in metastatic tumor lesions from melanoma patients compared to peripheral blood, *Cancer Immunology Immunotherapy*, 57, pp. 1795–1805.

Ji, D., Song, C., Li, Y., Xia, J., Wu, Y., Jia, J., Cui, X., Yu, S. and Gu, J. 2020. Combination of radiotherapy and suppression of Tregs enhances abscopal antitumor effect and inhibits metastasis in rectal cancer, *Journal of Immunotherapy of Cancer*, 8, p. e000826.

Ji, Z., Flaherty, K. T. and Tsao, H. 2012. Targeting the RAS pathway in melanoma, *Trends in Molecular Medicine*, 18, pp. 27–35.

Johannessen, C. M., Boehm, J. S., Kim, S. Y., Thomas, S. R., Wardwell, L., Johnson, L. A., Emery, C. M., Stransky, N., Cogdill, A. P., Barretina, J., Caponigro, G., Hieronymus, H., Murray, R. R., Salehi-Ashtiani, K., Hill, D. E., Vidal, M., Zhao, J. J., Yang, X., Alkan, O., Kim, S., Harris, J. L., Wilson, C. J., Myer, V. E., Finan, P. M., Root, D. E., Roberts, T. M., Golub, T., Flaherty, K. T., Dummer, R., Weber, B. L., Sellers, W. R., Schlegel, R., Wargo, J. A., Hahn, W. C. and Garraway, L. A. 2010. COT drives resistance to RAF inhibition through MAP kinase pathway reactivation, *Nature*, 468, pp. 968–972.

Johnson, M., Dudek, A. Z., Sukari, A., Call, J., Kunk, P. R., Lewis, K., Gainor, J. F., Sarantopoulos, J., Lee, P., Golden, A., Harney, A., Rothenberg, S. M., Zhang, Y. and Goldman, J. W. 2022. ARRY-382 in combination with pembrolizumab in patients with advanced solid tumors: Results from a phase 1b/2 study, *Clinical Cancer Research*, 28, pp. 2517–2526.

Kato, J., Hida, T., Someya, M., Sato, S., Sawada, M., Horimoto, K., Fujioka, M., Minowa, T., Matsui, Y., Tsuchiya, T., Kitagawa, M., Nakata, K., Sakata, K. I., Torigoe, T. and Uhara, H. 2019. Efficacy of combined radiotherapy and anti-programmed death 1 therapy in acral and mucosal melanoma, *Journal of Dermatology*, 46, pp. 328–333.

Kharouf, N., Flanagan, T. W., Hassan, S. Y., Shalaby, H., Khabaz, M., Hassan, S. L., Megahed, M., Haikel, Y., Santourlidis, S. and Hassan, M. 2023. Tumor microenvironment as a therapeutic target in melanoma treatment, *Cancers (Basel)*, 15, p. 3147.

Kim, A. and Cohen, M. S. 2016. The discovery of vemurafenib for the treatment of BRAF-mutated metastatic melanoma, *Expert Opinion in Drug Discovery*, 11, pp. 907–916.

Kim, H. J., Chang, J. S., Roh, M. R., Oh, B. H., Chung, K. Y., Shin, S. J. and Koom, W. S. 2019. Effect of radiotherapy combined with pembrolizumab on local tumor control in mucosal melanoma patients, *Frontiers in Oncology*, 9, p. 835.

Kim, J. H., Ahn, J. H. and Lee, M. 2017. Upregulation of MicroRNA-1246 is associated with BRAF inhibitor resistance in melanoma cells with mutant BRAF, *Cancer Research and Treatment*, 49, pp. 947–959.

Kim, K. H., Jung, M., Lee, H. J., Lee, S. J., Kim, M., Ahn, M. S., Choi, M. Y., Lee, N.-R., Shin, S. J. and Group, K. C. S. 2023. A phase II study on the efficacy of regorafenib in treating patients with c-KIT-mutated metastatic malignant melanoma that progressed after previous treatment (KCSG-UN-14-13), *European Journal of Cancer*, 193, p. 113312.

Koebel, C. M., Vermi, W., Swann, J. B., Zerafa, N., Rodig, S. J., Old, L. J., Smyth, M. J. and Schreiber, R. D. 2007. Adaptive immunity maintains occult cancer in an equilibrium state, *Nature*, 450, pp. 903–907.

Laborda-Illanes, A., Sanchez-Alcoholado, L., Dominguez-Recio, M. E., Jimenez-Rodriguez, B., Lavado, R., Comino-Méndez, I., Alba, E. and Queipo-Ortuño, M. I. 2020. Breast and gut microbiota action mechanisms in breast cancer pathogenesis and treatment, *Cancers*, 12, p. 2465.

Larkin, J., Chiarion-Sileni, V., Gonzalez, R., Grob, J. J., Cowey, C. L., Lao, C. D., Schadendorf, D., Dummer, R., Smylie, M. and Rutkowski, P. 2015. Combined nivolumab and ipilimumab or monotherapy in untreated melanoma, *New England Journal of Medicine*, 373, pp. 23–34.

Larkin, J., Chiarion-Sileni, V., Gonzalez, R., Grob, J.-J., Rutkowski, P., Lao, C. D., Cowey, C. L., Schadendorf, D., Wagstaff, J. and Dummer, R. 2019. Five-year survival with combined nivolumab and ipilimumab in advanced melanoma, *New England Journal of Medicine*, 381, pp. 1535–1546.

Laumonnier, F., Holbert, S., Ronce, N., Faravelli, F., Lenzner, S., Schwartz, C. E., Lespinasse, J., Van Esch, H., Lacombe, D., Goizet, C., Phan-Dinh Tuy, F., Van Bokhoven, H., Fryns, J. P., Chelly, J., Ropers, H. H., Moraine, C., Hamel, B. C. and Briault, S. 2005. Mutations in PHF8 are associated with X linked mental retardation and cleft lip/cleft palate, *Journal of Medical Genetics*, 42, pp. 780–786.

Lee, K., Luong, M., Shaw, H., Nathan, P., Bataille, V. and Spector, T. 2021. The gut microbiome: What the oncologist ought to know, *British Journal of Cancer*, 125, pp. 1197–1209.

Lee, N., Zakka, L. R., Mihm, M. C., Jr. and Schatton, T. 2016. Tumour-infiltrating lymphocytes in melanoma prognosis and cancer immunotherapy, *Pathology*, 48, pp. 177–187.

Lennartsson, J. and Rönnstrand, L. 2012. Stem cell factor receptor/c-Kit: From basic science to clinical implications, *Physiological Reviews*, 92, pp. 1619–1649.

Li, L. and Tian, Y. 2023. The role of metabolic reprogramming of tumor-associated macrophages in shaping the immunosuppressive tumor microenvironment, *Biomedicine & Pharmacotherapie*, 161, p. 114504.

Lian, T., Li, C. and Wang, H. 2019. Trametinib in the treatment of multiple malignancies harboring MEK1 mutations, *Cancer Treatment Reviews*, 81, p. 101907.

Limeta, A., Ji, B., Levin, M., Gatto, F. and Nielsen, J. 2020. Meta-analysis of the gut microbiota in predicting response to cancer immunotherapy in metastatic melanoma, *JCI Insight*, 5, p. e140940.

Liniker, E., Menzies, A. M., Kong, B. Y., Cooper, A., Ramanujam, S., Lo, S., Kefford, R. F., Fogarty, G. B., Guminski, A., Wang, T. W., Carlino, M. S., Hong, A. and Long, G. V. 2016. Activity and safety of radiotherapy with anti-PD-1 drug therapy in patients with metastatic melanoma, *Oncoimmunology*, 5, p. e1214788.

Liu, L., Cao, Y., Chen, C., Zhang, X., Mcnabola, A., Wilkie, D., Wilhelm, S., Lynch, M. and Carter, C. 2006. Sorafenib blocks the RAF/MEK/ERK pathway, inhibits tumor angiogenesis, and induces tumor cell apoptosis in hepatocellular carcinoma model PLC/PRF/5, *Cancer Research*, 66, pp. 11851–11858.

Liu, Q., Borcherding, N., Shao, P., Cao, H., Zhang, W. and Qi, H. H. 2019. Identification of novel TGF-β regulated genes with pro-migratory roles, *Biochimica et Biophysica Acta (BBA) – Molecular Basis of Disease*, 1865, p. 165537.

Liu, Y., Hu, L., Wu, Z., Yuan, K., Hong, G., Lian, Z., Feng, J., Li, N., Li, D., Wong, J., Chen, J., Liu, M., He, J. and Pang, X. 2023. Loss of PHF8 induces a viral mimicry response by activating endogenous retrotransposons, *Nature Communications*, 14, p. 4225.

Luebker, S. A. and Koepsell, S. A. 2019. Diverse mechanisms of BRAF inhibitor resistance in melanoma identified in clinical and preclinical studies, *Frontiers in Oncology*, 9, p. 268.

Ma, Q., Chen, Z., Jia, G., Lu, X., Xie, X. and Jin, W. 2015. The histone demethylase PHF8 promotes prostate cancer cell growth by activating the oncomiR miR-125b, *Onco Targets Therapy*, 8, pp. 1979–1988.

Ma, W., Mao, Q., Xia, W., Dong, G., Yu, C. and Jiang, F. 2019. Gut microbiota shapes the efficiency of cancer therapy, *Frontiers in Microbiology*, 10, p. 1050.

Ma, X., Wu, Y., Zhang, T., Song, H., Jv, H., Guo, W. and Ren, G. 2017. The clinical significance of c-Kit mutations in metastatic oral mucosal melanoma in China, *Oncotarget*, 8, pp. 82661–82673.

Maibach, F., Sadozai, H., Seyed Jafari, S. M., Hunger, R. E. and Schenk, M. 2020. Tumor-infiltrating lymphocytes and their prognostic value in cutaneous melanoma, *Frontiers in Immunology*, 11, p. 2105.

Makaranka, S., Scutt, F., Frixou, M., Wensley, K. E., Sharma, R. and Greenhowe, J. 2022. The gut microbiome and melanoma: A review, *Experimental Dermatology*, 31, pp. 1292–1301.

Matson, V., Fessler, J., Bao, R., Chongsuwat, T., Zha, Y., Alegre, M.-L., Luke, J. J. and Gajewski, T. F. 2018. The commensal microbiome is associated with anti-PD-1 efficacy in metastatic melanoma patients, *Science*, 359, pp. 104–108.

Mccann, T. S., Sobral, L. M., Self, C., Hsieh, J., Sechler, M. and Jedlicka, P. 2019. Biology and targeting of the Jumonji-domain histone demethylase family in childhood neoplasia: A preclinical overview, *Expert Opinion on Therapeutic Targets*, 23, pp. 267–280.

Miller, J. F. and Sadelain, M. 2015. The journey from discoveries in fundamental immunology to cancer immunotherapy, *Cancer Cell*, 27, pp. 439–449.

Mittal, D., Gubin, M. M., Schreiber, R. D. and Smyth, M. J. 2014. New insights into cancer immunoediting and its three component phases – elimination, equilibrium and escape, *Current Opinion in Immunology*, 27, pp. 16–25.

Mizuno, R., Kawada, K., Itatani, Y., Ogawa, R., Kiyasu, Y. and Sakai, Y. 2019. The role of tumor-associated neutrophils in colorectal cancer, *International Journal of Molecular Sciences*, 20, p. 529.

Montor, W. R., Salas, A. and Melo, F. H. M. 2018. Receptor tyrosine kinases and downstream pathways as druggable targets for cancer treatment: The current arsenal of inhibitors, *Molecular Cancer*, 17, p. 55.

Moubarak, R. S., De Pablos-Aragoneses, A., Ortiz-Barahona, V., Gong, Y., Gowen, M., Dolgalev, I., Shadaloey, S. A. A., Argibay, D., Karz, A., Von Itter, R., Vega-Sáenz De Miera, E. C., Sokolova, E., Darvishian, F., Tsirigos, A., Osman, I. and Hernando, E. 2022. The histone demethylase PHF8 regulates TGFβ signaling and promotes melanoma metastasis, *Science Advances*, 8, p. eabi7127.

Nazarian, R., Shi, H., Wang, Q., Kong, X., Koya, R. C., Lee, H., Chen, Z., Lee, M. K., Attar, N., Sazegar, H., Chodon, T., Nelson, S. F., Mcarthur, G., Sosman, J. A., Ribas, A. and Lo, R. S. 2010. Melanomas acquire resistance to B-RAF(V600E) inhibition by RTK or N-RAS upregulation, *Nature*, 468, pp. 973–977.

Nelson, B. E., Adashek, J. J., Lin, S. H. and Subbiah, V. 2023. The abscopal effect in patients with cancer receiving immunotherapy, *Med*, 4, pp. 233–244.

Nissan, M. H., Pratilas, C. A., Jones, A. M., Ramirez, R., Won, H., Liu, C., Tiwari, S., Kong, L., Hanrahan, A. J., Yao, Z., Merghoub, T., Ribas, A., Chapman, P. B., Yaeger, R., Taylor, B. S., Schultz, N., Berger, M. F., Rosen, N. and Solit, D. B. 2014. Loss of NF1 in cutaneous melanoma is associated with RAS activation and MEK dependence, *Cancer Research*, 74, pp. 2340–2350.

Norval, M. and Wright, C. Y. 2017. The Epidemiology of Cutaneous Melanoma in the White and Black African Population Groups in South Africa. In: Ward, W. H. and Farma, J. M. (eds.) *Cutaneous Melanoma: Etiology and Therapy*. Brisbane (AU): Codon Publications.

Oliver, D. E., Patel, K. R., Switchenko, J., Parker, D., Lawson, D. H., Delman, K. A., Kudchadkar, R. R. and Khan, M. K. 2016. Roles of adjuvant and salvage radiotherapy for desmoplastic melanoma, *Melanoma Research*, 26, pp. 35–41.

Pandesh, S., Haghjooy Javanmard, S., Shakeri-Zadeh, A. and Shokrani, P. 2021. Targeted photothermal therapy of melanoma in C57BL/6 mice using Fe(3)O(4)@Au core-shell nanoparticles and near-infrared laser, *Journal of Biomedical Physics & Engineering*, 11, pp. 29–38.

Papaccio, F., Kovacs, D., Bellei, B., Caputo, S., Migliano, E., Cota, C. and Picardo, M. 2021. Profiling cancer-associated fibroblasts in melanoma, *International Journal of Molecular Sciences,* 22, p. 7255.

Park, S. S., Dong, H., Liu, X., Harrington, S. M., Krco, C. J., Grams, M. P., Mansfield, A. S., Furutani, K. M., Olivier, K. R. and Kwon, E. D. 2015. PD-1 restrains radiotherapy-induced abscopal effect, *Cancer Immunology Research*, 3, pp. 610–619.

Patel, M., Eckburg, A., Gantiwala, S., Hart, Z., Dein, J., Lam, K. and Puri, N. 2021. Resistance to molecularly targeted therapies in melanoma, *Cancers (Basel)*, 13, p. 1115.

Petit, V., Raymond, J., Alberti, C., Pouteaux, M., Gallagher, S. J., Nguyen, M. Q., Aplin, A. E., Delmas, V. and Larue, L. 2019. C57BL/6 congenic mouse NRAS(Q61K) melanoma cell lines are highly sensitive to the combination of Mek and Akt inhibitors in vitro and in vivo, *Pigment Cell Melanoma Research*, 32, pp. 829–841.

Pham, D. D. M., Guhan, S. and Tsao, H. 2020. KIT and melanoma: Biological insights and clinical implications, *Yonsei Medical Journal*, 61, pp. 562–571.

Pollock, P. M., Harper, U. L., Hansen, K. S., Yudt, L. M., Stark, M., Robbins, C. M., Moses, T. Y., Hostetter, G., Wagner, U., Kakareka, J., Salem, G., Pohida, T., Heenan, P., Duray, P., Kallioniemi, O., Hayward, N. K., Trent, J. M. and Meltzer, P. S. 2003. High frequency of BRAF mutations in nevi, *Nature Genetics*, 33, pp. 19–20.

Poulikakos, P. I., Persaud, Y., Janakiraman, M., Kong, X., Ng, C., Moriceau, G., Shi, H., Atefi, M., Titz, B., Gabay, M. T., Salton, M., Dahlman, K. B., Tadi, M., Wargo, J. A., Flaherty, K. T., Kelley, M. C., Misteli, T., Chapman, P. B., Sosman, J. A., Graeber, T. G., Ribas, A., Lo, R. S., Rosen, N. and Solit, D. B. 2011. RAF inhibitor resistance is mediated by dimerization of aberrantly spliced BRAF(V600E), *Nature*, 480, pp. 387–390.

Priyanka, Abusalah, M. A. H., Chopra, H., Sharma, A., Mustafa, S. A., Choudhary, O. P., Sharma, M., Dhawan, M., Khosla, R., Loshali, A., Sundriyal, A. and Saini, J. 2023. Nanovaccines: A game changing approach in the fight against infectious diseases, *Biomedicine & Pharmacotherapy*, 167, p. 115597.

Qi, H. H., Sarkissian, M., Hu, G. Q., Wang, Z., Bhattacharjee, A., Gordon, D. B., Gonzales, M., Lan, F., Ongusaha, P. P., Huarte, M., Yaghi, N. K., Lim, H., Garcia, B. A., Brizuela, L., Zhao, K., Roberts, T. M. and Shi, Y. 2010. Histone H4K20/H3K9 demethylase PHF8 regulates zebrafish brain and craniofacial development, *Nature*, 466, pp. 503–507.

Raedler, L. A. 2015. Keytruda (Pembrolizumab): First PD-1 inhibitor approved for previously treated unresectable or metastatic melanoma, *American Health & Drug Benefits*, 8, pp. 96–100.

Rager, T., Eckburg, A., Patel, M., Qiu, R., Gantiwala, S., Dovalovsky, K., Fan, K., Lam, K., Roesler, C., Rastogi, A., Gautam, S., Dube, N., Morgan, B., Nasifuzzaman, S. M., Ramaswami, D., Gnanasekar, V., Smith, J., Merchant, A. and Puri, N. 2022. Treatment of metastatic melanoma with a combination of immunotherapies and molecularly targeted therapies, *Cancers (Basel)*, 14, p. 3779.

Reits, E. A., Hodge, J. W., Herberts, C. A., Groothuis, T. A., Chakraborty, M., Wansley, E. K., Camphausen, K., Luiten, R. M., De Ru, A. H., Neijssen, J., Griekspoor, A., Mesman, E., Verreck, F. A., Spits, H., Schlom, J., Van Veelen, P. and Neefjes, J. J. 2006. Radiation modulates the peptide repertoire, enhances MHC class I expression, and induces successful antitumor immunotherapy, *Journal of Experimental Medicine*, 203, pp. 1259–1271.

Relecom, A., Merhi, M., Inchakalody, V., Uddin, S., Rinchai, D., Bedognetti, D. and Dermime, S. 2021. Emerging dynamics pathways of response and resistance to PD-1 and CTLA-4 blockade: Tackling uncertainty by confronting complexity, *Journal of Experimental & Clinical Cancer Research*, 40, p. 74.

Roskoski, R., Jr. 2012. ERK1/2 MAP kinases: Structure, function, and regulation, *Pharmacological Research*, 66, pp. 105–143.

Routy, B., Gopalakrishnan, V., Daillère, R., Zitvogel, L., Wargo, J. A. and Kroemer, G. 2018a. The gut microbiota influences anticancer immunosurveillance and general health, *Nature Reviews Clinical Oncology*, 15, pp. 382–396.

Routy, B., Le Chatelier, E., Derosa, L., Duong, C. P., Alou, M. T., Daillère, R., Fluckiger, A., Messaoudene, M., Rauber, C. and Roberti, M. P. 2018b. Gut microbiome influences efficacy of PD-1-based immunotherapy against epithelial tumors, *Science*, 359, pp. 91–97.

Ryu, S., Youn, C., Moon, A. R., Howland, A., Armstrong, C. A. and Song, P. I. 2017. Therapeutic inhibitors against mutated BRAF and MEK for the treatment of metastatic melanoma, *Chonnam Medical Journal*, 53, pp. 173–177.

Saâda-Bouzid, E., Defaucheux, C., Karabajakian, A., Coloma, V. P., Servois, V., Paoletti, X., Even, C., Fayette, J., Guigay, J. and Loirat, D. 2017. Hyperprogression during anti-PD-1/PD-L1 therapy in patients with recurrent and/or metastatic head and neck squamous cell carcinoma, *Annals of Oncology*, 28, pp. 1605–1611.

Salzmann, M., Pawlowski, J., Loquai, C., Rafei-Shamsabadi, D. A., Meiss, F., Ugurel, S., Schadendorf, D., Meier, F., Enk, A. H. and Hassel, J. C. 2022. MEK inhibitors for pre-treated, NRAS-mutated metastatic melanoma: A multi-centre, retrospective study, *European Journal of Cancer*, 166, pp. 24–32.

Sarkisian, S. and Davar, D. 2018. MEK inhibitors for the treatment of NRAS mutant melanoma, *Drug Design, Development and Therapy*, 12, pp. 2553–2565.

Savoia, P., Fava, P., Casoni, F. and Cremona, O. 2019. Targeting the ERK signaling pathway in melanoma, *International Journal of Molecular Science,* 20, p. 1483.

Schatton, T., Schütte, U., Frank, N. Y., Zhan, Q., Hoerning, A., Robles, S. C., Zhou, J., Hodi, F. S., Spagnoli, G. C., Murphy, G. F. and Frank, M. H. 2010. Modulation of T-cell activation by malignant melanoma initiating cells, *Cancer Research*, 70, pp. 697–708.

Schellerer, V. S., Frenger, J., Merkel, S., Goehl, J., Kersting, S., Gruetzmann, R., Erdmann, M. and Foertsch, T. 2021. Results of isolated limb perfusion for metastasized malignant melanoma, *Surgical Oncology*, 38, p. 101603.

Shao, P., Liu, Q., Maina, P. K., Cui, J., Bair, T. B., Li, T., Umesalma, S., Zhang, W. and Qi, H. H. 2017. Histone demethylase PHF8 promotes epithelial to mesenchymal transition and breast tumorigenesis, *Nucleic Acids Research*, 45, pp. 1687–1702.

Shariev, A., Painter, N., Reeve, V. E., Haass, N. K., Rybchyn, M. S., Ince, F. A., Mason, R. S. and Dixon, K. M. 2022. PTEN: A novel target for vitamin D in melanoma, *Journal of Steroid Biochemistry and Molecular Biology*, 218, p. 106059.

Sharma, P., Hu-Lieskovan, S., Wargo, J. A. and Ribas, A. 2017. Primary, adaptive, and acquired resistance to cancer immunotherapy, *Cell*, 168, pp. 707–723.

Sheng, X., Yan, X., Chi, Z., Si, L., Cui, C., Tang, B., Li, S., Mao, L., Lian, B., Wang, X., Bai, X., Zhou, L., Kong, Y., Dai, J., Wang, K., Tang, X., Zhou, H., Wu, H., Feng, H., Yao, S., Flaherty, K. T. and Guo, J. 2019. Axitinib in combination with toripalimab, a humanized immunoglobulin G(4) monoclonal antibody against programmed cell death-1, in patients with metastatic mucosal melanoma: An open-label phase IB trial, *Journal of Clinical Oncology*, 37, pp. 2987–2999.

Shi, W. 2017. Radiation Therapy for Melanoma. In: Ward WH, Farma JM, editors. Cutaneous Melanoma: Etiology and Therapy [Internet]. Brisbane (AU): Codon Publications; 2017 Dec 21. Chapter 8. PMID: 29461772.

Shurin, M. R., Shurin, G. V., Lokshin, A., Yurkovetsky, Z. R., Gutkin, D. W., Chatta, G., Zhong, H., Han, B. and Ferris, R. L. 2006. Intratumoral cytokines/chemokines/growth factors and tumor infiltrating dendritic cells: Friends or enemies? *Cancer and Metastasis Reviews*, 25, pp. 333–356.

Siddiqui, B. A., Chapin, B. F., Jindal, S., Duan, F., Basu, S., Yadav, S. S., Gu, A. D., Espejo, A. B., Kinder, M., Pettaway, C. A., Ward, J. F., Tidwell, R. S. S., Troncoso, P., Corn, P. G., Logothetis, C. J., Knoblauch, R., Hutnick, N., Gottardis, M., Drake, C. G., Sharma, P. and Subudhi, S. K. 2023. Immune and pathologic responses in patients with localized prostate cancer who received daratumumab (anti-CD38) or edicotinib (CSF-1R inhibitor), *Journal for Immunotherapy of Cancer*, 11, p. e006262.

Siegel, P. M. and Massagué, J. 2003. Cytostatic and apoptotic actions of TGF-beta in homeostasis and cancer, *Nature Reviews Cancer*, 3, pp. 807–821.

Siewe, N. and Friedman, A. 2021. TGF-β inhibition can overcome cancer primary resistance to PD-1 blockade: A mathematical model, *PLOS ONE*, 16, p. e0252620.

Singh, S., Barik, D., Arukha, A. P., Prasad, S., Mohapatra, I., Singh, A. and Singh, G. 2023. Small molecule targeting immune cells: A novel approach for cancer treatment, *Biomedicines*, 11, p. 2621.

Sivan, A., Corrales, L., Hubert, N., Williams, J. B., Aquino-Michaels, K., Earley, Z. M., Benyamin, F. W., Man Lei, Y., Jabri, B. and Alegre, M.-L. 2015. Commensal bifidobacterium promotes antitumor immunity and facilitates anti-PD-L1 efficacy, *Science*, 350, pp. 1084–1089.

Sobhani, N., Tardiel-Cyril, D. R., Davtyan, A., Generali, D., Roudi, R. and Li, Y. 2021. CTLA-4 in regulatory T cells for cancer immunotherapy, *Cancers (Basel)*, 13, p. 1440.

Society, A. C. 2024. *Key Statistics for Melanoma Skin Cancer* [Online]. Available: https://www.cancer.org/cancer/types/melanoma-skin-cancer/about/key-statistics.html [Accessed May 19, 2024].

Solana, R., Casado, J. G., Delgado, E., Delarosa, O., Marín, J., Durán, E., Pawelec, G. and Tarazona, R. 2007. Lymphocyte activation in response to melanoma: Interaction of NK-associated receptors and their ligands, *Cancer Immunology Immunotherapy*, 56, pp. 101–109.

Sonis, S. T. 2004. The pathobiology of mucositis, *Nature Reviews Cancer*, 4, pp. 277–284.

Strizzi, L., Catalano, A., Vianale, G., Orecchia, S., Casalini, A., Tassi, G., Puntoni, R., Mutti, L. and Procopio, A. 2001. Vascular endothelial growth factor is an autocrine growth factor in human malignant mesothelioma, *Journal of Pathology*, 193, pp. 468–475.

Sun, C., Wang, L., Huang, S., Heynen, G. J., Prahallad, A., Robert, C., Haanen, J., Blank, C., Wesseling, J., Willems, S. M., Zecchin, D., Hobor, S., Bajpe, P. K., Lieftink, C., Mateus, C., Vagner, S., Grernrum, W., Hofland, I., Schlicker, A., Wessels, L. F., Beijersbergen, R. L., Bardelli, A., Di Nicolantonio, F., Eggermont, A. M. and Bernards, R. 2014. Reversible and adaptive resistance to BRAF(V600E) inhibition in melanoma, *Nature*, 508, pp. 118–122.

Sun, J. Y., Yin, T. L., Zhou, J., Xu, J. and Lu, X. J. 2020. Gut microbiome and cancer immunotherapy, *Journal of Cellular Physiology*, 235, pp. 4082–4088.

Tagliaferri, L., Lancellotta, V., Fionda, B., Mangoni, M., Casà, C., Di Stefani, A., Pagliara, M. M., D'aviero, A., Schinzari, G., Chiesa, S., Mazzarella, C., Manfrida, S., Colloca, G. F., Marazzi, F., Morganti, A. G., Blasi, M. A., Peris, K., Tortora, G. and Valentini, V. 2022. Immunotherapy and radiotherapy in melanoma: A multidisciplinary comprehensive review, *Human Vaccines & Immunotherapy*, 18, p. 1903827.

Tailor, A., Estephan, H., Parker, R., Woodhouse, I., Abdulghani, M., Nicastri, A., Jones, K., Salatino, S., Muschel, R., Humphrey, T., Giaccia, A. and Ternette, N. 2022. Ionizing radiation drives key regulators of antigen presentation and a global expansion of the immunopeptidome, *Molecular & Cellular Proteomics*, 21, p. 100410.

Takashima, A. and Faller, D. V. 2013. Targeting the RAS oncogene, *Expert Opinion on Therapeutic Targets*, 17, pp. 507–531.

Tawbi, H. A. 2023. *RELATIVITY-047 Update: Nivolumab/Relatlimab Provides PFS Benefit in Previously Untreated Advanced Melanoma* [Online]. ASCO Daily News. Available: https://dailynews.ascopubs.org/do/relativity-047-update-nivolumab-relatlimab-provides-pfs-benefit-previously-untreated [Accessed July 26, 2024].

Tawbi, H. A., Schadendorf, D., Lipson, E. J., Ascierto, P. A., Matamala, L., Castillo Gutiérrez, E., Rutkowski, P., Gogas, H. J., Lao, C. D., De Menezes, J. J., Dalle, S., Arance, A., Grob, J. J., Srivastava, S., Abaskharoun, M., Hamilton, M., Keidel, S., Simonsen, K. L., Sobiesk, A. M., Li, B., Hodi, F. S. and Long, G. V. 2022. Relatlimab and nivolumab versus nivolumab in untreated advanced melanoma, *New England Journal of Medicine*, 386, pp. 24–34.

Teixeira, A. F., Ten Dijke, P. and Zhu, H. J. 2020. On-target anti-TGF-β therapies are not succeeding in clinical cancer treatments: What are remaining challenges? *Frontiers in Cell and Developmental Biology*, 8, p. 605.

Tian, J. and Quek, C. 2024. Understanding the tumor microenvironment in melanoma patients with in-transit metastases and its impacts on immune checkpoint immunotherapy responses, *International Journal of Molecular Sciences*, 25, p. 4243.

Tod, B. M., Kellett, P. E., Singh, E., Visser, W. I., Lombard, C. J. and Wright, C. Y. 2019. The incidence of melanoma in South Africa: An exploratory analysis of National Cancer Registry data from 2005 to 2013 with a specific focus on melanoma in black Africans, *South African Medical Journal*, 109, pp. 246–253.

Todd, J. R., Scurr, L. L., Becker, T. M., Kefford, R. F. and Rizos, H. 2014. The MAPK pathway functions as a redundant survival signal that reinforces the PI3K cascade in c-Kit mutant melanoma, *Oncogene*, 33, pp. 236–245.

Tonneau, M., Elkrief, A., Pasquier, D., Del Socorro, T. P., Chamaillard, M., Bahig, H. and Routy, B. 2021. The role of the gut microbiome on radiation therapy efficacy and gastrointestinal complications: A systematic review, *Radiotherapy and Oncology*, 156, pp. 1–9.

Twyman-Saint Victor, C., Rech, A. J., Maity, A., Rengan, R., Pauken, K. E., Stelekati, E., Benci, J. L., Xu, B., Dada, H., Odorizzi, P. M., Herati, R. S., Mansfield, K. D., Patsch, D., Amaravadi, R. K., Schuchter, L. M., Ishwaran, H., Mick, R., Pryma, D. A., Xu, X., Feldman, M. D., Gangadhar, T. C., Hahn, S. M., Wherry, E. J., Vonderheide, R. H. and Minn, A. J. 2015. Radiation and dual checkpoint blockade activate non-redundant immune mechanisms in cancer, *Nature*, 520, pp. 373–377.

Usyk, M., Pandey, A., Hayes, R. B., Moran, U., Pavlick, A., Osman, I., Weber, J. S. and Ahn, J. 2021. Bacteroides vulgatus and Bacteroides dorei predict immune-related adverse events in immune checkpoint blockade treatment of metastatic melanoma, *Genome Medicine*, 13(1), p. 11.

Van Herpen, C. M. L., Agarwala, S. S., Hauschild, A., Berking, C., Beck, J. T., Schadendorf, D., Jansen, R., Queirolo, P., Ascierto, P. A., Blank, C. U., Heinrich, M. C., Pal, R. R., Derti, A., Antona, V., Nauwelaerts, H., Zubel, A. and Dummer, R. 2019. Biomarker results from a phase II study of MEK1/2 inhibitor binimetinib (MEK162) in patients with advanced NRAS- or BRAF-mutated melanoma, *Oncotarget*, 10, pp. 1850–1859.

Vanni, I., Tanda, E. T., Dalmasso, B., Pastorino, L., Andreotti, V., Bruno, W., Boutros, A., Spagnolo, F. and Ghiorzo, P. 2020. Non-BRAF mutant melanoma: Molecular features and therapeutical implications, *Frontiers in Molecular Bioscience*, 7, p. 172.

Vétizou, M., Pitt, J. M., Daillère, R., Lepage, P., Waldschmitt, N., Flament, C., Rusakiewicz, S., Routy, B., Roberti, M. P. and Duong, C. P. 2015. Anticancer immunotherapy by CTLA-4 blockade relies on the gut microbiota, *Science*, 350, pp. 1079–1084.

Viaud, S., Saccheri, F., Mignot, G., Yamazaki, T., Daillère, R., Hannani, D., Enot, D. P., Pfirschke, C., Engblom, C. and Pittet, M. J. 2013. The intestinal microbiota modulates the anticancer immune effects of cyclophosphamide, *Science*, 342, pp. 971–976.

Wang, W., Cheng, B. and Yu, Q. 2022. Cancer-associated fibroblasts as accomplices to confer therapeutic resistance in cancer, *Cancer Drug Resistance*, 5, pp. 889–901.

Wang, Y., Dembowsky, K., Chevalier, E., Stüve, P., Korf-Klingebiel, M., Lochner, M., Napp, L. C., Frank, H., Brinkmann, E., Kanwischer, A., Bauersachs, J., Gyöngyösi, M., Sparwasser, T. and Wollert, K. C. 2019. C-X-C motif chemokine receptor 4 blockade promotes tissue repair after myocardial infarction by enhancing regulatory T cell mobilization and immune-regulatory function, *Circulation*, 139, pp. 1798–1812.

Wei, X., Mao, L., Chi, Z., Sheng, X., Cui, C., Kong, Y., Dai, J., Wang, X., Li, S., Tang, B., Lian, B., Yan, X., Bai, X., Zhou, L., Guo, J. and Si, L. 2019. Efficacy evaluation of imatinib for the treatment of melanoma: Evidence from a retrospective study, *Oncology Research*, 27, pp. 495–501.

Wellbrock, C. and Hurlstone, A. 2010. BRAF as therapeutic target in melanoma, *Biochemical Pharmacology*, 80, pp. 561–567.

Wesolowski, R., Sharma, N., Reebel, L., Rodal, M. B., Peck, A., West, B. L., Marimuthu, A., Severson, P., Karlin, D. A., Dowlati, A., Le, M. H., Coussens, L. M. and Rugo, H. S. 2019. Phase Ib study of the combination of pexidartinib (PLX3397), a CSF-1R inhibitor, and paclitaxel in patients with advanced solid tumors, *Therapeutic Advances in Medical Oncology*, 11, p. 1758835919854238.

Wilson, M. A. and Schuchter, L. M. 2016. Chemotherapy for melanoma, *Melanoma*, 167, pp. 209–229.

Wu, C., Mao, Y., Wang, X., Li, P. and Tang, B. 2022. Deep-tissue fluorescence imaging study of reactive oxygen species in a tumor microenvironment, *Analytical Chemistry*, 94, pp. 165–176.

Wu, H.-J. and Wu, E. 2012. The role of gut microbiota in immune homeostasis and autoimmunity, *Gut Microbes*, 3, pp. 4–14.

Xiao, Y. and Yu, D. 2021. Tumor microenvironment as a therapeutic target in cancer, *Pharmacology & Therapy*, 221, p. 107753.

Xie, N., Shen, G., Gao, W., Huang, Z., Huang, C. and Fu, L. 2023. Neoantigens: Promising targets for cancer therapy, *Signal Transduction and Targeted Therapy*, 8, p. 9.

Xu, C., Chen, Y.-P., Du, X.-J., Liu, J.-Q., Huang, C.-L., Chen, L., Zhou, G.-Q., Li, W.-F., Mao, Y.-P. and Hsu, C. 2018. Comparative safety of immune checkpoint inhibitors in cancer: Systematic review and network meta-analysis, *BMJ*, 363, p. k4226.

Xu, J.-Y., Liu, M.-T., Tao, T., Zhu, X. and Fei, F.-Q. 2021. The role of gut microbiota in tumorigenesis and treatment, *Biomedicine & Pharmacotherapy*, 138, p. 111444.

Xu, Y., Li, W., Lin, S., Liu, B., Wu, P. and Li, L. 2023. Fibroblast diversity and plasticity in the tumor microenvironment: Roles in immunity and relevant therapies, *Cell Communication and Signaling*, 21, p. 234.

Yan, J., Wu, X., Yu, J., Yu, H., Xu, T., Brown, K. M., Bai, X., Dai, J., Ma, M., Tang, H., Si, L., Chi, Z., Sheng, X., Cui, C., Kong, Y. and Guo, J. 2018. Analysis of NRAS gain in 657 patients with melanoma and evaluation of its sensitivity to a MEK inhibitor, *European Journal of Cancer*, 89, pp. 90–101.

Yang, X., Guo, Y., Chen, C., Shao, B., Zhao, L., Zhou, Q., Liu, J., Wang, G., Yuan, W. and Sun, Z. 2021. Interaction between intestinal microbiota and tumour immunity in the tumour microenvironment, *Immunology*, 164, pp. 476–493.

Yao, M., Liu, X., Qian, Z., Fan, D., Sun, X., Zhong, L. and Wu, P. 2023. Research progress of nanovaccine in anti-tumor immunotherapy, *Frontiers in Oncology*, 13, p. 1211262.

Yu, Q., Xie, J., Li, J., Lu, Y. and Liao, L. 2019. Clinical outcomes of BRAF plus MEK inhibition in melanoma: A meta-analysis and systematic review, *Cancer Medicine*, 8, pp. 5414–5424.

Yuan, J., Ginsberg, B., Page, D., Li, Y., Rasalan, T., Gallardo, H. F., Xu, Y., Adams, S., Bhardwaj, N., Busam, K., Old, L. J., Allison, J. P., Jungbluth, A. and Wolchok, J. D. 2011. CTLA-4 blockade increases antigen-specific CD8(+) T cells in prevaccinated patients with melanoma: Three cases, *Cancer Immunology Immunotherapy*, 60, pp. 1137–1146.

Zanotto-Filho, A., Rajamanickam, S., Loranc, E., Masamsetti, V. P., Gorthi, A., Romero, J. C., Tonapi, S., Gonçalves, R. M., Reddick, R. L., Benavides, R., Kuhn, J., Chen, Y. and Bishop, A. J. R. 2018. Sorafenib improves alkylating therapy by blocking induced inflammation, invasion and angiogenesis in breast cancer cells, *Cancer Letters*, 425, pp. 101–115.

Zhang, Y. and Ertl, H. C. 2016. Depletion of FAP+ cells reduces immunosuppressive cells and improves metabolism and functions CD8+T cells within tumors, *Oncotarget*, 7, pp. 23282–99.

Zhang, X., Fang, X., Gao, Z., Chen, W., Tao, F., Cai, P., Yuan, H., Shu, Y., Xu, Q., Sun, Y. and Gu, Y. 2014. Axitinib, a selective inhibitor of vascular endothelial growth factor receptor, exerts an anticancer effect in melanoma through promoting antitumor immunity, *Anticancer Drugs*, 25, pp. 204–211.

Zhao, X. and Shao, C. 2020. Radiotherapy-mediated immunomodulation and anti-tumor abscopal effect combining immune checkpoint blockade, *Cancers (Basel)*, 12, p. 2762.

Zhong, J., Yan, W., Wang, C., Liu, W., Lin, X., Zou, Z., Sun, W. and Chen, Y. 2022. BRAF inhibitor resistance in melanoma: Mechanisms and alternative therapeutic strategies, *Current Treatment Options in Oncology*, 23, pp. 1503–1521.

Zhou, L., Yang, K., Andl, T., Wickett, R. R. and Zhang, Y. 2015. Perspective of targeting cancer-associated fibroblasts in melanoma, *Journal of Cancer*, 6, pp. 717–726.

Zhou, Q., Jin, X., Zhao, Y., Wang, Y., Tao, M., Cao, Y. and Yin, X. 2024. Melanoma-associated fibroblasts in tumor-promotion flammation and antitumor immunity: Novel mechanisms and potential immunotherapeutic strategies, *Human Molecular Genetics*, 33, pp. 1186–1193.

Zhou, S., Lu, J., Liu, S., Shao, J., Liu, Z., Li, J. and Xiao, W. 2023. Role of the tumor microenvironment in malignant melanoma organoids during the development and metastasis of tumors, *Frontiers in Cell and Developmental Biology*, 11, p. 1166916.

Zodwa, D., Thandeka, K., Rodney, H., Mpho, C. and Zilungile, M.-K. 2016. Current Immunotherapeutic Treatments in Colon Cancer. In: Luis, R. (ed.) *Colorectal Cancer*. Rijeka: IntechOpen.

Zou, J., Lei, T., Guo, P., Yu, J., Xu, Q., Luo, Y., Ke, R. and Huang, D. 2019. Mechanisms shaping the role of ERK1/2 in cellular senescence (review), *Molecular Medicine Reports*, 19, pp. 759–770.

Zou, W. and Chen, L. 2008. Inhibitory B7-family molecules in the tumour microenvironment, *Nature Reviews Immunology*, 8, pp. 467–477.

7 Integrating Genomics and Proteomics

A Multi-Omics Approach to Melanoma Treatment

Rodney Hull and Zodwa Dlamini
SAMRC Precision Oncology Research Unit (PORU), DSTI/NRF SARChI Chair in Precision Oncology and Cancer Prevention (POCP), Pan African Cancer Research Institute (PACRI), University of Pretoria, Pretoria, South Africa

Thulo Molefi
Department of Medical Oncology, Faculty of Health Sciences, Steve Biko Academic Hospital, University of Pretoria, Pretoria, South Africa

Mark Jose
Life Fourways Hospital, Sandton, South Africa

Kamal Veer Saini
Fortrea Inc., Durham, NC, USA
and
Addenbrooke's Hospital, Cambridge University Hospitals NHS Foundation Trust, Cambridge, UK

INTRODUCTION

The risk of developing melanoma is influenced by environmental factors such as exposure to UV, life experiences such as infection by HPV, and, most importantly for this chapter, genetic alterations and mutations. The influence of UV exposure is one of the most important risk factors for most forms of melanoma. Exposure to UV through the use of artificial sources, such as sunbeds or intermittent sun exposure, or a history of sunburns, leads to increased levels of DNA damage (Garbe et al., 2010; O'Neill and Scoggins, 2019). A family history of melanoma is another important risk factor. Current tools utilized to diagnose melanoma include clinical history and assessment, examining both the personal and family history of melanoma occurrence and risk factors. These risk factors include a Fitzpatrick skin type, a history of childhood sunburns, the presence of multiple naevi, the presence of dysplastic naevi syndrome, and the identification of suspicious lesions. These suspicious lesions are assessed using methods such as the ABCDE rule, the Menzies method, and the presence of an odd—"Ugly duckling" mole. These assessments can be made using various diagnostic methods such as imaging techniques (dermoscopy) and the analysis of biopsy material using immunohistochemical markers for melanoma diagnosis and genomic and proteomic markers. Some of the genomic markers include genes such as BRAF, NRAS, NF1, TERT, and CDKN2A15. Proteomics markers include annexin, vimentin, and H4 (Teh et al., 2023). The genetic variations that are characteristic

DOI: 10.1201/9781003511625-7

of melanomas can lead to an individual having a gene expression profile that increases the risk of developing melanoma or through genetic mutations being inherited (Psaty et al., 2010).

These genetic changes resulting from DNA damage or through the inheritance of mutations led to studies that aimed to identify genetic markers for an increased risk of developing melanoma or a pattern of genetic changes that can be used to diagnose and characterize melanomas. This has also led to the creation of algorithms that can be employed by artificial intelligence (AI) to analyze large data sets to identify these patterns, leading to the rapid diagnosis of melanomas (Valenti et al., 2021). Even though the use of these algorithms and genetic biomarkers has improved diagnosis, there is still room for improvement, as many melanomas are still diagnosed at a late stage, resulting in poor survival and a poor prognosis. These genetic mutations can alter the ability of the skin to resist the damaging effects of UV light. Genetic mutations that are particularly important in this respect include *braf*. The BRAF protein controls the proliferation of melanocytes through the regulation of the expression of cell cycle inhibitors of kinase 4A (INK4A) (Miller et al., 2006).

Apart from examining the changes in gene sequences, the expression level of various proteins can also be used as important biomarkers for melanoma. For example, protein components of the tumor microenvironment. These include proteins such as lymphocyte cytosolic protein 2, autophagy, beclin 1, regulator 1, loricrin, nicotinamide N-methyltransferase, and TBC (Georgescu et al., 2022). Not only are these proteins useful as diagnostic or prognostic biomarkers, but also the study of the expression of these proteins may lead to the identification of new signaling pathways, potential biomarkers, and new therapeutic targets (Das et al., 2023). The advances made in the use of omics technologies have allowed for the identification of new biomarkers for a great variety of disorders, including cancer. In 2019, it was reported that more than 51,100 biomarkers for various cancers had been identified through the use of a wide range of omics approaches (Donnelly et al., 2019). Finally, metabolomics, microbiomics, and epigenomics have led to the identification of biomarkers in the form of cancer-specific metabolites, microbial populations, and epigenetic changes. Genomics has led to the identification of biomarkers using DNA isolated from tumor cells and tissues as well as circulating tumor DNA (ctDNA). Transcriptomics has identified biomarkers from tumor cell mRNA as well as from non-coding RNA such as mir-RNA. Proteomics has allowed for the identification of cancer-specific protein populations, shedding light on the phenotype of these cancers (Tsimberidou et al., 2022).

The most important development for the advancement of cancer genomics has been the advent of next-generation sequencing (NGS). This technology allows to detect and sequence multiple mutations that drive cancer across multiple samples simultaneously. This can be achieved through whole genome or whole transcriptome sequencing or the use of assays for specific genes (de Unamuno Bustos et al., 2017). Proteomics has advanced mainly through improvements in mass spectrometry, which has been the principal technology for protein sequencing for many years. Shotgun sequencing, otherwise known as bottom-up proteomics, is the most commonly used technique. Chromatographic methods are normally used to separate the sample into individual peptides, which are fed into the mass spec. Previously, this was mainly achieved through the use of 2D PAGE. Individual proteins are excised from the gel and then analyzed using the mass spectrometer. These methods aim to reduce sample complexity to more comprehensively characterize the proteome (Su et al., 2022).

GENOMICS

Approximately 10% of melanoma patients report that they have a family history of malignancy with a relative who has been diagnosed with the disease. The contribution of heritable melanoma risk genes to the development of melanoma is an important factor even though most mutations and genetic changes that contribute to the development and progression of melanoma are somatic (Artomov et al., 2017; Read et al., 2016; Soura et al., 2016). A multidisciplinary study involving genomic and transcriptomic techniques demonstrated a consecutive order of mutations (signaling pathways involved in MAPK, telomerase, cell cycle, chromatin, p53, and PI3K) that occur in the progression to malignant melanoma, suggesting evolution from premalignant lesions, as well as possible biomarkers (Shain et al., 2018). Currently, mutations in genes, such as CDKN2A, CDK4,

BAP1, POT1, ACD, TERF2IP, and TERT, are known to increase the chances of developing melanoma. It has been found that mutations in these genes account for only 50% of familial melanoma cases, and the genetic basis of the remaining 50% remains unknown (Newton-Bishop et al., 2020; Soura et al., 2016). **Table 7.1** lists genes that have been found to have mutations associated with melanoma and provides a list of genes and the type or stage of the disease they are associated with.

TABLE 7.1
Genes Commonly Mutated in Melanomas

Gene	Tissue/Sample	Reference
5-hmC	Lower levels of melanoma Higher in naevi	Salgado et al. (2020)
Akt3	Melanoma progression biomarker	Wouters et al. (2017)
Arx	Primary melanoma	Duan et al. (2018)
Bap1	Germline variants novel non-sense mutations associated with cutaneous and ocular melanoma	Artomov et al. (2017)
	Braf	
BRAFV600E	Low mutational load in naevi	Colebatch et al. (2019)
	Dysplastic naevi with a lower mutational load than melanoma	Melamed et al. (2017)
Braf (mutant)	Primary melanoma in specific genetic subtypes	Kunz et al. (2018)
	Benign naevi	Shain et al. (2018)
	Can be used as a marker to classify melanoma into one of four subtypes due to it being the most common mutation	The Cancer Genome Atlas (2015)
Braf (Wild type)	Benign naevi in specific genetic subtypes	Kunz et al. (2018)
BRAF/MEK inhibitor resistance signatures	In specific genetic subtypes of benign naevi and primary melanoma	Kunz et al. (2018)
	Cdkn2a	
Cdkn2a	Germline variants truncated variants associated with cutaneous and ocular melanoma	Artomov et al. (2017)
Cdkn2a mutations	Absent in dysplastic naevi present in melanoma	Melamed et al. (2017)
CNV	Different frequency in Chinese melanoma patients compared to Western melanoma patients	Luo et al. (2020)
Ddb2	Primary melanoma	Duan et al. (2018)
Dock8	SNPs associated with naevus count and/or melanoma risk	Duffy et al. (2018)
Ephx3	Melanoma progression biomarker	Wouters et al. (2017)
Fam208b	SNPs associated with naevus count and/or melanoma risk	Duffy et al. (2018)
Fmn1	SNPs associated with naevus count and/or melanoma risk	Duffy et al. (2018)
Gib2	Melanoma progression biomarker	Wouters et al. (2017)
Gprc5a	SNPs associated with naevus count and/or melanoma risk	Duffy et al. (2018)
Hdac4	SNPs associated with naevus count and/or melanoma risk	Duffy et al. (2018)
Hoxa9	Melanoma progression biomarker	Wouters et al. (2017)
Kittlg	SNPs associated with naevus count and/or melanoma risk	Duffy et al. (2018)
Mapk	Altered signaling pathways in transition from benign naevi to melanoma	Shain et al. (2018)
Mc1r	Germline variants splice donor mutations associated with cutaneous and ocular melanoma	Artomov et al. (2017)
Meox2	Melanoma progression and prognostic biomarker	Wouters et al. (2017)
Mitf	In specific genetic subtypes of benign naevi and primary melanoma	Kunz et al. (2018)
Mbp	Primary melanoma	Duan et al. (2018)
NFIC	SNPs associated with naevus count and/or melanoma risk	Duffy et al. (2018)
NF1	Absent in dysplastic naevi present in melanoma	Melamed et al. (2017)
	Can be used as a marker to classify melanoma into one of four subtypes due to it being the most common mutation	The Cancer Genome Atlas (2015)

(Continued)

TABLE 7.1 *(Continued)*
Genes Commonly Mutated in Melanomas

Gene	Tissue/Sample	Reference
	Nras	
NRASQ61K	Low mutational load in naevi	Colebatch et al. (2019)
NRAS Q61R	Low mutational load in naevi	Colebatch et al. (2019)
	Dysplastic naevi with a lower mutational load than melanoma	Melamed et al. (2017)
NRAS mutations	In specific genetic subtypes of benign naevi and primary melanoma and lower mutational prevalence on other subtypes	Kunz et al. (2018)
	Intermediate lesions	Shain et al. (2018)
Olig3	Melanoma prognostic biomarker	Wouters et al. (2017)
p53	Altered signaling pathways in transition from benign naevi to melanoma	Shain et al. (2018)
	Absent in dysplastic naevi present in melanoma	Melamed et al. (2017)
	Advanced primary melanoma	Shain et al. (2018)
	Malignant melanoma	Shain et al. (2018)
P12k	Altered signaling pathways in transition from benign naevi to melanoma	Shain et al. (2018)
Pon3	Melanoma progression biomarker	Wouters et al. (2017)
	Advanced primary melanomas	Shain et al. (2018)
Pot1	Germline variants splice donor mutations associated with cutaneous and ocular melanoma	Artomov et al. (2017)
Pten	Absent in dysplastic naevi present in melanoma	Melamed et al. (2017)
Rac1	Absent in dysplastic naevi present in melanoma	Melamed et al. (2017)
Rbp1	Melanoma progression biomarker	Wouters et al. (2017)
Serpine	melanoma progression biomarker	Wouters et al. (2017)
Syne2	SNPs associated with naevus count and/or melanoma risk	Duffy et al. (2018)
Tbc1d16	Melanoma progression biomarker	Wouters et al. (2017)
Telomerase	Altered signaling pathways in transition from benign naevi to melanoma	Shain et al. (2018)
Tert promoter mutations	Acquired naevi subclones	Colebatch et al. (2019)
	Melanoma *in situ*	Shain et al. (2018)
Tfap2b	Melanoma progression biomarker	Wouters et al. (2017)
Twist1	Melanoma progression biomarker	Wouters et al. (2017)
UVR	Acquired naevi subclones	Colebatch et al. (2019)

Abbreviations: 5hmC, *5-hydroxymethylcytosine*; ARX, Aristaless-related homeobox; CNV, copy number variations; DDB2, Damage-specific DNA binding protein 2; MBP, Myelin basic protein; UVR, UV radiation-induced DNA damage.

Mutations in BRAF, KRAS, and NRAS

The genes commonly mutated in melanoma are components of specific signaling pathways, including the receptor tyrosine kinase (RTK), phosphatidylinositol-3-kinase (PI(3)K), retinoblastoma (RB), p53, Wnt, and NF-kB pathways (Pimiento et al., 2013). The *braf* gene is so commonly mutated in melanoma (approximately 60% of melanomas), to the extent that it is one of the most commonly used biomarkers for the disease and is a druggable target for the treatment of melanoma. BRAF plays a role in the MAP kinase signaling pathway. In this pathway, it is found downstream of RAS. Where it initiates the MAPK signaling cascade that results in the activation of ERK (**Figure 7.1**) (Kondoh and Nishida, 2007). BEAF is a member of the RAF protein family, all of which can phosphorylate MEK. BRAF is unique as it has the strongest capacity to activate the kinase signaling pathway. The activation of MEK/MAPK-ERK pathways results in the activation of genes involved in cell proliferation, differentiation, and apoptosis. This pathway is activated by various stimuli molecules such as cytokines, growth factors, hormones, and environmental stressors (Whitmarsh, 2007).

BRAF normally forms a homodimer through the interaction of the protein's kinase domains. These dimers are the enzymatically active form under normal conditions and phosphorylate downstream targets (Bollag et al., 2012). Mutations in the *braf* gene are categorized into three separate classes (Yao et al., 2017). Class I mutations result in a BRAF monomer that is constitutively active. Class II mutations result in BRAF dimers that are constitutively active, and class

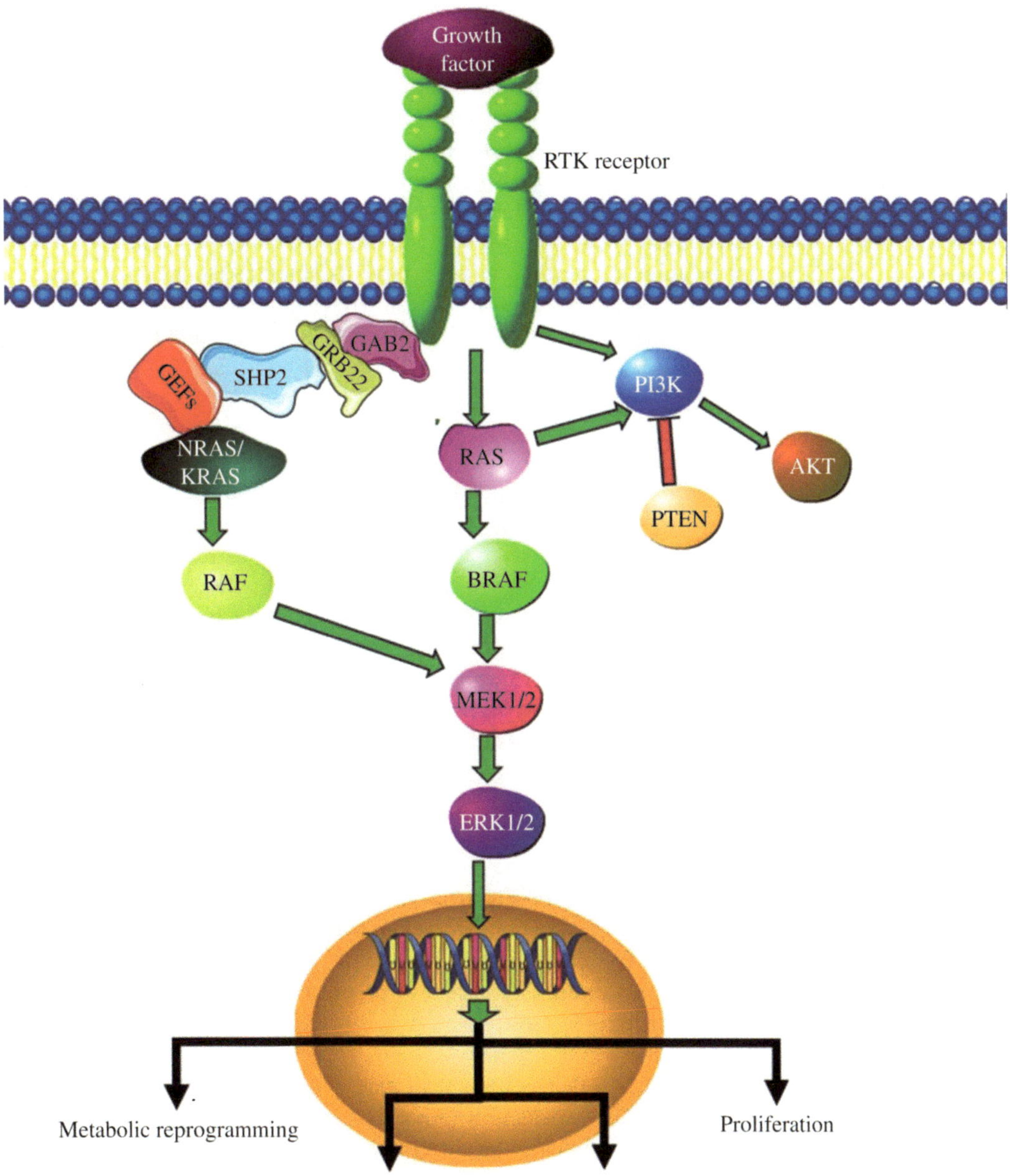

FIGURE 7.1 BRAF, KRAS, and NRAS signaling pathways: The BRAF protein is a proto-oncogene that plays a role in initiating the MEK ERK signaling pathway, which stimulates cell growth. In melanoma, mutations in the *braf* gene lead to a protein that is constitutively active, leading to increased cell proliferation, metabolic reprogramming, differentiation, and cell growth. The same is true of the KRAS and NRAS proteins, which initiate the MEK ERK pathway through a separate signaling pathway initiated through receptor tyrosine kinase signaling.

III mutations have decreased activity or are inactive (Lin et al., 2019). Mutations in *braf* are also associated with melanomas that originate in areas of the skin that receive high doses of UV in the form of sunlight. In other words, areas of the skin are commonly damaged through sunburn (Houben et al., 2004).

Mutant BRAF protein is constitutively active, resulting in continued activation of the MAPK cascade and ERK, resulting in continuous proliferative signaling. BRAF is a good drug target since most melanomas only contain *braf* mutations without having concomitant mutations in other genes in this signaling pathway, such as *kras* and *nras*. However, *pten* and *braf* mutations are found to occur together in up to 10% of all melanomas (Guhan et al., 2021; Newton-Bishop et al., 2020; Pimiento et al., 2013). Mutations in RAS family members, located upstream of BRAF, such as KRAS and NRAS, were some of the genes initially identified to be mutated in melanoma. These small GTP-binding proteins are known to play an important role in signaling pathways that control proliferative differentiation and can result in metabolic reprogramming. As such *kras* mutations are found in 20–30% of melanomas, making them the second most common mutation associated with the development and progression of melanomas. The presence of NRAS mutant proteins is common in aggressive melanomas isolated from elderly patients with UV-damaged skin (Guhan et al., 2021). These NRAS mutant melanomas are more aggressive than BRAF mutant melanomas, with greater Breslow thickness and higher rates of proliferation (Pimiento et al., 2013).

Microphthalmia-Associated Transcription Factor

Another gene that is commonly mutated in melanoma is the microphthalmia-associated transcription factor (*mitf*). This is a melanocyte-specific transcription factor and plays a crucial role in the normal development of melanocytes, ensuring the survival of the melanocyte cell lineage. MITF can activate and regulate the expression of over 100 target genes, and as such, it can regulate differentiation, proliferation, migration, senescence, and initiate survival signaling in melanocytes by inducing the expression of proteins such as BCL2A1, BCL2, and BIRC7 (**Figure 7.2**) (Hartman and Czyz, 2013, 2015b). Transcripts of *mitf* can be alternately spliced to give rise to several isoforms with different N-termini and are expressed in different tissues, with the shortest isoform being expressed solely in melanocytes and melanoma cells (Tassabehji et al., 1994), as is a variant known as the MITF-Model, which contains two in-frame deletions (Wang et al., 2010). The protein forms a homodimer with another MITF or a heterodimer with MiT (Hemesath et al., 1994).

Mutations known to occur within the *mitf* gene include single base substitutions (Hartman and Czyz, 2015a), single nucleotide polymorphisms (Garraway et al., 2005), and a gain-of-function oncogenic $MITF^{E318K}$ variant that is present in familial melanoma patients (Bertolotto et al., 2011; Yokoyama et al., 2011). Mutant MITF acts as a specific type of oncogene known as a lineage-survival oncogene, contributing to abnormal and excessive proliferation of melanocytes. BRAF, KRAS, and NRAS mutants are oncogenic due to them gaining new oncogenic activities, while MITF mutant proteins lose their ability to be regulated. These deregulated proteins then over activate downstream proliferative signaling that is present in normal melanocytes (Pimiento et al., 2013). Increased expression of MITF is associated with a poor prognosis and the development of chemoresistance (Lee et al., 2024). Alterations in the alternative splicing of the *mitf* mRNA are also altered in melanoma. Some of these splice variants can aberrantly activate MEK1-pathway without accompanying *braf* or *kras* mutations (Primot et al., 2010). The regulation of MITF activity is controlled through various signaling pathways that control its transcription and subcellular localization. These include the WNT, CREB, MAPK, p21, and alpha MSH pathways. Mutations in the individual components of these pathways, such as SOX10 (sex-determining region Y-box 10), have been identified in some melanomas. In some cases, *mitf* and *sox10* mutations occur in a mutually exclusive manner (Cronin et al., 2009).

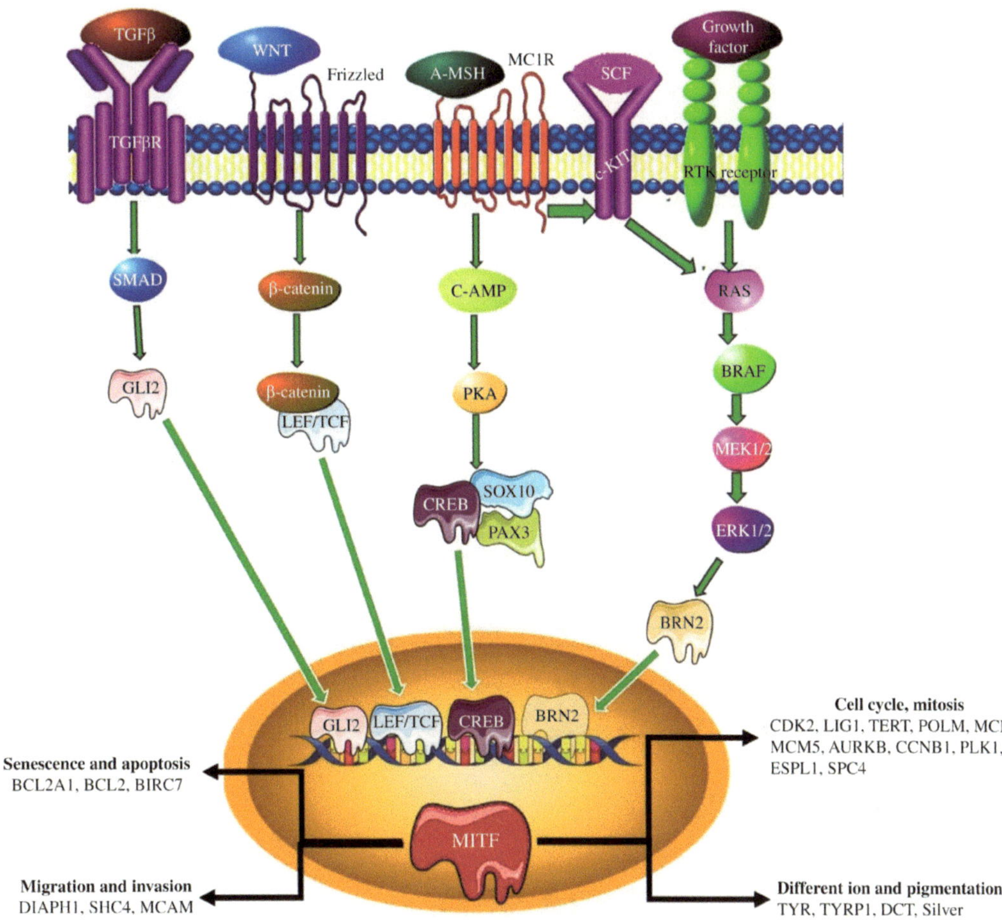

FIGURE 7.2 **Microphthalmia-associated transcription factor (MITF) signaling pathways.** MITF is a transcription factor that is activated by multiple signaling pathways. Once activated, MITF initiates the transcription of various genes that activate progression through the cell cycle, and regulates the expression of genes involved in the development survival and function of melanocytes. MITF forms a dimer to bind DNA and acts as a transcription factor for a plethora of target genes.

Mixed Cancer Syndromes (MCS)

Mixed cancer syndromes (MCS) are familial conditions related to a single or multiple genetic mutations that can predispose individuals to develop various cancers. The hereditary causes of melanomas have been found to be linked to specific patterns of mutations and malignancies. This has resulted in the development of the term melanoma tumor syndromes (Soura et al., 2016). Melanoma is one of the various malignancies that is linked to the BAP1 tumor predisposition syndrome (BAP1-TPDS). This syndrome is inherited, with the majority of those with the syndrome having parents with the syndrome as well. This syndrome centers around mutations in the tumor suppressor gene, BRCA1 associated protein 1 (*bap1*). Melanoma is the third most common type of cancer associated with mutations in this gene (Pilarski et al., 2022). The inactivation of BAP1 due to mutations in the *bap1* gene gives rise to BAP1-inactivated melanocytoma (BIM). BAP1 is a deubiquitinase that plays a role in regulating multiple cellular activities, including cell cycle regulation, chromatin remodeling, DNA damage response, differentiation, senescence, and cell death (**Figure 7.3A**) (Wiesner et al., 2011). In many of these processes, BAP1 plays a role in mitotic spindle formation, and its inactivation in cancer cells can contribute to mitotic abnormalities and chromosomal instability

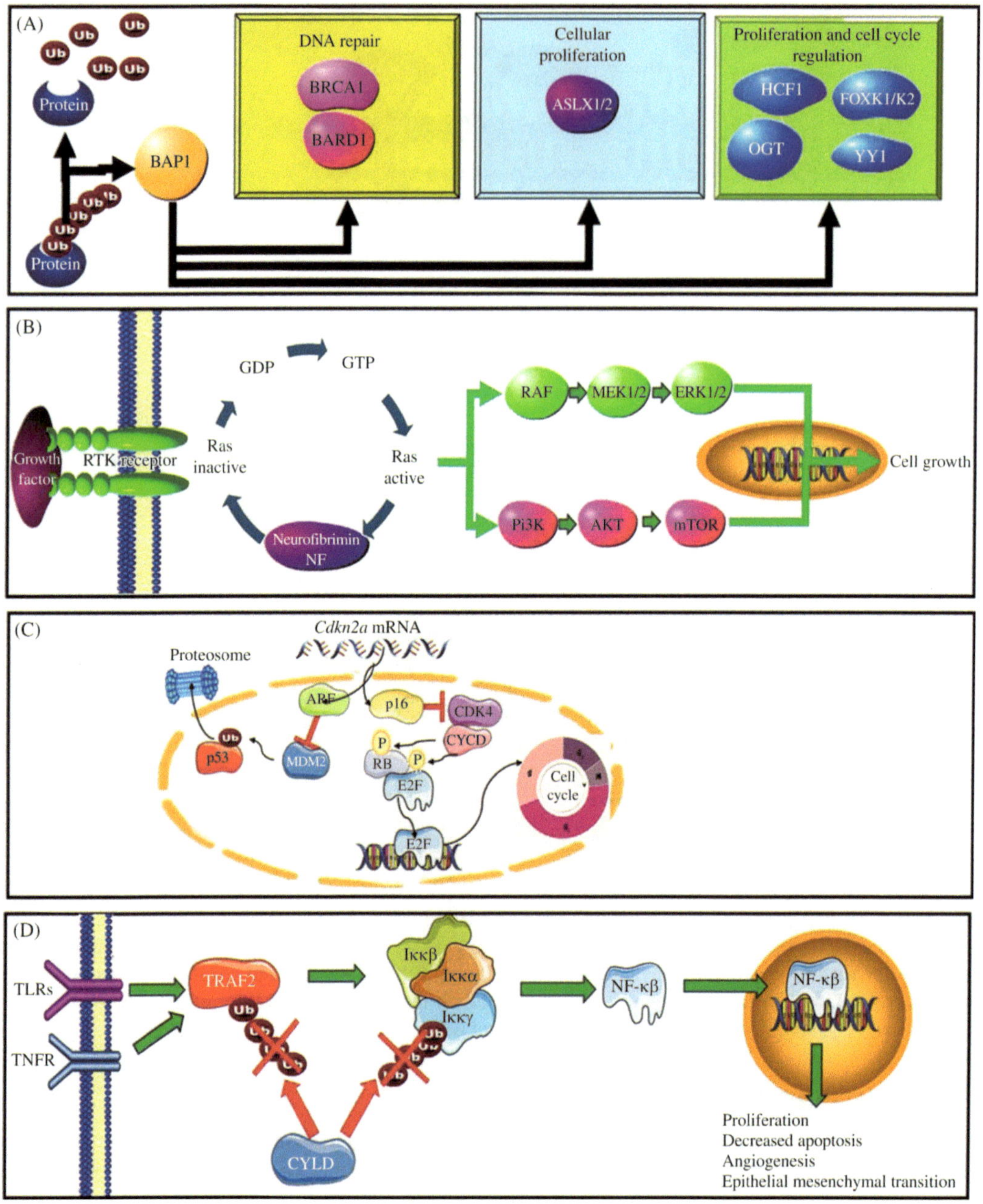

FIGURE 7.3 Signaling in mixed cancer syndromes (MCS). (A) BAP1 tumor predisposition syndrome. BRCA1 associated protein-1 (ubiquitin carboxy-terminal functions as a deubiquitinating enzyme and regulates the amount of ubiquitinated Histone H2A Nucleosomes bound to their promoters and regulates gene expression. (B) Neurofibromatosis 1 (NF1) Signaling pathway. NF1 negatively regulates the ability of the RAS protein to activate the MEK signaling pathway. (C) Familial atypical multiple mole-melanoma (FAMMM) syndrome involves mutations in the *csjn2a* gene, which is spliced to give rise to two gene products. One of which ARF negatively regulates a negative regulator of the tumor suppressor p53. The other protein product, p16, regulates the activity of the E2F transcription factor, which induces the expression of genes that promote progression through the cell cycle. Another gene that is mutated in this pathway is *cycdk4*. (D) CYLD cutaneous syndrome (CCS) is a deubiquitylation enzyme that negatively regulates the activation of NF-κβ.

(Patel et al., 2017; Zarrizi et al., 2014). Mutations in other genes are also found in this syndrome. These commonly include mutations in *braf* and less often in *kras* and *nras* (Donati et al., 2020).

Another mutation leading to its own tumor predisposition syndrome is mutations in the protection of telomerase 1 (*pot1*), which is inherited through autosomal dominant inheritance. The POT1-TPD syndrome leads to an increase in the lifetime risk of melanoma (Henry et al., 2022). In addition to regulating telomere function, POT1 inhibits the DNA damage response pathway from being activated incorrectly (Aramburu et al., 2020, 2022). Mutations in the *pot1* gene resulted in altered telomere length and the development of cancer (Simonin-Wilmer et al., 2023).

Neurofibromatosis 1 (NF1), a disorder that is inherited through autosomal dominant inheritance. The disorder mainly affects the nervous system, but it is also associated with pathologies in other tissues, making it a multisystem disorder. Previously it was known as von Recklinghausen's disease, and along with neurofibromatosis 2, these syndromes can predispose individuals to benign and malignant tumors (Tamura, 2021). NF1 manifests as cutaneous and skeletal abnormalities, and in terms of visible phenotype, it can cause pigment spots and freckles of skinfolds (Uusitalo et al., 2015). NF1 is an autosomal dominant inherited disorder, and I linked to aggressive tumors that are more likely to have a poor prognosis (Friedman, 1993; Guhan et al., 2021). NF1 is the result of mutations in *neurofibromin*. This gene is large and consists of 57 constitutive exons, which are known to give rise to three differently spliced variants (Gutmann et al., 1991). Neurofibromin is active in the Ras pathway, where it acts as a negative regulator of the Ras pathway and as such plays a role in the regulation of cell survival, proliferation, and differentiation (**Figure 7.3B**) (Peltonen et al., 2017).

The first syndrome described as being associated with melanoma is familial atypical multiple mole-melanoma (FAMMM syndrome), which was described as early as 1820. The syndrome is associated with an extremely high nevus count. The patient also has a family history of melanoma (Soura et al., 2016). FAMMM syndrome-associated melanomas are more prone to superficial spreading and invasive nodular melanomas, which are more deadly and aggressive (Ford et al., 1995). This syndrome is associated with germline missense or nonsense mutations in *cdkn2a*. The *cdkn2a* mRNA is alternately spliced to give rise to two proteins, p16 and p14ARF. Both these proteins act as tumor suppressor proteins by either suppressing the transcription of genes that promote G1-to-S transition or preventing the degradation of p53 (Figure 7.3C) (Marzuka-Alcalá et al., 2014). Another gene that is commonly mutated in the FAMMM syndrome is cyclin dependent kinase 4 (*cdk4*). Mutations in this gene are far rarer than mutations in *cdkn2a4* (Puntervoll et al., 2013). CDK4 is the direct target for p16, which inhibits its ability to bind to CYCD, which in turn phosphorylates RB, leading to RB releasing the transcription factor E2F. The mutant variants of CDK4 are unable to bind to p16 **(Figure 7.3C)** (Molven et al., 2005).

CYLD cutaneous syndrome (CCS) is another genetic syndrome associated with multiple skin cancers including melanoma, cylindromas, spiradenomas, trichoepitheliomas, and (infrequently) membranous basal cell adenoma of the salivary gland. This syndrome is caused by germline mutations of *cylindromatosis* (*cyld*) (Dubois and Rajan, 1993). CYLD is a deubiquitinase and acts as a tumor suppressor, and its expression is suppressed in malignant melanoma by the SNAIL1 transcriptional repressor. Decreased CTKD expression or activity is associated with increased proliferation, increased migration, accelerated tumor growth, and development of tumors at an earlier age (de Jel et al., 2019). CYLD regulates genes involved in proliferation, migration, and angiogenesis (**Figure 7.3D**) (Dubois and Rajan, 1993).

PROTEOMICS

Proteomics involves studying proteins on a large scale and normally refers to the characterization of the entire protein population of a cell, tissue organ, or even organism. The proteome represents the observed phenotype and is the result of all genomic, transcriptomic and epigenomic changes, alterations, and interactions. As such the proteome can be considered as a more appropriate means of studying the final phenotype of a tumor (Gil et al., 2019). Traditionally, proteomics was a far less attractive route for the identification of new biomarkers. This was due to the comparative difficulty involved in the application of high-throughput techniques to the proteome. This is largely due to the chemical composition of proteins contributing to the difficulty in the qualitative and quantitative analysis of proteins. Initial proteomic studies relied on low-throughput techniques such as immunohistochemistry and western blot. These techniques were limited in that they examined single proteins and required the existence of antibodies to that protein (Macklin et al., 2020). Immunohistochemistry is used in the diagnosis and classification of melanomas through the use of antibodies against various proteins, such as the S100 family, Ki-67, preferentially expressed antigen in melanoma (PRAME), HMB45, and SOX10. These proteins all serve as biomarkers for advanced or metastatic melanoma, and there are no biomarkers that are currently used for the diagnosis of early-stage melanoma using immunohistochemistry (Hessler et al., 2020).

In addition to this, the accuracy of diagnoses or clinical stratification of heterogeneous melanomas requires the use of patterns of the expression of multiple biomarkers. This is especially true since the progression of melanoma may require mutations in multiple genes, leading to the expression of multiple altered proteins or aberrant protein expression patterns. As such, diagnosis and characterization would require expression data for multiple protein biomarkers (Shain et al., 2018). The detection and use of protein biomarkers, as well as the study of proteomics, have been revolutionized by the development of new high-throughput techniques. These include protein microarrays and advanced mass spectroscopy techniques, which allow for molecular and proteomic analysis. This has allowed for the characterization of the whole protein complement of specific specimens, tissues, or cells. Samples can also be enriched for specific populations of proteins (Macklin et al., 2020; Sabel et al., 2011).

These techniques can lead to the generation of a large quantity of data, and bioinformatic tools are required to identify protein expression patterns. There are three main bioinformatic workflows that are used to analyze this data. The first of these is the data-dependent acquisition (DDA/IDA) workflow. This involves data that are collected by the mass spectrometer randomly, discarding some while collecting others. Or it will rely on the user to scan and collect data based on user-defined criteria (Defossez et al., 2023). The second common workflow is targeted multiple or selective reaction monitoring (MRM/SRM). This technique targets individual peptide sequences to establish the presence and level of proteins that contain these peptide sequences (Fu et al., 2016). The final commonly used technique for the bioinformatic analysis of mass spectrometry data is data-independent acquisition (DIA). This method uses a second stage of mass spectrometry to analyze a specific subset of ions that fall within a range of mass/charge ratios (Ludwig et al., 2018). DIA is especially useful when being used to discover novel proteins, which in turn allows for the identification of new signaling pathways that play a role in the development and progression of melanoma.

Table 7.2 reviews some melanoma proteomic studies over the past 10 years (2015–2024). The table shows a general shift in the type of study. Earlier studies focused on a smaller number of proteins examining expression changes in a smaller number of proteins. Later studies have shifted to a high-throughput analysis of whole proteomes. Large-scale studies using mass spectrometry to examine whole proteomes of melanoma with or without 2D PAGE have identified novel proteins from metastatic melanoma. These studies have led to the identification of various biomarkers for the progression from primary to malignant metastatic melanoma, such as MDA-9 and GRP78 (Guan et al., 2015); differential expression of FASN and 14-3-3ε (Dowling et al., 2016), serum markers such as RGN, STX7, MTHFD1L, S100A6 (Byström et al., 2017) as well as serum vitronectin and dermcidin (Ortega-Martínez et al., 2016).

The upregulation of V-type proteins, cell adhesion, transporter, and exchanger proteins was identified as a biomarker for poor prognosis (Zila et al., 2018). Other potential prognostic biomarkers include vimentin, nestin, fibronectin, annexin A1, dipeptidyl peptidase IV, and histone H2A1B. These biomarkers may also serve as treatment targets (Aebersold and Mann, 2016). While markers for specific types of melanomas have been identified, such as collagen α3 (VI) and HSPβ1 as biomarkers for uveal metastasis (Trilla-Fuertes et al., 2019).

TABLE 7.2
Proteomic Studies of Melanoma in the Past Ten Years

	Samples					Methods			
Study Details	**FFPE**	**Cell Lines**	**Blood**	**Fresh Tissue**			**DDA**	**DIA**	**Reference**
Identified 13,176 protein-coding genes correlated with 366,172 peptides, 52,000 phosphorylation sites, and 4,400 acetylation sites. The study also reported 12,751 gene products	X	X	X		Malignant melanoma	LC-MS/MS	X	X	Betancourt et al. (2021)
Identified 18 peptides unique to benign naevi and 197 peptides unique to malignant melanoma	X				Benign naevi Malignant melanoma	MSI			Casadonte et al. (2021)
8,100 proteins identified in melanoma cell lines		X			Malignant melanoma	LC-MS.MS		X	Gao et al. (2021)
Identified 2,750 proteins, 16 of which whose expression is different between malignant and non-malignant melanoma	X				Primary melanoma	LC-MS			Shapanis et al. (2020)
Creation of HGMS classification model to distinguish between benign naevi and malignant melanoma	X				Benign naevi Malignant melanoma	HGMS/ MS–MALDI-TOF			Lazova et al. (2020)
Identified 6,000 proteins with variable expression levels between primary and metastatic tumors		X		X	Primary and Metastatic melanoma	LC-MS/MS	X		Gil et al. (2019)
Identified 2,527 unique proteins with ectosomes as metastatic uveal melanoma biomarkers		X			Primary uveal melanoma	LC-MS/MS	X		Surman et al. (2019)
Identified 4,006 protein groups, and relationship between genomic mutation and proteomics identified 17 proteins identified to be expressed in samples with different genetic mutations (*braf, nraf*)	X				Primary melanoma	LC-MS/MS	X		Trilla-Fuertes et al. (2019)
Identified 10 antibodies that can be used as diagnostic method for early melanoma			X		Malignant melanoma	Protein microarray			Zaenker et al. (2018)
Identified 5,977 proteins that play a role in epithelial-mesenchymal transition	X			X	Metastatic melanoma	LC-MS/MS	X		Zila et al. (2018)

(Continued)

TABLE 7.2 *(Continued)*
Proteomic Studies of Melanoma in the Past Ten Years

	Samples					Methods			
Study Details	**FFPE**	**Cell Lines**	**Blood**	**Fresh Tissue**			**DDA**	**DIA**	**Reference**
MSI can be used as a diagnostic tool	X				Benign naevus Metastatic melanoma	MSI			Lazova et al. (2017)
Identification of diagnostic proteins in the blood			X		Malignant melanoma	IC-MS			Byström et al. (2017)
Progression of melanoma predicted by serum proteins			X		Melanoma *in situ* Malignant melanoma	LC-MS/MS			Ortega-Martínez et al. (2016)
Identification of pathways that may lead to progression to metastatic melanoma	X				Melanoma *in situ* Malignant melanoma	LC-MS/MS			Dowling et al. (2016)
Prognostic markers for metastatic melanoma				X	Primary melanoma Metastatic melanoma	MALDI-TOF MS			Guan et al. (2015)
Potential markers for uveal melanoma progression				X	Uveal primary metastatic melanoma	LC-MS/MS			Trilla-Fuertes et al. (2019)

PROTEOGENOMICS

Since proteins are the downstream products of the genome and transcriptome, the relationship between genomic changes and accompanying changes in the proteome is obvious. For instance, Neurofibromin is normally expressed ubiquitously across tissues and cell types. This expression changes across different tissues. In a percentage of melanoma (~18%) the expression of Neurofibromin is completely absent, while it is merely reduced in the majority of melanomas. This decrease in the expression of the protein occurs in melanomas with both *braf* and *neurofibromin* mutations (Maertens et al., 2013). Immunohistochemical analysis of melanoma biopsies demonstrated both decreases in the expression of BAP1 as well as decreased nuclear staining. BIM syndrome is also associated with clumps of inactive BAP1 proteins. While some of these changes in BAP1 expression are associated with mutations in the *bap1* gene, there are other cases where the loss of nuclear BAP1 expression is not associated with mutations in both alleles of *bap1* (Wiesner et al., 2012). This could potentially be due to epigenetic changes or genomic mutations that fall outside of the coding region that have not been identified (Wiesner et al., 2012). Genomic changes can be used to predict the primary structure of the protein, i.e., the amino acid sequence. Proteomic analysis can be used to determine characteristics of the protein, such as post-translation modifications. The determination of differences in the expression levels of proteins across different tissues or cell locations and how these change with the development and progression of disease is also a vital function of proteomics (Kuhlman and Bradley, 2019). However, other proteomic influences on the final phenotype are difficult to predict. These include characteristics that rely on protein-protein interaction and environmental effects and stimuli. The similar interrelated information shared across the genome, transcriptome, and proteome needs to be integrated with each other as well as with complementary information (Zhu et al., 2024).

The field of proteogenomics aims to integrate the various data obtained from genomic, transcriptomic, and proteomic analysis. This includes information related to the identification of aspects within these omics and other datasets, both qualitative and quantitative data. This information can be used to identify mutations and/or single amino acid variants associated with the stage, subtype, and treatment response of melanoma, thereby allowing the disease progression to be tracked and the outcome to be predicted. The use of standard proteomic methods cannot identify many of the sequence variants, such as the identification of DNA sequence variants (mutations, SNPs, etc.), splice variants, single amino acid polymorphisms, and the generation of splice junction peptides. This information requires the integration of this omics data, due to the fact that the interpretation of proteomics data relies on databases that contain the canonical sequences. These databases include Uniprot, Ensembl, and SwissProt. Even databases that contain different proteoforms, such as Uniprot and Trembl, only contain a limited number of variants. In this context, the canonical protein sequence is the longest protein sequence, the sequence of the most abundantly expressed variant or protein-coding gene. Canonical sequence data from these databases can be supplemented with sequence data from other databases such as CanProVar1.2 (Li et al., 2010; Zhang et al., 2017), VarCards3 (Li et al., 2018), and COSMIC4 (Forbes et al., 2017).

In addition to this, alternate frame translation can be used to identify new protein-coding sequences and therefore the amino acid sequence of these new variants. These alternate frames include the use of six-frame translation in genomic DNA sequences where the three possible reading frames are translated in both directions on the strand. Alternate three reading frames can only be applied in one direction (Zhu et al., 2018). Yet another technique to analyze the integrated data is to use the genomic and transcriptomic data from a single sample to predict the protein sequence variants (Low et al., 2013).

The identification of mutations that are expressed at the protein/phenotype level only occurs once in every million base pairs in melanoma (Motwani and Eccles, 2021). This makes these altered proteins extremely valuable for various applications, such as biomarkers or drug targets. For instance, these altered protein variants allow for the development of drug resistance, a growing problem in the treatment of melanoma. Proteogenomics would facilitate the identification of variants associated with the development of resistance, allowing for these variants to be targeted to counter resistance or as biomarkers to detect and track the development of resistance to particular treatments (Mani et al., 2022). For example, although the targeting of mutant BRAF and KRAS in malignant melanoma using drugs such as vemurafenib or dabrafenib is an effective treatment strategy, patients rapidly develop resistance to these drugs. The basis of this development likely relies on the development of proteins with somatic mutations (Salemi et al., 2018). By using a proteogenomic approach, protein variants created by coding mutations were identified in cell lines derived from malignant melanoma. These protein sequences were identified by combining exonic and proteomic data while minimizing false negatives and positives. Initially, proteomic data were analyzed to identify amino acid sequence changes in samples obtained from lymph node metastatic melanomas. This led to the identification of numerous proteins with single amino acid changes. Members of the poly ADP-ribose polymerases (the PARP protein family) were amongst those identified. These proteins play a role in the replication of DNA, mRNA transcription, and chromatin modification in these processes (Salemi et al., 2018).

The presence of these mutations and single amino acid substitutions in PARPs was identified using MS/MS peptide spectra. One of the mutations detected in PARP-4 involves a threonine being substituted for a proline residue at position 1328 and an alanine for a threonine at position 1265. In PARP-9, a mutation was identified resulting in a change from a tyrosine to a cysteine at position 493 (Kamaletdinova et al., 2019). PARP inhibitors are known to effectively target BRCA1/2-deficient cancers and are therefore considered as an effective cancer treatment and are being investigated for the treatment of melanomas (Musella et al., 2018; Papeo et al., 2013; Plummer et al., 2013). These PARP mutations also demonstrate the concept of synthetic lethality, where a cell can survive the effects of a single mutation but not the co-occurrence of multiple mutations is lethal for the cell (Helleday, 2011). PARP inhibitors also increase the effectiveness of DNA-damaging agents (Musella et al., 2018). Resistance to PARP inhibitors has been observed, and the aforementioned single amino acid mutations are implicated in the development of this resistance (Montoni et al., 2013; Schlacher, 2017).

Establishing the role of these mutations in melanoma development and progression relies on linking the genetic mutations to changes in protein expression levels and function. This relies on co-expression correlation analysis between the presence of the mutation and changes in protein expression levels and activity. Due to post-transcriptional regulation, regulation of translation, post-translational modification, and mRNA and protein degradation, there is only a mid-level correlation between genomic sequence changes and the phenotype (Schwanhäusser et al., 2011). Various statistical methods have been developed to identify somatic or germline mutations or chromosomal aberrations that can change the expression levels of the protein and identify the role of these changes in melanoma development, diagnosis, and progression. Multivariate statistics perform dimension reduction to integrate various heterogeneous omics molecular profiles. These statistics are then used to create a model to predict various outcomes such as survival or treatment efficiency. The models for diagnosis are, such as melanoma classification and staging. Some of these multivariate statistical tests include non-negative matrix factorization algorithm (Ray et al., 2017), joint non-negative matrix factorization (Zhang et al., 2011), and the mixOmics R package (Rohart et al., 2017).

A useful gene expression analysis method involves the creation of compound co-expression networks using correlation or partial correlation. These networks contain clusters of co-expressed genes grouped by biological function in a hierarchical function. That is more specific functions that contribute to a larger, more generalized function. This is known as functional coherence (van Dam et al., 2018). Another useful type of model is the Graphical Gaussian Model (GGM). The Network-based Integration of Multi-omics Data (NetICS) prioritizes cancer gene mutations and expression data in a computational framework to integrate diverse types of omics data. This tool builds a directed functional interaction network to classify events that contribute to the development and progression of cancer (Dimitrakopoulos et al., 2018).

OTHER OMICS

Genomics and proteomics are not the only important omics technologies that are being studied for the diagnosis, prognosis, monitoring, and treatment of melanoma. Microbiomics describes the populations of various microbes that are present within the patient. This is due to the microbiome altering the immune response, while the skin microbiome changes in response to the development and progression of melanoma.

Epigenomics

Epigenetic factors such as DNA methylation are important factors in regulating gene expression and linking genes to protein expression. Epigenomics is the omics study involved in the characterization of all the epigenetic modifications within the cell (Hatzimichael et al., 2014; Hsu et al., 2021).

DNA methylation is now thought to drastically alter protein expression and influence the development of various diseases such as cancer (Fernandez et al., 2012; Jones and Baylin, 2002). Methylation of DNA is associated with the silencing of genes, regardless of whether these genes are tumor suppressors or oncogenes. Decreased methylation is associated with genomic instability that can potentially activate oncogenes (Litovkin et al., 2015; Paska and Hudler, 2015; Weisenberger, 2014). Genome-wide expression studies have shown that the melanoma is associated with abnormal methylation. Potentially these altered methylation patterns can be used as biomarkers for melanoma diagnosis, treatment, and progression (Fu et al., 2017). Genes that are hypermethylated in melanoma include *line01, cldn11, tert, mgmt, kit, tnf, mitf, rassf6, rassf10, cpx3, mmp9, synpo2, cdkn1c, lxn, asc, col11a1, socs1, caspase 8, cdh1, mgmt., rar-b2, cita-piv, sos2, tnfrsf10c, tpm1, tpm3, cdkn2a, dppiv, frzb, socs3, thbs1,* and *tm* (Fu et al., 2017). DNA methylation can also be used as a prognostic biomarker for individuals with stage III melanoma. The level of methylation using genome-wide methylation profiles can be used to separate patients into a group with a more favorable outcome and a group with a less favorable survival outcome. The group with the more favorable outcome was characterized by a lower density of DNA methylation (Sigalotti et al., 2012).

Specific histone variants also play a specific role in melanoma. These variants are macroH2A, H2A.Z, and H3.3. MacroH2A plays a role in the regulation of genes that play a role in cell proliferation, and as such, it suppresses melanoma development and progression (Konstantinov et al., 2016). In melanoma, the expression of MacroH2A is suppressed or even lost (Kapoor et al., 2010). Conversely, the expression of H2A.Z.2 and H3.3 is increased in melanoma, where they promote the expression of genes responsible for the proliferation of melanoma (Ávila-López et al., 2021). Noncoding RNAs (ncRNAs) regulate the expression of genes in various ways; microRNAs typically regulate the stability and translation of mRNA, and long noncoding RNAs (lncRNAs) modulate gene expression in various ways, including regulating translation, protein activity and stability, and protein localization, among others. Studies have revealed a large number of lncRNAs that are upregulated in melanoma and a lower number of lncRNAs that were downregulated in melanoma (Guo et al., 2021). The lncRNA SAMMSON is associated with the expression of MITF and is present at higher levels in melanoma (Leucci et al., 2016). Other lncRNAs that are massively overexpressed in melanoma include UCA1 and MALAT-1. It has also been noted that the levels of these lncRNAs are associated with the stage of melanoma (Lazăr et al., 2020).

The expression of a large number of miRNAs was altered in melanoma (Neagu et al., 2020). RNA sequencing of benign and malignant naevi revealed six miRNAs that could be used to differentiate benign naevi from melanoma. These included MIR31-5P; MIR21-5P; MIR211-5P; MIR125A-5P; MIR125B-5P; and MIR100-5P (Torres et al., 2020). The miRNAs let-7e, miR-99b, miR-100, miR-125a, miR-125b, miR-146a, and miR-146b were implicated in the resistance of melanoma to immunotherapy (Huber et al., 2018). The miRNA, miR-221-3p, shows a distinctive pattern of expression in different stages of melanoma, with levels being higher in stage IV than in stage I. Following surgical removal of melanoma tissue, the levels of this miRNA were observed to decrease (Kanemaru et al., 2011).

Microbiomics

It has become apparent that the patient's microbiome plays an important role in the development and progression of cancer, with the microbiome now being considered as a component of the tumor microenvironment. The interactions between cancer cells and the microbiome can influence the metabolism of cancer cells and can also influence the progression and metastasis of the cancer and change the response of the cancer to various treatments (Kovács et al., 2020; Zhao and Hu, 2020). Commensal microbes present in the tissue and where the tumor is, as well as microbes within the tumor's microenvironment, can interact directly with the tumor. The microbes present throughout the body can also affect the tumor through the release of microbial metabolites that can influence the tumor (Xavier et al., 2020).

The most abundant and diverse microbiome in the human body is located in the gut. Through interactions with the immune system and the secretion of microbial metabolites, the gut microbiota can either promote the development of melanoma, or the microbiota may play a protective role against the development of melanoma. This depends on the makeup of the microbial population. Dysbiosis describes a disruption in the normal microbial makeup of the microbiome and is characterized by an increase in harmful microbes and a decrease in beneficial ones. In addition to this, dysbiosis normally represents a decrease in the biodiversity of the gut microbiome. The presence of specific species of bacteria or their metabolites can be used as biomarkers for melanoma progression and prognosis. In addition to this, changing the composition of the microbiome through the use of probiotics or fecal microbial transplants are potential therapeutic strategies to treat melanoma (Kumar et al., 2022).

Additionally, it has become apparent that the skin commensal microbiome plays an important role in promoting or altering skin immunity. The ability of the skin microbiome to promote the immune system may protect an individual against skin inflammatory disorders, infections, wounds, and skin cancer. The influence of the gut microbiome on melanoma is well-studied, while the role of the skin microbiome is less studied and less well understood (Byrd et al., 2018). Altering the composition of the skin microbiome may have a potential therapeutic role in either protecting individuals from developing melanoma or treating melanoma. This can be achieved through the use of health-promoting strains from the microbiome of oral or topical probiotics (Michielin et al., 2019).

Initial studies indicated that the diversity of the skin microbiome is lower in those patients with melanoma compared to those who had melanocytic nevi (Salava et al., 2016). Later studies confirmed that the composition of the skin microbiome is significantly altered in those with melanoma and that the melanoma microbiome was less diverse than the normal skin microbiome (Makaranka et al., 2022). Some of these changes include an increase in the abundance of bacteria of the genera Fusobacterium and Trueperella in melanoma samples. While bacteria of the genus Corynebacterium are associated with the progression of acral melanoma (Kallini et al., 2013). Probiotics and prebiotics have also been shown to play a role in protecting the skin from skin damage caused by UVR (Patra et al., 2020). Probiotics injected into or applied topically to melanomas may lead to the alteration of the tumor's immune microenvironment (Mattia et al., 2018).

RESEARCH DIAGNOSIS, TREATMENT, AND PERSONALIZED MEDICINE

The integration of data from various omics sources, along with the addition of data such as a patient's medical history, demographic, socioeconomic status, and information from the scientific, opens the door to the development of precision medicine for melanoma management. This data could be used to personalize the diagnosis, prognosis, management, and treatment of melanoma for specific populations or even individuals (Valenti et al., 2021). This integration becomes even more complex when it became apparent that multi-omics data cannot be just gathered from a sample representing the whole patient but needs to represent the multi-omics data from the tumor, the tumor microenvironment, the normal tissue surrounding the tissue, and the microenvironment of this surrounding tissue. Omic data also needs to be collected and integrated from sources such as the gut microbiome. This would allow for the modeling of the complex interactions that occur between these various tissues and their microenvironments (Valenti et al., 2021). A large number of genetic mutations and the resulting altered proteins lead to changes in the signaling pathways and molecular interactions within and between these various tissues and microenvironments making the identification of patterns within this data extremely complex in melanoma (Falcone et al., 2020). Figure 7.4 summarizes the use of multi-omic techniques in the research and application of knowledge concerning the underlying molecular causes of melanoma as well as the various ways in which omics technologies can be used to manage the disease. AI is a promising tool to facilitate this integration due to the complex and diverse nature of all this data. Here the AI will use machines and deep learning algorithms to sort, classify, and reduce the complexity of the data. Eventually, AI can learn to recognize patterns within the data that can be associated with various melanoma types, treatment responses, and outcomes, as well as the survival chances of a patient (Poalelungi et al., 2023).

Screening, Diagnosis, and Prognosis

As previously mentioned, one of the main aims of multi-omics research is the identification of biomarkers, whose presence, absence, or expression level can be used to identify patterns that can be used to detect, treat, and manage melanoma. Biomarkers can be used for screening, an important strategy to manage melanoma, as this can identify individuals who are prone to developing multiple melanomas. They can also be used for diagnosis and staging, especially since Breslow thickness and ulceration, the current staging methods, have been proven to be inadequate (Sabel et al., 2011). For instance, melanoma can be differentiated from other cancers using biomarkers such as S100, MART-1, gp100/HMB45, HMB-45, MART-1/Melan-A, tyrosinase, and MITF. S100 is considered to be the most accurate of these markers (Ohsie et al., 2008). Biomarkers can also be used to distinguish benign melanocytic tumors from malignant ones. In this case, the most useful biomarker at present is Ki67. Biomarkers can also be used to stage melanomas, with lactate dehydrogenase (LDH) being used as a marker for stage IV melanoma and, as such, can be used as a prognostic biomarker. Its presence in the serum also means obtaining samples to detect it is noninvasive (Sabel et al., 2011).

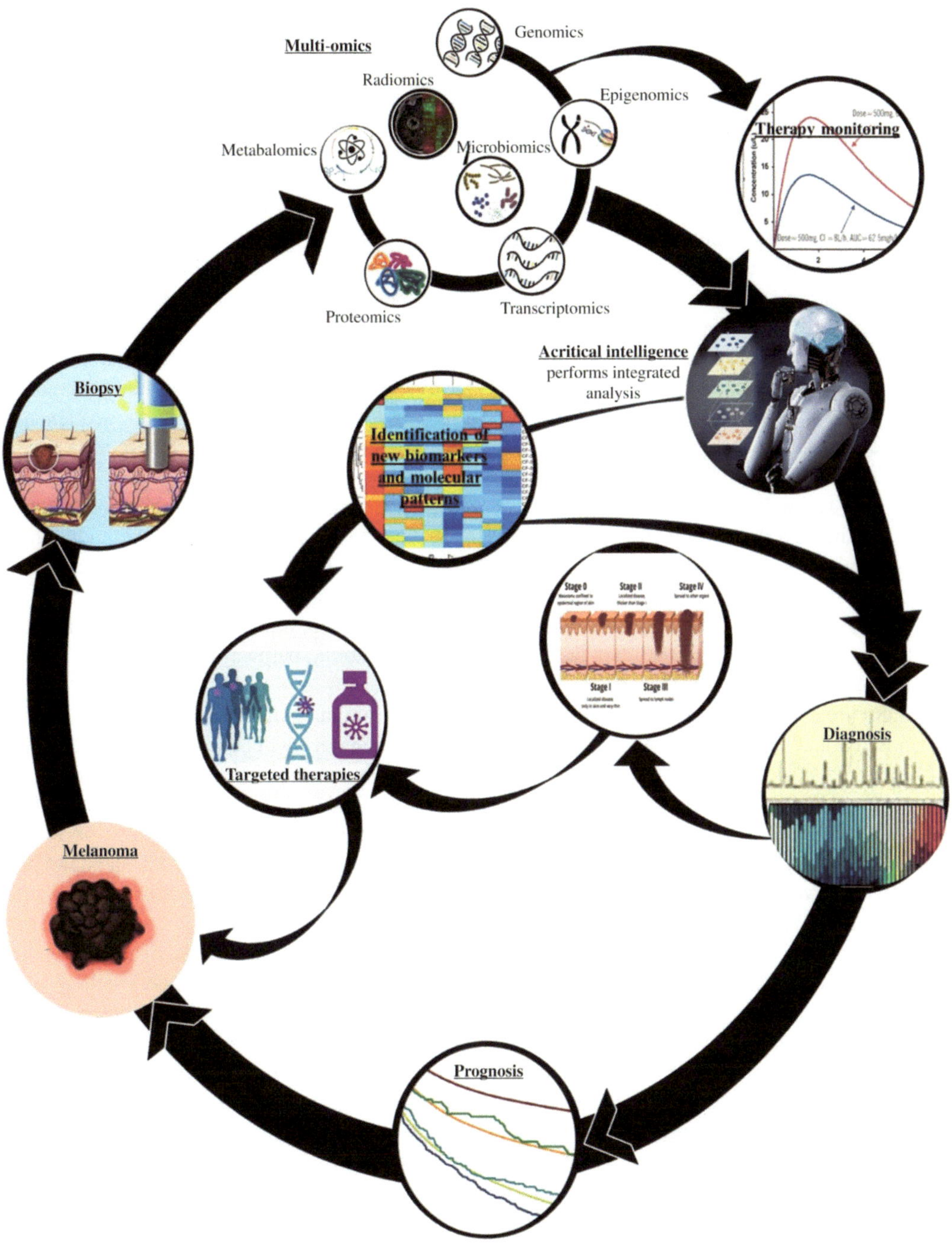

FIGURE 7.4 The application of multi-omics in the research and management of melanoma. Patient biopsies are analyzed using various omics technologies. These results are analyzed by AI. In a research setting, the AI can identify new biomarkers or molecular patterns specific to melanoma types or stages. These can then be used to develop new targeted therapies. In a clinical setting, the AI can identify diagnostic markers to diagnose the disease. The patient's melanoma is assigned a type and staged using these diagnostic markers. At this stage, the correct targeted therapy can be applied based on the stage and type of melanoma. Biomarkers can also be used to make a prognosis. The response to treatment can be monitored by taking another biopsy and performing more omics tests. This collected material can also feed back into the research stream.

Treatment and Research

Selecting the appropriate treatment strategy involves establishing the speed at which the disease is progressing, whether metastasis has occurred, and being able to predict any adverse drug reactions (ADRs). More aggressive melanoma requires more aggressive treatments, such as extra surgical procedures, adjuvant therapies, or the use of different combinations of drugs to increase effectiveness and decrease toxicity. Traditional methods of grouping patients resulted in what was thought to be a homogenous group that would respond in the same way. In reality, each patient is an individual with different genetics, molecular patterns, and risk factors (Sabel et al., 2011). The ability of genetic variations to influence the outcomes of pharmacological treatments means that the identification of the variants and the association with treatment outcomes can improve the safety and efficacy of pharmacological treatments. Personalized medicine in this case would be the use of integrated data (multi-omic as well as other data) to determine what would inform the clinician as to what treatment should be given to a specific patient. Melanomas have genetic changes that dictate the progression and response to treatment of the cancer, but the variations within the germline genetic sequence of the patient must also be taken into consideration when predicting the patient's response to a specific drug (Kang et al., 2020; Wheeler et al., 2013).

Another technology that has advanced research in understanding the heterogeneity of melanoma and the underlying molecular patterns driving melanoma is single-cell omics methods. These techniques can be applied to the field of pharmaco-omics. This field uses the genetic or functional makeup of diseased tissues to guide the implementation of personalized therapeutic strategies for patients. For instance, Raman spectro-microscopy uses spatial mapping of metabolites within a cell to identify new drug targets that can alter signaling and metabolic pathways in a series of patient-derived melanoma cell lines (Du et al., 2020).

ADRs are a leading cause of mortality and illness in melanoma patients, and ADRs are defined by an individual's genotype, age, and gender. They are also obviously dependent on the drug being administered as well as what combinations of drugs are being used and the influence of drug-drug interactions. Finally, they are dependent on the tumor itself, what mutations or changes have driven carcinogenesis and continue to contribute to the progression of the disease (Jenkins and Fisher, 2021). Pharmacogenomics (PGx) combines pharmacology and genomics to try and understand how an individual would process or respond to specific drugs and inform the healthcare provider on the best treatment. Since drug treatments are based on the underlying mechanisms that drive the disease, many of the drugs used to treat melanoma target the BRAF pathway. These drugs are known to have predictable responses to treatment across patients but are also known to be less than ideal when it comes to effective responses across different patients. In contrast, immunotherapies used to target melanoma are unpredictable in their adverse effects but are a more effective treatment (Helgadottir et al., 2018; Jenkins and Fisher, 2021; Tarhini et al., 2019).

The greater understanding of the underlying biology of melanoma can be greatly increased through the use of multi-omic methods to identify new genes, gene products, and key molecular pathways that play a role in melanoma development and progression. The design of drugs to target these differences between normal tissue and melanoma can play a significant role in the effective treatment of melanoma (Griewank et al., 2014; Valenti et al., 2021).

LIMITATIONS

One of the main limitations in omics research is the quality of the nucleic or proteins extracted from samples. In many cases, biomolecules that are present at lower levels may be absent from or under-represented in the sample. This used to be a greater problem when formalin-fixed paraffin-embedded (FFPE) samples were used. This is especially true for proteomic studies where the formaldehyde can interfere with the protein extraction and the quality of the extracted proteins due to crosslinking and fixation. However, techniques to reliably extract protein samples for proteomic analysis have been developed (Magdeldin and Yamamoto, 2012; Shields et al., 2016).

In terms of limitations in the acquisition of proteomic data obtained through mass spectrometry, DIA has distinct advantages over DDA, being able to analyze a large number of proteins, similar to DDA, but with the added ability to be as sensitive as targeted mass spectrometry. However, the complex MS/MS spectra generated by DIA are difficult to interpret. Methods that have been proposed to solve this include windowed DIA methods. These involve segmenting the mass charge spectra. Following these statistical methods, like Pearson's distribution, to analyze mass charge spectra over a specific range, reducing spectral complexity (Lou and Shui, 2024). The collection, analysis, and storage of multi-omic data leads to concerns regarding the privacy of patient data and ethical issues surrounding its use. These issues are increased when AI is used to automate the analysis of this data, as clinicians and patients cannot always be sure as to what the AI is doing by acting as a black box.

The development of targeted therapies has been guided by the identification of the genetic and proteomic profiles involved in the development of melanoma as well as its malignant transformation to identify novel therapeutic targets (Bhatia et al., 2009; Domingues et al., 2018). Targeted therapies based on the use of omics data may have drawbacks that arise due to an incomplete understanding of the diverse interactions they take part in. One of the most promising treatments for melanoma is the use of BRAF inhibitors. The toxicity of therapies targeting BRAF can be increased by the use of radiation therapy (Patel et al., 2020). Another drawback to the use of these targeted therapies is the development of resistance during treatment (Luke et al., 2017; Schadendorf et al., 2018). In patients with metastatic melanoma, treatment with novel targeted therapies has led to an improved prognosis for these patients; however, the duration of the effective response to these treatments is limited due to the development of resistance (Davis et al., 2019). Melanoma, like all cancers, is a complex and heterogeneous disease that changes over time. The disease can be influenced by factors such as changes in protein expression influenced by changes in the metabolome, microbiome, cancer and normal tissue, population, environmental, and socioeconomic influences (Su et al., 2022). These problems require the identification of new biomarkers and potential targets as well as a greater understanding of the signaling pathways these molecules take part in.

CONCLUSION

Multi-omics technologies are proving to be a powerful tool for the identification of new biomarkers and therapeutic targets for the diagnosis, treatment, and study of melanoma. As in the Central Dogma, genomics provides the starting point for the study of the molecular basis of melanoma, while the proteome is the endpoint representing the observable phenotype resulting from the individual's genetic code. While the study of genomics and proteomics on their own provides useful information that can be applied to the effective prevention and management of melanoma, the integration of proteomics and genomics will give a more comprehensive overview of the molecular mechanisms involved in the development and progression of melanoma. However, other layers of gene expression regulation exist between the genome and the proteome. These include the epigenome (DNA modifications that do not affect the gene sequence), the transcriptome, the metabolome (chemicals that are by-products of metabolism), and finally the microbiome. The integrated analysis of the genome and the proteome, known as proteogenomics, accompanied with the integration of information from other omics sources such as metabolomics, epigenomics, and microbiomics, will allow researchers to be able to identify the molecular and physiological changes that drive melanoma development and progression.

This integrated approach allows for the identification of biomarkers that can be used to screen individuals and identify high-risk individuals who can then take steps to prevent the development of melanoma. Biomarkers can also be identified for use in the diagnosis, staging, and classification of melanoma. The classification and staging of melanoma will help in the selection of the appropriate treatment strategy and inform the clinician as to the probable outcome and prognosis. When applied to treatment, the biomarkers identified through multi-omics can be used to monitor treatment response and be used to fine-tune treatment plans. Since these biomarkers are molecules or microbes whose levels or abundance are different between healthy skin, benign naevi, primary melanoma, and metastatic melanoma, they can also be used to identify the molecular pathways involved in the various stages and types of melanomas. This provides a new avenue for the development of treatments that target either these molecular pathways or the individual components of the various signaling pathways. The integration of the complex data obtained from the various omics technologies requires the development and application of new AI models that use machine learning and deep learning algorithms. All these large complex datasets and analysis techniques will guide research into the underlying causes and drivers of melanoma into a new promising era.

REFERENCES

Aebersold, R. and Mann, M. 2016. Mass-spectrometric exploration of proteome structure and function, *Nature*, 537, pp. 347–355.

Aramburu, T., Kelich, J., Rice, C. and Skordalakes, E. 2022. POT1-TPP1 binding stabilizes POT1, promoting efficient telomere maintenance, *Computational and Structural Biotechnology Journal*, 20, pp. 675–684.

Aramburu, T., Plucinsky, S. and Skordalakes, E. 2020. POT1-TPP1 telomere length regulation and disease, *Computational and Structural Biotechnology Journal*, 18, pp. 1939–1946.

Artomov, M., Stratigos, A. J., Kim, I., Kumar, R., Lauss, M., Reddy, B. Y., Miao, B., Daniela Robles-Espinoza, C., Sankar, A., Njauw, C. N., Shannon, K., Gragoudas, E. S., Marie Lane, A., Iyer, V., Newton-Bishop, J. A., Timothy Bishop, D., Holland, E. A., Mann, G. J., Singh, T., Daly, M. J. and Tsao, H. 2017. Rare variant, Gene-based association study of hereditary melanoma using whole-exome sequencing, *Journal of the National Cancer Institute*, 109, p. djx083.

Ávila-López, P. A., Guerrero, G., Nuñez-Martínez, H. N., Peralta-Alvarez, C. A., Hernández-Montes, G., Álvarez-Hilario, L. G., Herrera-Goepfert, R., Albores-Saavedra, J., Villegas-Sepúlveda, N., Cedillo-Barrón, L., Montes-Gómez, A. E., Vargas, M., Schnoor, M., Recillas-Targa, F. and Hernández-Rivas, R. 2021. H2A.Z overexpression suppresses senescence and chemosensitivity in pancreatic ductal adenocarcinoma, *Oncogene*, 40, pp. 2065–2080.

Bertolotto, C., Lesueur, F., Giuliano, S., Strub, T., De Lichy, M., Bille, K., Dessen, P., D'hayer, B., Mohamdi, H., Remenieras, A., et al. 2011. A SUMOylation-defective MITF germline mutation predisposes to melanoma and renal carcinoma, *Nature*, 480, pp. 94–98.

Betancourt, L. H., Gil, J., Sanchez, A., Doma, V., Kuras, M., Murillo, J. R., Velasquez, E., Çakir, U., Kim, Y., Sugihara, Y., Parada, I. P., et al. 2021. The human melanoma proteome atlas-complementing the melanoma transcriptome, *Clinical and Translational Medicine*, 11, p. e451.

Bhatia, S., Tykodi, S. S. and Thompson, J. A. 2009. Treatment of metastatic melanoma: An overview, *Oncology (Williston Park)*, 23, pp. 488–496.

Bollag, G., Tsai, J., Zhang, J., Zhang, C., Ibrahim, P., Nolop, K. and Hirth, P. 2012. Vemurafenib: The first drug approved for BRAF-mutant cancer, *Nature Reviews. Drug Discovery*, 11, pp. 873–886.

Byrd, A. L., Belkaid, Y. and Segre, J. A. 2018. The human skin microbiome, *Nature Reviews. Microbiology*, 16, pp. 143–155.

Byström, S., Fredolini, C., Edqvist, P. H., Nyaiesh, E. N., Drobin, K., Uhlén, M., Bergqvist, M., Pontén, F. and Schwenk, J. M. 2017. Affinity proteomics exploration of melanoma identifies proteins in serum with associations to T-stage and recurrence, *Translational Oncology*, 10, pp. 385–395.

Casadonte, R., Kriegsmann, M., Kriegsmann, K., Hauk, I., Meliß, R. R., Müller, C. S. L. and Kriegsmann, J. 2021. Imaging mass spectrometry-based proteomic analysis to differentiate melanocytic nevi and malignant melanoma, *Cancers (Basel)*, 13, p. 3197.

Colebatch, A. J., Ferguson, P., Newell, F., Kazakoff, S. H., Witkowski, T., Dobrovic, A., Johansson, P. A., Saw, R. P., Stretch, J. R. and Mcarthur, G. A. 2019. Molecular genomic profiling of melanocytic nevi, *Journal of Investigative Dermatology*, 139, pp. 1762–1768.

Cronin, J. C., Wunderlich, J., Loftus, S. K., Prickett, T. D., Wei, X., Ridd, K., Vemula, S., Burrell, A. S., Agrawal, N. S., Lin, J. C., Banister, C. E., Buckhaults, P., Rosenberg, S. A., Bastian, B. C., Pavan, W. J. and Samuels, Y. 2009. Frequent mutations in the MITF pathway in melanoma, *Pigment Cell and Melanoma Research*, 22, pp. 435–444.

Das, S., Dey, M. K., Devireddy, R. and Gartia, M. R. 2023. Biomarkers in cancer detection, diagnosis, and prognosis, *Sensors (Basel)*, 24, p. 37.

Davis, L. E., Shalin, S. C. and Tackett, A. J. 2019. Current state of melanoma diagnosis and treatment, *Cancer Biology & Therapy*, 20, pp. 1366–1379.

de Jel, M. M., Schott, M., Lamm, S., Neuhuber, W., Kuphal, S. and Bosserhoff, A.-K. 2019. Loss of CYLD accelerates melanoma development and progression in the Tg(Grm1) melanoma mouse model, *Oncogenesis*, 8, p. 56.

de Unamuno Bustos, B., Murria Estal, R., Pérez Simó, G., De Juan Jimenez, I., Escutia Muñoz, B., Rodríguez Serna, M., Alegre De Miquel, V., Llavador Ros, M., Ballester Sánchez, R., Nagore Enguídanos, E., Palanca Suela, S. and Botella Estrada, R. 2017. Towards personalized medicine in melanoma: Implementation of a clinical next-generation sequencing panel, *Scientific Reports,* 7, p. 495.

Defossez, E., Bourquin, J., Von Reuss, S., Rasmann, S. and Glauser, G. 2023. Eight key rules for successful data-dependent acquisition in mass spectrometry-based metabolomics, *Mass Spectrometry Reviews*, 42, pp. 131–143.

Dimitrakopoulos, C., Hindupur, S. K., Häfliger, L., Behr, J., Montazeri, H., Hall, M. N. and Beerenwinkel, N. 2018. Network-based integration of multi-omics data for prioritizing cancer genes, *Bioinformatics*, 34(14): pp. 2441–2448.

Domingues, B., Lopes, J. M., Soares, P. and Pópulo, H. 2018. Melanoma treatment in review, *ImmunoTargets and Therapy*, 7, pp. 35–49.

Donati, M., Kastnerova, L., Cempírková, D., Vaněček, T., Michal, M. and Kazakov, D. V. 2020. Vulvar pigmented epithelioid melanocytoma with a novel HTT-PKN1 fusion: A case report, *The American Journal of Dermatopathology*, 42, pp. 544–546.

Donnelly, D., 3rd, Aung, P. P. and Jour, G. 2019. The "-OMICS" facet of melanoma: Heterogeneity of genomic, proteomic and metabolomic biomarkers, *Seminars in Cancer Biology*, 59, pp. 165–174.

Dowling, P., Moran, B., Mcauley, E., Meleady, P., Henry, M., Clynes, M., Mcmenamin, M., Leonard, N., Monks, M., Wynne, B., Ormond, P. and Larkin, A. 2016. Quantitative label-free mass spectrometry analysis of formalin-fixed, paraffin-embedded tissue representing the invasive cutaneous malignant melanoma proteome, *Oncology Letters*, 12, pp. 3296–3304.

Du, Y., Lv, G., Jing, C., Liu, J. and Liu, J. 2020. ZNF750 inhibits the proliferation and invasion of melanoma cells through modulating the Wnt/b-catenin signaling pathway, *Folia histochemica et cytobiologica*, 58, pp. 255–263.

Duan, H., Jiang, K., Wei, D., Zhang, L., Cheng, D., Lv, M., Xu, Y. and He, A. 2018. Identification of epigenetically altered genes and potential gene targets in melanoma using bioinformatic methods, *OncoTargets and Therapy*, 11, pp. 9–15.

Dubois, A. and Rajan, N. 1993. CYLD Cutaneous Syndrome. In: Adam, M. P., Feldman, J., Mirzaa, G. M., Pagon, R. A., Wallace, S. E., Bean, L. J. H., Gripp, K. W. and Amemiya, A. (eds.) *GeneReviews®*. Seattle (WA): University of Washington, Seattle.

Duffy, D. L., Zhu, G., Li, X., Sanna, M., Iles, M. M., Jacobs, L. C., Evans, D. M., Yazar, S., Beesley, J., Law, M. H., Kraft, P., Visconti, A., Taylor, J. C., Liu, F., et al. 2018. Novel pleiotropic risk loci for melanoma and nevus density implicate multiple biological pathways, *Nature Communications*, 9, p. 4774.

Falcone, I., Conciatori, F., Bazzichetto, C., Ferretti, G., Cognetti, F., Ciuffreda, L. and Milella, M. 2020. Tumor microenvironment: Implications in melanoma resistance to targeted therapy and immunotherapy, *Cancers (Basel)*, 12, p. 2870.

Fernandez, A. F., Huidobro, C. and Fraga, M. F. 2012. De novo DNA methyltransferases: Oncogenes, tumor suppressors, or both? *Trends in Genetics*, 28, pp. 474–479.

Forbes, S. A., Beare, D., Boutselakis, H., Bamford, S., Bindal, N., Tate, J., Cole, C. G., Ward, S., Dawson, E., Ponting, L., Stefancsik, R., Harsha, B., Kok, C. Y., Jia, M., Jubb, H., Sondka, Z., Thompson, S., De, T. and Campbell, P. J. 2017. COSMIC: Somatic cancer genetics at high-resolution, *Nucleic Acids Research*, 45, pp. D777–D783.

Ford, D., Bliss, J. M., Swerdlow, A. J., Armstrong, B. K., Franceschi, S., Green, A., Holly, E. A., Mack, T., Mackie, R. M., and Osterlind, A. 1995. Risk of cutaneous melanoma associated with a family history of the disease. The International Melanoma Analysis Group (IMAGE), *International Journal of Cancer*, 62, pp. 377–381.

Friedman, J. M. 1993. Neurofibromatosis 1. In: Adam, M. P., Feldman, J., Mirzaa, G. M., Pagon, R. A., Wallace, S. E., Bean, L. J. H., Gripp, K. W. and Amemiya, A. (eds.) *GeneReviews®*. Seattle (WA): University of Washington, Seattle.

Fu, Q., Chen, Z., Zhang, S., Parker, S. J., Fu, Z., Tin, A., Liu, X. and Van Eyk, J. E. 2016. Multiple and selective reaction monitoring using triple quadrupole mass spectrometer: Preclinical large cohort analysis, *Methods in Molecular Biology*, 1410, pp. 249–264.

Fu, S., Wu, H., Zhang, H., Lian, C. G. and Lu, Q. 2017. DNA methylation/hydroxymethylation in melanoma, *Oncotarget*, 8, pp. 78163–78173.

Gao, E., Li, W., Wu, C., Shao, W., Di, Y. and Liu, Y. 2021. Data-independent acquisition-based proteome and phosphoproteome profiling across six melanoma cell lines reveals determinants of proteotypes, *Molecular Omics*, 17, pp. 413–425.

Garbe, C., Peris, K., Hauschild, A., Saiag, P., Middleton, M., Spatz, A., Grob, J. J., Malvehy, J., Newton-Bishop, J., Stratigos, A., Pehamberger, H. and Eggermont, A. 2010. Diagnosis and treatment of melanoma: European consensus-based interdisciplinary guideline, *European Journal of Cancer*, 46, pp. 270–283.

Garraway, L. A., Widlund, H. R., Rubin, M. A., Getz, G., Berger, A. J., Ramaswamy, S., Beroukhim, R., Milner, D. A., Granter, S. R., Du, J., Lee, C., Wagner, S. N., Li, C., Golub, T. R., Rimm, D. L., Meyerson, M. L., Fisher, D. E. and Sellers, W. R. 2005. Integrative genomic analyses identify MITF as a lineage survival oncogene amplified in malignant melanoma, *Nature*, 436, pp. 117–122.

Georgescu, S. R., Mitran, C. I., Mitran, M. I., Matei, C., Constantin, C., Neagu, M. and Tampa, M. 2022. Apprising diagnostic and prognostic biomarkers in cutaneous melanoma-persistent updating, *Journal of Personalized Medicine*, 12, p. 1506.

Gil, J., Betancourt, L. H., Pla, I., Sanchez, A., Appelqvist, R., Miliotis, T., Kuras, M., Oskolas, H., Kim, Y., Horvath, Z., Eriksson, J., Berge, E., Burestedt, E., Jönsson, G., Baldetorp, B., Ingvar, C., Olsson, H., Lundgren, L., Horvatovich, P., Murillo, J. R., Sugihara, Y., Welinder, C., Wieslander, E., Lee, B., Lindberg, H., Pawłowski, K., Kwon, H. J., Doma, V., Timar, J., Karpati, S., Szasz, A. M., Németh, I. B., Nishimura, T., Corthals, G., Rezeli, M., Knudsen, B., Malm, J. and Marko-Varga, G. 2019. Clinical protein science in translational medicine targeting malignant melanoma, *Cell Biology and Toxicology*, 35, pp. 293–332.

Griewank, K. G., Scolyer, R. A., Thompson, J. F., Flaherty, K. T., Schadendorf, D. and Murali, R. 2014. Genetic alterations and personalized medicine in melanoma: Progress and future prospects, *Journal of the National Cancer Institute*, 106, p. djt435.

Guan, M., Chen, X., Ma, Y., Tang, L., Guan, L., Ren, X., Yu, B., Zhang, W. and Su, B. 2015. MDA-9 and GRP78 as potential diagnostic biomarkers for early detection of melanoma metastasis, *Tumour Biology*, 36, pp. 2973–2982.

Guhan, S., Klebanov, N. and Tsao, H. 2021. Melanoma genomics: A state-of-the-art review of practical clinical applications, *British Journal of Dermatology*, 185, pp. 272–281.

Guo, W., Wang, H. and Li, C. 2021. Signal pathways of melanoma and targeted therapy, *Signal Transduction and Targeted Therapy*, 6, p. 424.

Gutmann, D. H., Wood, D. L. and Collins, F. S. 1991. Identification of the neurofibromatosis type 1 gene product, *Proceedings of the National Academy of Sciences of the United States of America*, 88, pp. 9658–9662.

Hartman, M. L. and Czyz, M. 2013. Anti-apoptotic proteins on guard of melanoma cell survival, *Cancer Letters*, 331, pp. 24–34.

Hartman, M. L. and Czyz, M. 2015a. MITF in melanoma: Mechanisms behind its expression and activity, *Cellular and Molecular Life Sciences*, 72, pp. 1249–1260.

Hartman, M. L. and Czyz, M. 2015b. Pro-survival role of MITF in melanoma, *Journal of Investigative Dermatology*, 135, pp. 352–358.

Hatzimichael, E., Lagos, K., Sim, V. R., Briasoulis, E. and Crook, T. 2014. Epigenetics in diagnosis, prognostic assessment and treatment of cancer: An update, *EXCLI Journal*, 13, pp. 954–976.

Helgadottir, H., Rocha Trocoli Drakensjö, I. and Girnita, A. 2018. Personalized medicine in malignant melanoma: Towards patient tailored treatment, *Frontiers in Oncology*, 8, p. 202.

Helleday, T. 2011. The underlying mechanism for the PARP and BRCA synthetic lethality: Clearing up the misunderstandings, *Molecular Oncology*, 5(4): pp. 387–393.

Hemesath, T. J., Steingrímsson, E., Mcgill, G., Hansen, M. J., Vaught, J., Hodgkinson, C. A., Arnheiter, H., Copeland, N. G., Jenkins, N. A. and Fisher, D. E. 1994. Microphthalmia, a critical factor in melanocyte development, defines a discrete transcription factor family, *Genes & Development,* 8, pp. 2770–2780.

Henry, M. L., Osborne, J. and Else, T. 2022. POT1 Tumor Predisposition. In: Adam, M. P., Feldman, J., Mirzaa, G. M., Pagon, R. A., Wallace, S. E., Bean, L. J. H., Gripp, K. W. and Amemiya, A. (eds.) *GeneReviews®*. Seattle (WA): University of Washington, Seattle.

Hessler, M., Jalilian, E., Xu, Q., Reddy, S., Horton, L., Elkin, K., Manwar, R., Tsoukas, M., Mehregan, D. and Avanaki, K. 2020. Melanoma biomarkers and their potential application for in vivo diagnostic imaging modalities, *International Journal of Molecular Sciences,* 21, p. 9583.

Houben, R., Becker, J. C., Kappel, A., Terheyden, P., Bröcker, E. B., Goetz, R. and Rapp, U. R. 2004. Constitutive activation of the Ras-Raf signaling pathway in metastatic melanoma is associated with poor prognosis, *Journal of Carcinogenesis*, 3, p. 6.

Hsu, C. J., Meers, O., Buschbeck, M. and Heidel, F. H. 2021. The role of MacroH2A histone variants in cancer, *Cancers (Basel)*, 13, p. 3003.

Huber, V., Vallacchi, V., Fleming, V., Hu, X., Cova, A., Dugo, M., Shahaj, E., Sulsenti, R., Vergani, E., Filipazzi, P., De Laurentiis, A., Lalli, L., Di Guardo, L., Patuzzo, R., Vergani, B., Casiraghi, E., Cossa, M., Gualeni, A., Bollati, V., Arienti, F., De Braud, F., Mariani, L., Villa, A., Altevogt, P., Umansky, V., Rodolfo, M. and Rivoltini, L. 2018. Tumor-derived microRNAs induce myeloid suppressor cells and predict immunotherapy resistance in melanoma, *Journal of Clinical Investigation*, 128, pp. 5505–5516.

Jenkins, R. W. and Fisher, D. E. 2021. Treatment of advanced melanoma in 2020 and beyond, *Journal of Investigative Dermatology*, 141, pp. 23–31.

Jones, P. A. and Baylin, S. B. 2002. The fundamental role of epigenetic events in cancer, *Nature Reviews. Genetics*, 3, pp. 415–428.

Kallini, J. R., Jain, S. K. and Khachemoune, A. 2013. Lentigo maligna: Review of salient characteristics and management, *American Journal of Clinical Dermatology*, 14, pp. 473–480.

Kamaletdinova, T., Fanaei-Kahrani, Z. and Wang, Z. Q. 2019. The enigmatic function of PARP1: From PARylation activity to PAR readers, *Cells*, 8, p. 1625.

Kanemaru, H., Fukushima, S., Yamashita, J., Honda, N., Oyama, R., Kakimoto, A., Masuguchi, S., Ishihara, T., Inoue, Y., Jinnin, M. and Ihn, H. 2011. The circulating microRNA-221 level in patients with malignant melanoma as a new tumor marker, *Journal of Dermatological Sciences*, 61, pp. 187–193.

Kang, H., Li, J., Wu, M., Shen, L. and Hou, L. 2020. Building a pharmacogenomics knowledge model toward precision medicine: Case study in melanoma, *JMIR Medical Informatics*, 8, p. e20291.

Kapoor, A., Goldberg, M. S., Cumberland, L. K., Ratnakumar, K., Segura, M. F., Emanuel, P. O., Menendez, S., Vardabasso, C., Leroy, G., Vidal, C. I., Polsky, D., Osman, I., Garcia, B. A., Hernando, E. and Bernstein, E. 2010. The histone variant macroH2A suppresses melanoma progression through regulation of CDK8, *Nature*, 468, pp. 1105–1109.

Kondoh, K. and Nishida, E. 2007. Regulation of MAP kinases by MAP kinase phosphatases, *Biochimica et Biophysica Acta*, 1773, pp. 1227–1237.

Konstantinov, N. K., Ulff-Møller, C. J. and Dimitrov, S. 2016. Histone variants and melanoma: Facts and hypotheses, *Pigment Cell & Melanoma Research*, 29, pp. 426–433.

Kovács, T., Mikó, E., Ujlaki, G., Sári, Z. and Bai, P. 2020. The microbiome as a component of the tumor microenvironment, *Advances in Experimental Medicine and Biology*, 1225, pp. 137–153.

Kuhlman, B. and Bradley, P. 2019. Advances in protein structure prediction and design, *Nature Reviews Molecular Cell Biology*, 20, pp. 681–697.

Kumar, P., Brazel, D., Derogatis, J., Valerin, J. B. G., Whiteson, K., Chow, W. A., Tinoco, R. and Moyers, J. T. 2022. The cure from within? A review of the microbiome and diet in melanoma, *Cancer Metastasis Reviews*, 41, pp. 261–280.

Kunz, M., Löffler-Wirth, H., Dannemann, M., Willscher, E., Doose, G., Kelso, J., Kottek, T., Nickel, B., Hopp, L., Landsberg, J., Hoffmann, S., Tüting, T., Zigrino, P., Mauch, C., Utikal, J., Ziemer, M., Schulze, H. J., Hölzel, M., Roesch, A., Kneitz, S., Meierjohann, S., Bosserhoff, A., Binder, H. and Schartl, M. 2018. RNA-seq analysis identifies different transcriptomic types and developmental trajectories of primary melanomas, *Oncogene*, 37, pp. 6136–6151.

Lazăr, A. D., Dinescu, S. and Costache, M. 2020. The non-coding landscape of cutaneous malignant melanoma: A possible route to efficient targeted therapy, *Cancers (Basel)*, 12, p. 3378.

Lazova, R., Smoot, K., Anderson, H., Powell, M. J., Rosenberg, A. S., Rongioletti, F., Pilloni, L., D'hallewin, S., Gueorguieva, R., Tantcheva-Poór, I., Obadofin, O., Camacho, C., Hsi, A., Kluger, H. H., Fadare, O. and Seeley, E. H. 2020. Histopathology-guided mass spectrometry differentiates benign nevi from malignant melanoma, *Journal of Cutaneous Pathology*, 47, pp. 226–240.

Lazova, R., Yang, Z., El Habr, C., Lim, Y., Choate, K. A., Seeley, E. H., Caprioli, R. M. and Yangqun, L. 2017. Mass spectrometry imaging can distinguish on a proteomic level between proliferative nodules within a benign congenital nevus and malignant melanoma, *The American Journal of Dermatopathology*, 39, pp. 689–695.

Lee, A., Lim, J. and Lim, J.-S. 2024. Emerging roles of MITF as a crucial regulator of immunity, *Experimental & Molecular Medicine*, 56, pp. 311–318.

Leucci, E., Vendramin, R., Spinazzi, M., Laurette, P., Fiers, M., Wouters, J., Radaelli, E., Eyckerman, S., Leonelli, C., Vanderheyden, K., Rogiers, A., Hermans, E., Baatsen, P., Aerts, S., Amant, F., Van Aelst, S., Van Den Oord, J., De Strooper, B., Davidson, I., Lafontaine, D. L., Gevaert, K., Vandesompele, J., Mestdagh, P. and Marine, J. C. 2016. Melanoma addiction to the long non-coding RNA SAMMSON, *Nature*, 531, pp. 518–522.

Li, J., Duncan, D. T. and Zhang, B. 2010. CanProVar: A human cancer proteome variation database, *Human Mutations*, 31, pp. 219–228.

Li, J., Shi, L., Zhang, K., Zhang, Y., Hu, S., Zhao, T., Teng, H., Li, X., Jiang, Y., Ji, L. and Sun, Z. 2018. VarCards: An integrated genetic and clinical database for coding variants in the human genome, *Nucleic Acids Research*, 46, pp. D1039–D1048.

Lin, Q., Zhang, H., Ding, H., Qian, J., Lizaso, A., Lin, J., Han-Zhang, H., Xiang, J., Li, Y. and Zhu, H. 2019. The association between BRAF mutation class and clinical features in BRAF-mutant Chinese non-small cell lung cancer patients, *Journal of Translational Medicine*, 17, p. 298.

Litovkin, K., Van Eynde, A., Joniau, S., Lerut, E., Laenen, A., Gevaert, T., Gevaert, O., Spahn, M., Kneitz, B., Gramme, P., Helleputte, T., Isebaert, S., Haustermans, K. and Bollen, M. 2015. DNA methylation-guided prediction of clinical failure in high-risk prostate cancer, *PLOS ONE*, 10, p. e0130651.

Lou, R. and Shui, W. 2024. Acquisition and analysis of DIA-based proteomic data: A comprehensive survey in 2023, *Molecular & Cellular Proteomics*, 23, p. 100712.

Low, T. Y., van Heesch, S., van den Toorn, H., Giansanti, P., Cristobal, A., Toonen, P., Schafer, S., Hübner, N., van Breukelen, B., Mohammed, S., et al. 2013. Quantitative and qualitative proteome characteristics extracted from in-depth integrated genomics and proteomics analysis, *Cell Reports*, 5(5), pp. 1469–1478.

Ludwig, C., Gillet, L., Rosenberger, G., Amon, S., Collins, B. C. and Aebersold, R. 2018. Data-independent acquisition-based SWATH-MS for quantitative proteomics: A tutorial, *Molecular Systems Biology*, 14, p. e8126.

Luke, J. J., Flaherty, K. T., Ribas, A. and Long, G. V. 2017. Targeted agents and immunotherapies: Optimizing outcomes in melanoma, *Nature Reviews. Clinical Oncology*, 14, pp. 463–482.

Luo, Y., Zhang, Z., Liu, J., Li, L., Xu, X., Yao, X., Dai, Z., Wang, X., Yang, S., Wu, H., Bu, J., Wu, Y., Xiang, T. and Li, X. 2020. Characterizations of gene alterations in melanoma patients from Chinese population, *Biomed Research International*, 2020, p. 6096814.

Macklin, A., Khan, S. and Kislinger, T. 2020. Recent advances in mass spectrometry based clinical proteomics: Applications to cancer research, *Clinical Proteomics*, 17, p. 17.

Maertens, O., Johnson, B., Hollstein, P., Frederick, D. T., Cooper, Z. A., Messiaen, L., Bronson, R. T., Mcmahon, M., Granter, S., Flaherty, K., Wargo, J. A., Marais, R. and Cichowski, K. 2013. Elucidating distinct roles for NF1 in melanomagenesis, *Cancer Discovery*, 3, pp. 338–349.

Magdeldin, S. and Yamamoto, T. 2012. Toward deciphering proteomes of formalin-fixed paraffin-embedded (FFPE) tissues, *Proteomics*, 12, pp. 1045–1058.

Makaranka, S., Scutt, F., Frixou, M., Wensley, K. E., Sharma, R. and Greenhowe, J. 2022. The gut microbiome and melanoma: A review, *Experimental Dermatology*, 31, pp. 1292–1301.

Mani, D. R., Krug, K., Zhang, B., Satpathy, S., Clauser, K. R., Ding, L., Ellis, M., Gillette, M. A. and Carr, S. A. 2022. Cancer proteogenomics: Current impact and future prospects, *Cancer*, 22, pp. 298–313.

Marzuka-Alcalá, A., Gabree, M. J. and Tsao, H. 2014. Melanoma susceptibility genes and risk assessment, *Methods in Molecular Biology*, 1102, pp. 381–393.

Mattia, G., Puglisi, R., Ascione, B., Malorni, W., Carè, A. and Matarrese, P. 2018. Cell death-based treatments of melanoma: Conventional treatments and new therapeutic strategies, *Cell Death & Disease*, 9, p. 112.

Melamed, R. D., Aydin, I. T., Rajan, G. S., Phelps, R., Silvers, D. N., Emmett, K. J., Brunner, G., Rabadan, R. and Celebi, J. T. 2017. Genomic characterization of dysplastic nevi unveils implications for diagnosis of melanoma, *Journal of Investigative Dermatology*, 137, pp. 905–909.

Michielin, O., Van Akkooi, A. C. J., Ascierto, P. A., Dummer, R. and Keilholz, U. 2019. Cutaneous melanoma: ESMO Clinical Practice Guidelines for diagnosis, treatment and follow-up, *Annals of Oncology*, 30, pp. 1884–1901.

Miller, E., Barnea, Y., Karin, E., Leshem, D., Weiss, J., Leider-Trejo, L. and Schneebaum, S. 2006. Sentinel lymph node biopsy in the diagnosis and treatment of multicentric malignant melanoma of the penis, *The Israel Medical Association Journal*, 8, pp. 292–293.

Molven, A., Grimstvedt, M. B., Steine, S. J., Harland, M., Avril, M. F., Hayward, N. K. and Akslen, L. A. 2005. A large Norwegian family with inherited malignant melanoma, multiple atypical nevi, and CDK4 mutation, *Genes, Chromosomes & Cancer*, 44, pp. 10–18.

Montoni, A., Robu, M., Pouliot, E. and Shah, G. M.. 2013. Resistance to PARP-inhibitors in cancer therapy. *Frontiers in Pharmacology*, 4: p. 18.

Motwani, J. and Eccles, M. R. 2021. Genetic and genomic pathways of melanoma development, invasion and metastasis, *Genes (Basel)*, 12, p. 1543.

Musella, A., Bardhi, E., Marchetti, C., Vertechy, L., Santangelo, G., Sassu, C., Tomao F., Rech, F., D'Amelio, R., Monti, M., et al. 2018. Rucaparib: An emerging parp inhibitor for treatment of recurrent ovarian cancer, *Cancer Treatment Reviews*, 66: pp. 7–14.

Neagu, M., Constantin, C., Cretoiu, S. M. and Zurac, S. 2020. miRNAs in the diagnosis and prognosis of skin cancer, *Frontiers in Cell and Developmental Biology*, 8, p. 71.

Newton-Bishop, J., Bishop, D. T. and Harland, M. 2020. Melanoma genomics, *Acta Dermato-Venereologica*, 100, p. adv00138.

O'neill, C. H. and Scoggins, C. R. 2019. Melanoma, *Journal of Surgical Oncology*, 120, pp. 873–881.

Ohsie, S. J., Sarantopoulos, G. P., Cochran, A. J. and Binder, S. W. 2008. Immunohistochemical characteristics of melanoma, *Journal of Cutaneous Pathology*, 35, pp. 433–444.

Ortega-Martínez, I., Gardeazabal, J., Erramuzpe, A., Sanchez-Diez, A., Cortés, J., García-Vázquez, M. D., Pérez-Yarza, G., Izu, R., Luís Díaz-Ramón, J., De La Fuente, I. M., Asumendi, A. and Boyano, M. D. 2016. Vitronectin and dermcidin serum levels predict the metastatic progression of AJCC I-II early-stage melanoma, *International Journal of Cancer*, 139, pp. 1598–1607.

Papeo, G., Casale, E., Montagnoli, A. and Cirla, A.2013. PARP inhibitors in cancer therapy: An update, *Expert Opinion on Therapeutic Patents*, 23(4): pp. 503–514.

Paska, A. V. and Hudler, P. 2015. Aberrant methylation patterns in cancer: A clinical view, *Biochemia Medica (Zagreb)*, 25, pp. 161–176.

Patel, H., Yacoub, N., Mishra, R., White, A., Long, Y., Alanazi, S. and Garrett, J. T. 2020. Current advances in the treatment of BRAF-mutant melanoma, *Cancers (Basel)*, 12, p. 482.

Patel, S. J., Sanjana, N. E., Kishton, R. J., Eidizadeh, A., Vodnala, S. K., Cam, M., Gartner, J. J., Jia, L., Steinberg, S. M., Yamamoto, T. N., Merchant, A. S., Mehta, G. U., Chichura, A., Shalem, O., Tran, E., Eil, R., Sukumar, M., Guijarro, E. P., Day, C. P., Robbins, P., Feldman, S., Merlino, G., Zhang, F. and Restifo, N. P. 2017. Identification of essential genes for cancer immunotherapy, *Nature*, 548, pp. 537–542.

Patra, V., Gallais Sérézal, I. and Wolf, P. 2020. Potential of skin microbiome, pro- and/or pre-biotics to affect local cutaneous responses to UV exposure, *Nutrients*, 12, p. 1795.

Peltonen, S., Kallionpää, R. A. and Peltonen, J. 2017. Neurofibromatosis type 1 (NF1) gene: Beyond café au lait spots and dermal neurofibromas, *Experimental Dermatology*, 26, pp. 645–648.

Pilarski, R., Carlo, M. I., Cebulla, C. and Abdel-Rahman, M. 2022. BAP1 Tumor Predisposition Syndrome. In: Adam, M. P., Feldman, J., Mirzaa, G. M., Pagon, R. A., Wallace, S. E., Bean, L. J. H., Gripp, K. W. and Amemiya, A. (eds.) *GeneReviews®*. Seattle (WA): University of Washington, Seattle.

Pimiento, J. M., Larkin, E. M., Smalley, K. S., Wiersma, G. L., Monks, N. R., Fedorenko, I. V., Peterson, C. A. and Nickoloff, B. J. 2013. Melanoma genotypes and phenotypes get personal, *Laboratory Investigation*, 93, pp. 858–867.

Plummer, R., Lorigan, P., Steven, N., Scott, L., Middleton, M. R., Wilson, R.H., Mulligan, E., Curtin, N., Wang, D., Dewji, R., et al. 2013. A phase II study of the potent PARP inhibitor, Rucaparib (PF-01367338, AG014699), with temozolomide in patients with metastatic melanoma demonstrating evidence of chemopotentiation, *Cancer Chemotherapy and Pharmacology*, 71(5): pp. 1191–1199.

Poalelungi, D. G., Musat, C. L., Fulga, A., Neagu, M., Neagu, A. I., Piraianu, A. I. and Fulga, I. 2023. Advancing patient care: How artificial intelligence is transforming healthcare, *Journal of Personalized Medicine*, 13, p. 1214.

Primot, A., Mogha, A., Corre, S., Roberts, K., Debbache, J., Adamski, H., Dreno, B., Khammari, A., Lesimple, T., Mereau, A., Goding, C. R. and Galibert, M. D. 2010. ERK-regulated differential expression of the Mitf 6a/b splicing isoforms in melanoma, *Pigment Cell & Melanoma Research*, 23, pp. 93–102.

Psaty, E. L., Scope, A., Halpern, A. C. and Marghoob, A. A. 2010. Defining the patient at high risk for melanoma, *International Journal of Dermatology*, 49, pp. 362–376.

Puntervoll, H. E., Yang, X. R., Vetti, H. H., Bachmann, I. M., Avril, M. F., Benfodda, M., Catricalà, C., Dalle, S., Duval-Modeste, A. B., Ghiorzo, P., Grammatico, P., Harland, M., Hayward, N. K., Hu, H. H., Jouary, T., Martin-Denavit, T., Ozola, A., Palmer, J. M., Pastorino, L., Pjanova, D., Soufir, N., Steine, S. J., Stratigos, A. J., Thomas, L., Tinat, J., Tsao, H., Veinalde, R., Tucker, M. A., Bressac-De Paillerets, B., Newton-Bishop, J. A., Goldstein, A. M., Akslen, L. A. and Molven, A. 2013. Melanoma prone families with CDK4 germline mutation: Phenotypic profile and associations with MC1R variants, *Journal of Medical Genetics*, 50, pp. 264–270.

Ray, B., Liu, W. and Fenyö, D. 2017. Adaptive multiview nonnegative matrix factorization algorithm for integration of multimodal biomedical data, *Cancer Informatics*, 16: p. 1176935117725727.

Read, J., Wadt, K. A. and Hayward, N. K. 2016. Melanoma genetics, *Journal of Medical Genetics*, 53, pp. 1–14.

Rohart, F., Gautier, B., Singh, A. and KA, L. C. 2017. mixOmics: An R package for 'omics feature selection and multiple data integration, *PLoS Computational Biology*, 13(11): p. e1005752.

Sabel, M. S., Liu, Y. and Lubman, D. M. 2011. Proteomics in melanoma biomarker discovery: Great potential, many obstacles, *International Journal of Proteomics*, 2011, p. 181890.

Salava, A., Aho, V., Pereira, P., Koskinen, K., Paulin, L., Auvinen, P. and Lauerma, A. 2016. Skin microbiome in melanomas and melanocytic nevi, *European Journal of Dermatology*, 26, pp. 49–55.

Salemi, R., Falzone, L., Madonna, G., Polesel, J., Cinà, D., Mallardo, D., Ascierto, P. A., Libra, M. and Candido, S. 2018. MMP-9 as a candidate marker of response to BRAF inhibitors in melanoma patients with BRAF(V600E) mutation detected in circulating-free DNA, *Frontiers in Pharmacology,* 9: p. 856.

Salgado, C., Oosting, J., Janssen, B., Kumar, R., Gruis, N. and Van Doorn, R. 2020. Genome-wide characterization of 5-hydoxymethylcytosine in melanoma reveals major differences with nevus, *Genes Chromosomes Cancer*, 59, pp. 366–374.

Schadendorf, D., Van Akkooi, A. C. J., Berking, C., Griewank, K. G., Gutzmer, R., Hauschild, A., Stang, A., Roesch, A. and Ugurel, S. 2018. Melanoma, *Lancet*, 392, pp. 971–984.

Schlacher, K. 2017. PARPi focus the spotlight on replication fork protection in cancer, *Nature Cell Biology*, 19(11): pp. 1309–1310.

Schwanhäusser, B., Busse, D., Li, N., Dittmar, G., Schuchhardt, J., Wolf, J., Chen, W. and Selbach, M. 2011. Global quantification of mammalian gene expression control, *Nature*, 473(7347): pp. 337–342.

Shain, A. H., Joseph, N. M., Yu, R., Benhamida, J., Liu, S., Prow, T., Ruben, B., North, J., Pincus, L., Yeh, I., Judson, R. and Bastian, B. C. 2018. Genomic and transcriptomic analysis reveals incremental disruption of key signaling pathways during melanoma evolution, *Cancer Cell*, 34, pp. 45–55.e4.

Shapanis, A., Lai, C., Sommerlad, M., Parkinson, E., Healy, E. and Skipp, P. 2020. Proteomic profiling of archived tissue of primary melanoma identifies proteins associated with metastasis, *International Journal of Molecular Sciences*, 21.

Shields, B. D., Tackett, A. J. and Shalin, S. C. 2016. Proteomics and melanoma: A current perspective, *Global Dermatology*, 3, pp. 366–370.

Sigalotti, L., Covre, A., Fratta, E., Parisi, G., Sonego, P., Colizzi, F., Coral, S., Massarut, S., Kirkwood, J. M. and Maio, M. 2012. Whole genome methylation profiles as independent markers of survival in stage IIIC melanoma patients, *Journal of Translational Medicine*, 10, p. 185.

Simonin-Wilmer, I., Ossio, R., Leddin, E. M., Harland, M., Pooley, K. A., Martil De La Garza, M. G., Obolenski, S., Hewinson, J., Wong, C. C., Iyer, V., Taylor, J. C., Newton-Bishop, J. A., Bishop, D. T., Cisneros, G. A., Iles, M. M., Adams, D. J. and Robles-Espinoza, C. D. 2023. Population-based analysis of POT1 variants in a cutaneous melanoma case-control cohort, *Journal of Medical Genetics*, 60, pp. 692–696.

Soura, E., Eliades, P. J., Shannon, K., Stratigos, A. J. and Tsao, H. 2016. Hereditary melanoma: Update on syndromes and management: Genetics of familial atypical multiple mole melanoma syndrome, *Journal of the American Academy of Dermatology*, 74, pp. 395–407; quiz 408–10.

Su, T., Zhong, Y., Zeng, W., Zhang, Y., Wang, S., Cheng, J., Yang, H., Wei, Y. and Gong, M. 2022. A comparative study of data-dependent acquisition and data-independent acquisition in proteomics analysis of clinical lung cancer tissues constrained by blood contamination, *Proteomics. Clinical Applications*, 16, p. e2000099.

Surman, M., Hoja-Łukowicz, D., Szwed, S., Kędracka-Krok, S., Jankowska, U., Kurtyka, M., Drożdż, A., Lityńska, A., Stępień, E. and Przybyło, M. 2019. An insight into the proteome of uveal melanoma-derived ectosomes reveals the presence of potentially useful biomarkers, *International Journal of Molecular Sciences,* 20, p. 3789.

Tamura, R. 2021. Current understanding of neurofibromatosis type 1, 2, and schwannomatosis, *International Journal of Molecular Science*, 22, p. 5850.

Tarhini, A., Mcdermott, D., Ambavane, A., Gupte-Singh, K., Aponte-Ribero, V., Ritchings, C., Benedict, A., Rao, S., Regan, M. M. and Atkins, M. 2019. Clinical and economic outcomes associated with treatment sequences in patients with BRAF-mutant advanced melanoma, *Immunotherapy*, 11, pp. 283–295.

Tassabehji, M., Newton, V. E. and Read, A. P. 1994. Waardenburg syndrome type 2 caused by mutations in the human microphthalmia (MITF) gene, *Nature Genetics*, 8, pp. 251–255.

Teh, R., Azimi, A., Pupo, G. M., Ali, M., Mann, G. J. and Fernández-Peñas, P. 2023. Genomic and proteomic findings in early melanoma and opportunities for early diagnosis, *Experimantal Dermatology*, 32, pp. 104–116.

The Cancer Genome Atlas. 2015. Genomic classification of cutaneous melanoma, *Cell*, 161, pp. 1681–1696.

Torres, R., Lang, U. E., Hejna, M., Shelton, S. J., Joseph, N. M., Shain, A. H., Yeh, I., Wei, M. L., Oldham, M. C., Bastian, B. C. and Judson-Torres, R. L. 2020. MicroRNA ratios distinguish melanomas from nevi, *Journal of Investigative Dermatology*, 140, pp. 164–173.e7.

Trilla-Fuertes, L., Gámez-Pozo, A., Prado-Vázquez, G., Zapater-Moros, A., Díaz-Almirón, M., Fortes, C., Ferrer-Gómez, M., López-Vacas, R., Parra Blanco, V., Márquez-Rodas, I., Soria, A., Fresno Vara, J. and Espinosa, E. 2019. Melanoma proteomics suggests functional differences related to mutational status, *Scientific Reports,* 9, p. 7217.

Tsimberidou, A. M., Fountzilas, E., Bleris, L. and Kurzrock, R. 2022. Transcriptomics and solid tumors: The next frontier in precision cancer medicine, *Seminars in Cancer Biology*, 84, pp. 50–59.

Uusitalo, E., Leppävirta, J., Koffert, A., Suominen, S., Vahtera, J., Vahlberg, T., Pöyhönen, M., Peltonen, J. and Peltonen, S. J. T. J. O. I. D. 2015. Incidence and mortality of neurofibromatosis: A total population study in Finland, *Journal of Investigative Dermatology*, 135, pp. 904–906.

Valenti, F., Falcone, I., Ungania, S., Desiderio, F., Giacomini, P., Bazzichetto, C., Conciatori, F., Gallo, E., Cognetti, F., Ciliberto, G., Morrone, A. and Guerrisi, A. 2021. Precision medicine and melanoma: Multi-omics approaches to monitoring the immunotherapy response, *International Journal of Molecular Science*, 22, p. 3837.

Van Dam, S., Võsa, U., Van Der Graaf, A., Franke, L. and De Magalhães, J. P. 2018. Gene co-expression analysis for functional classification and gene-disease predictions, *Briefings in Bioinformatics*, 19, pp. 575–592.

Wang, Y., Radfar, S., Liu, S., Riker, A. I. and Khong, H. T. 2010. Mitf-Mdel, a novel melanocyte/melanoma-specific isoform of microphthalmia-associated transcription factor-M, as a candidate biomarker for melanoma, *BMC Medicine*, 8, p. 14.

Weisenberger, D. J. 2014. Characterizing DNA methylation alterations from The Cancer Genome Atlas, *Journal of Clinical Investigation*, 124, pp. 17–23.

Wheeler, H. E., Maitland, M. L., Dolan, M. E., Cox, N. J. and Ratain, M. J. 2013. Cancer pharmacogenomics: Strategies and challenges, *Nature Reviews. Genetics*, 14, pp. 23–34.

Whitmarsh, A. J. 2007. Regulation of gene transcription by mitogen-activated protein kinase signaling pathways, *Biochimica et Biophysica Acta*, 1773, pp. 1285–1298.

Wiesner, T., Fried, I., Ulz, P., Stacher, E., Popper, H., Murali, R., Kutzner, H., Lax, S., Smolle-Jüttner, F., Geigl, J. B. and Speicher, M. R. 2012. Toward an improved definition of the tumor spectrum associated with BAP1 germline mutations, *Journal of Clinical Oncology*, 30, pp. e337–e340.

Wiesner, T., Obenauf, A. C., Murali, R., Fried, I., Griewank, K. G., Ulz, P., Windpassinger, C., Wackernagel, W., Loy, S., Wolf, I., Viale, A., Lash, A. E., Pirun, M., Socci, N. D., Rütten, A., Palmedo, G., Abramson, D., Offit, K., Ott, A., Becker, J. C., Cerroni, L., Kutzner, H., Bastian, B. C. and Speicher, M. R. 2011. Germline mutations in BAP1 predispose to melanocytic tumors, *Nature Genetics*, 43, pp. 1018–1021.

Wouters, J., Vizoso, M., Martinez-Cardus, A., Carmona, F. J., Govaere, O., Laguna, T., Joseph, J., Dynoodt, P., Aura, C., Foth, M., Cloots, R., Van Den Hurk, K., Balint, B., Murphy, I. G., Mcdermott, E. W., Sheahan, K., Jirström, K., Nodin, B., Mallya-Udupi, G., Van Den Oord, J. J., Gallagher, W. M. and Esteller, M. 2017. Comprehensive DNA methylation study identifies novel progression-related and prognostic markers for cutaneous melanoma, *BMC Medicine*, 15, p. 101.

Xavier, J. B., Young, V. B., Skufca, J., Ginty, F., Testerman, T., Pearson, A. T., Macklin, P., Mitchell, A., Shmulevich, I., Xie, L., Caporaso, J. G., Crandall, K. A., Simone, N. L., Godoy-Vitorino, F., Griffin, T. J., Whiteson, K. L., Gustafson, H. H., Slade, D. J., Schmidt, T. M., Walther-Antonio, M. R. S., Korem, T., Webb-Robertson, B. M., Styczynski, M. P., Johnson, W. E., Jobin, C., Ridlon, J. M., Koh, A. Y., Yu, M., Kelly, L. and Wargo, J. A. 2020. The cancer microbiome: Distinguishing direct and indirect effects requires a systemic view, *Trends in Cancer*, 6, pp. 192–204.

Yao, Z., Yaeger, R., Rodrik-Outmezguine, V. S., Tao, A., Torres, N. M., Chang, M. T., Drosten, M., Zhao, H., Cecchi, F., Hembrough, T., Michels, J., Baumert, H., Miles, L., Campbell, N. M., De Stanchina, E., Solit, D. B., Barbacid, M., Taylor, B. S. and Rosen, N. 2017. Tumours with class 3 BRAF mutants are sensitive to the inhibition of activated RAS, *Nature*, 548, pp. 234–238.

Yokoyama, S., Woods, S. L., Boyle, G. M., Aoude, L. G., Macgregor, S., Zismann, V., Gartside, M., Cust, A. E., Haq, R., Harland, M., Taylor, J. C., Duffy, D. L., Holohan, K., Dutton-Regester, K., Palmer, J. M., Bonazzi, V., Stark, M. S., Symmons, J., Law, M. H., Schmidt, C., Lanagan, C., O'connor, L., Holland, E. A., Schmid, H., Maskiell, J. A., Jetann, J., Ferguson, M., Jenkins, M. A., Kefford, R. F., Giles, G. G., Armstrong, B. K., Aitken, J. F., Hopper, J. L., Whiteman, D. C., Pharoah, P. D., Easton, D. F., Dunning, A. M., Newton-Bishop, J. A., Montgomery, G. W., Martin, N. G., Mann, G. J., Bishop, D. T., Tsao, H., Trent, J. M., Fisher, D. E., Hayward, N. K. and Brown, K. M. 2011. A novel recurrent mutation in MITF predisposes to familial and sporadic melanoma, *Nature*, 480, pp. 99–103.

Zaenker, P., Lo, J., Pearce, R., Cantwell, P., Cowell, L., Lee, M., Quirk, C., Law, H., Gray, E. and Ziman, M. 2018. A diagnostic autoantibody signature for primary cutaneous melanoma, *Oncotarget*, 9, pp. 30539–30551.

Zarrizi, R., Menard, J. A., Belting, M. and Massoumi, R. 2014. Deubiquitination of γ-tubulin by BAP1 prevents chromosome instability in breast cancer cells, *Cancer Research*, 74, pp. 6499–6508.

Zhang, L., Chen, Z., Zheng, M. and He, X. 2011. Robust non-negative matrix factorization, *Frontiers of Electrical and Electronic Engineering in China*, **6**(2): pp. 192–200.

Zhang, M., Wang, B., Xu, J., Wang, X., Xie, L., Zhang, B., Li, Y. and Li, J. 2017. CanProVar 2.0: An updated database of human cancer proteome variation, *Journal of Proteome Research*, 16, pp. 421–432.

Zhao, K. and Hu, Y. 2020. Microbiome harbored within tumors: A new chance to revisit our understanding of cancer pathogenesis and treatment, *Signal Transduction and Targeted Therapy*, 5, p. 136.

Zhu, Y., Orre, L. M., Johansson, H. J., Huss, M., Boekel, J., Vesterlund, M., Fernandez-Woodbridge, A., Branca, R. M. M. and Lehtiö, J. 2018. Publisher Correction: Discovery of coding regions in the human genome by integrated proteogenomics analysis workflow, *Nature Communications*, 9(1), p. 1852.

Zhu, Q. M., Hsu, Y. H., Lassen, F. H., Macdonald, B. T., Stead, S., Malolepsza, E., Kim, A., Li, T., Mizoguchi, T., Schenone, M., Guzman, G., Tanenbaum, B., Fornelos, N., Carr, S. A., Gupta, R. M., Ellinor, P. T. and Lage, K. 2024. Protein interaction networks in the vasculature prioritize genes and pathways underlying coronary artery disease, *Communications Biology*, 7, p. 87.

Zila, N., Bileck, A., Muqaku, B., Janker, L., Eichhoff, O. M., Cheng, P. F., Dummer, R., Levesque, M. P., Gerner, C. and Paulitschke, V. 2018. Proteomics-based insights into mitogen-activated protein kinase inhibitor resistance of cerebral melanoma metastases, *Clinical Proteomics*, 15, p. 13.

8 Next-Generation Imaging Technologies

Revolutionizing Melanoma Monitoring and Assessment

Lloyd Mabonga, Richard Khanyile, and Zodwa Dlamini
SAMRC/UP Precision Oncology Research Unit, DSTI/NRF SARChI Chair in Precision Oncology (POCP) and Cancer Prevention, Pan African Cancer Research Institute (PACRI), University of Pretoria, Pretoria, South Africa

Edward Ngwenya
ARWYP Medical Centre, Kempton Park, South Africa

Ian C. Chikanza
Rheumatology & Immunology (Adult & Paediatric), International Arthritis & Hypermobility Center, Harley Street Clinic, London, UK
and
Faculty of Medicine, Catholic University
Department of Pediatrics & Child Health, University of Zimbabwe, Harare, Zimbabwe

INTRODUCTION

Melanoma presents significant challenges in early detection and accurate diagnosis. It originates in the melanocytes, the cells responsible for producing melanin, the pigment that gives skin its color (Fakhoury et al., 2024). Unlike other forms of skin cancer, melanoma is particularly dangerous because it is more likely to metastasize to other parts of the body if not detected and treated aggressively early. While it accounts for a small percentage of skin cancer cases, it is responsible for most skin cancer-related deaths (Boutros et al., 2024). The incidence of melanoma has been rising steadily over the past few decades, making it a significant public health concern, not only in Africa but also globally. Risk factors for developing melanoma include excessive exposure to ultraviolet (UV) radiation from the sun or tanning beds, having fair skin, a history of sunburns, a large number of moles, and a family history of the disease (Boutros et al., 2024; Fakhoury et al., 2024). Early detection is crucial, as melanoma can often be treated effectively if caught in its initial stages. As shown in **Table 8.1**, the "ABCDE" rule is the mnemonic used for the early detection of melanoma. The rule helps individuals recognize potential warning signs in moles or skin lesions that could indicate the presence of melanoma (Fakhoury et al., 2024). However, the gold standard of management is surgical removal of the tumor, which can be curative if the cancer has not spread (Bouton et al., 2024). Monitoring and assessment of melanoma are critical components in managing the disease, both for early detection and for monitoring after treatment to catch any recurrence. Effective monitoring involves a combination of self-examinations, professional skin examinations, and various diagnostic tools and procedures (Smith et al., 2024).

DOI: 10.1201/9781003511625-8

TABLE 8.1
The "ABCDE" Rule of Early Detection in Melanoma

Characteristic	Description	Significance	Reference
A **Asymmetry** 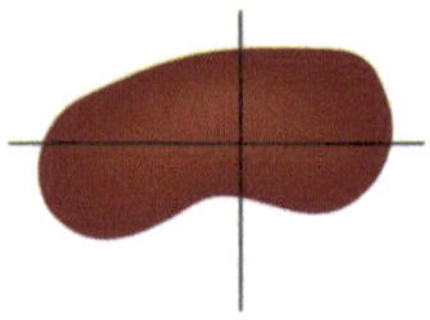	One-half of the mole or lesion does not match the other half.	Benign moles are typically symmetrical. Asymmetry can be a sign of abnormal cell growth, which is characteristic of melanoma.	Fakhoury et al. (2024)
B **Border** 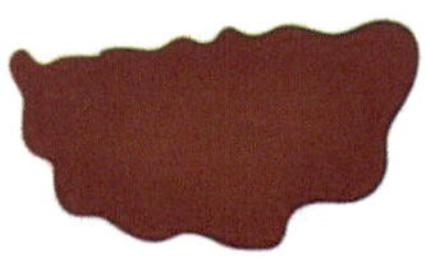	The edges of the mole are irregular, ragged, notched, or blurred.	Healthy moles usually have smooth, even borders. Uneven or poorly defined borders may indicate skin cancer.	Fakhoury et al. (2024)
C **Color** 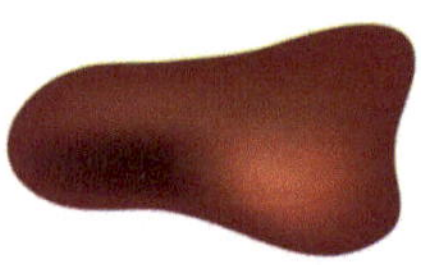	The mole has multiple colors, such as different shades of brown, black, red, white, or blue.	A single, uniform color is typical of benign moles. Multiple colors or an uneven distribution of color can be a warning sign of melanoma.	Fakhoury et al. (2024)
D **Diameter** 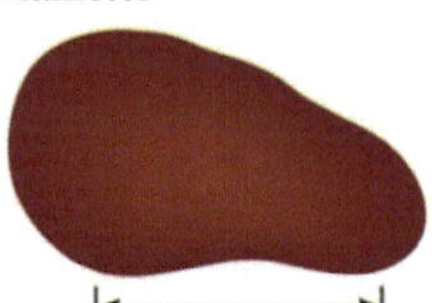	The mole is larger than 6 mm in diameter (about the size of a pencil eraser).	While melanomas can be smaller, they are often larger than 6 mm when diagnosed. Any increase in size should be evaluated.	Fakhoury et al. (2024)
E **Evolving** 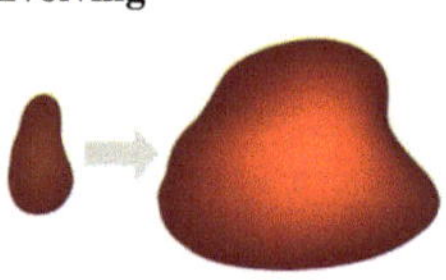	The mole is changing in size, shape, and color, or is becoming symptomatic (e.g., itching, bleeding).	Changes in a mole over time, such as growth or the development of new symptoms, can indicate malignancy and should prompt further investigation.	Fakhoury et al. (2024)

Regular skin self-examinations (SSE) are a key part of monitoring for melanoma. Individuals are encouraged to become familiar with their skin and to regularly check for any new moles or changes in existing moles (Manne et al., 2024). Dermatologists recommend regular professional skin examinations, especially for individuals at higher risk of melanoma. During these examinations, a dermatologist will thoroughly check the skin for any suspicious lesions and may use tools like dermatoscopes to examine moles more closely. If a suspicious lesion is found, further assessment is necessary to determine if it is melanoma (Manne et al., 2024). The primary method for diagnosing melanoma is a biopsy, where a sample of the suspicious lesion is removed and examined under a microscope. After a biopsy, the tissue is examined by a pathologist to determine the presence of cancer cells and to assess features such as the depth of invasion, which helps stage the melanoma (Ojukwu et al., 2024). For more advanced cases where there is concern about spread, imaging tests such as X-rays, computed tomography (CT) scans, magnetic resonance imaging (MRI) scans, or positron emission tomography (PET) scans may be used to check for metastasis. For individuals who have been treated for melanoma, regular follow-up appointments are crucial to monitor for recurrence (Manne et al., 2024; Ojukwu et al., 2024).

Traditional diagnostic approaches, such as visual examinations and biopsies, often fall short in detecting melanoma at its earliest and most treatable stages. These limitations underscore the urgent need for advanced imaging technologies that can provide more precise, noninvasive, and comprehensive assessments (Ojukwu et al., 2024). Effective monitoring and assessment are vital in the fight against melanoma, improving early detection rates, and ensuring timely intervention, which significantly improves the prognosis for individuals with this serious form of skin cancer (Ojukwu et al., 2024; Smith et al., 2024). The advent of next-generation imaging technologies marks a significant leap forward in melanoma monitoring and assessment (Lee et al., 2022). These innovative tools, including enhanced dermatoscopy, reflectance confocal microscopy (RCM), optical coherence tomography (OCT), multiphoton microscopy (MPM), and cutting-edge molecular imaging techniques like PET and photoacoustic imaging (PAI) (**Figure 8.1**), offer detailed visualization of skin lesions at both macroscopic and microscopic levels (McGale et al., 2023). These technologies enable clinicians to detect melanoma earlier, differentiate benign from malignant lesions more accurately, and monitor treatment responses effectively (Lee et al., 2022; McGale et al., 2023).

The integration of artificial intelligence (AI) and machine learning (ML) with these imaging technologies is transforming the landscape of melanoma diagnostics (McGale et al., 2023). AI algorithms and ML models, trained on vast datasets of imaging data, can identify patterns and features indicative of melanoma with remarkable precision, reducing diagnostic errors and enhancing clinical decision-making (McGale et al., 2023; Smith et al., 2024). This chapter sets the stage for a comprehensive exploration of next-generation imaging technologies in melanoma care. It explores how next-generation approaches are revolutionizing melanoma monitoring and assessment. The chapter expounds on the latest tools that enhance our ability to track and evaluate melanoma progression, from advanced imaging modalities to AI-driven analyses.

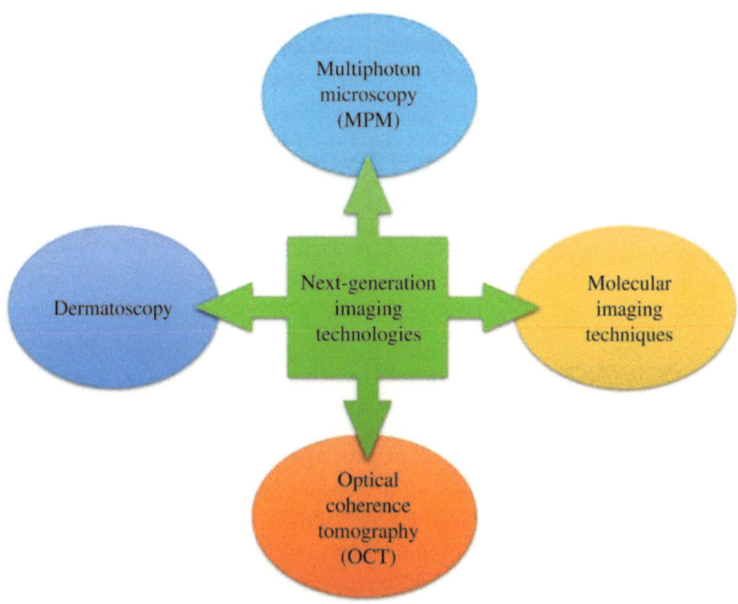

FIGURE 8.1 Next-generation imaging technologies used in melanoma monitoring and assessment. These technologies enable clinicians to detect melanoma earlier, differentiate benign from malignant lesions more accurately, and monitor treatment responses effectively.

DERMATOSCOPY AND REFLECTANCE CONFOCAL MICROSCOPY

Dermatoscopy

Dermatoscopy, also known as dermoscopy or epiluminescence microscopy, is a noninvasive diagnostic tool used extensively in the monitoring and assessment of melanoma (Jitian Mihulecea et al., 2023). Dermatoscopy allows for the detailed examination of pigmented and nonpigmented skin lesions, which can aid in the early detection of melanoma and other skin cancers. It provides a magnified view of the skin's surface, significantly improving the visualization of skin lesions (Holmes et al., 2018). Enhanced by polarized light, this technique allows dermatologists to examine skin structures not visible to the naked eye. Digital dermatoscopy integrates image analysis software, which helps in the storage, comparison, and detailed examination of lesions over time, aiding in early detection and monitoring of changes that might indicate malignancy (Wolner et al., 2017). Dermatoscopes typically provide 10× magnification and use polarized or non-polarized light to enhance the visualization of skin structures. This helps in identifying subtle features that are not visible to the naked eye (Jitian Mihulecea et al., 2023).

Contact dermatoscopy involves placing the device directly on the skin, often with a liquid interface (e.g., alcohol or oil) to reduce reflection (Holmes et al., 2018; Wolner et al., 2017). Non-contact dermatoscopy uses polarized light to achieve the same effect without skin contact. Dermatoscopy reveals various structures and colors within a lesion, which can help differentiate between benign and malignant growths (Jitian Mihulecea et al., 2023). It is crucial for monitoring patients at high risk for melanoma. Regular dermatoscopic examinations allow for the early detection of changes in existing lesions and the identification of new suspicious lesions (Jitian Mihulecea et al., 2023). In digital dermatoscopy, images of lesions are stored and compared over time to detect subtle changes that may indicate malignancy. Sequential digital dermoscopy imaging (SDDI) involves taking dermatoscopic images of lesions at regular intervals to monitor changes (Wolner et al., 2017).

Dermatoscopy increases the likelihood of detecting melanoma at an early, more treatable stage. It enhances diagnostic accuracy compared to visual inspection alone and provides a noninvasive method for monitoring and assessing skin lesions (Jitian Mihulecea et al., 2023). Digital dermatoscopy allows for detailed documentation and follow-up. However, despite the many benefits, dermatoscopy has limitations. The accuracy of dermatoscopy depends on the clinician's expertise and experience with dermatoscopy. There can be variability in interpretation among different clinicians, and it can still produce false positives and negatives (Wolner et al., 2017). Nonetheless, dermatoscopy is an invaluable tool in the monitoring and assessment of melanoma, offering detailed visualization of skin lesions that enhances early detection and accurate diagnosis. By utilizing dermatoscopic criteria and algorithms, clinicians can better differentiate between benign and malignant lesions, leading to improved patient outcomes. Regular monitoring with dermatoscopy, particularly in high-risk individuals, is essential for the early identification and treatment of melanoma (Holmes et al., 2018; Jitian Mihulecea et al., 2023).

Reflectance Confocal Microscopy

RCM is an advanced, noninvasive imaging technique used in dermatology for the in vivo examination of the skin at a cellular resolution (Liu et al., 2024). It plays a significant role in the monitoring and assessment of melanoma, offering detailed images of skin lesions that aid in the early detection and accurate diagnosis of melanoma and other skin cancers (Venturi et al., 2024). RCM provides cellular-level resolution images of the skin in a noninvasive manner. The technology is particularly useful for evaluating ambiguous lesions that are challenging to diagnose through dermatoscopy alone (Waddell et al., 2018). RCM's ability to provide real-time, high-resolution images of the epidermis and upper dermis enables the identification of characteristic features of melanoma, such as atypical melanocytes and architectural disarray, without the need for a biopsy (Liu et al., 2024). RCM provides high-resolution images comparable to histological examination, allowing for the visualization of skin structures and cells in real time. It is noninvasive, which means it can be used repeatedly for monitoring without causing any harm to the patient (Waddell et al., 2018).

RCM can image skin layers up to 200–300 micrometers deep, covering the epidermis and superficial dermis. It is a reflectance-based imaging technique that utilizes the reflectance of light from natural skin chromophores like melanin and keratin to create contrast in the images (Venturi et al., 2024). RCM helps identify specific features of melanoma in different skin layers. The key diagnostic characteristics of melanoma that are identified using RCM include (1) disorganization of the keratinocyte architecture in the epidermis, (2) presence of atypical melanocytes, which appear larger and with irregular shapes, scattered within the epidermis and at the dermo-epidermal junction (DEJ), (3) melanocytes are scattered individually or in nests within the upper layers of the epidermis, a hallmark of melanoma, (4) large, bright, dendritic cells indicative of melanocytes can be seen spreading into the epidermis, (5) irregular and disrupted appearance of the DEJ with atypical cells, (6) irregularly shaped nests of melanocytes at the DEJ or in the dermis, which are brighter due to higher reflectance, and (7) presence of atypical cells and structures in the superficial dermis (Liu et al., 2024; Waddell et al., 2018).

RCM is particularly valuable for monitoring patients at high risk of melanoma and for follow-up of suspicious lesions. It establishes a baseline image of a lesion to compare with future images, helping detect subtle changes over time (Waddell et al., 2018). RCM facilitates regular imaging sessions that allow for the monitoring of changes in lesions, aiding in the early detection of malignant transformation. It helps assess the effectiveness of treatments by monitoring changes in lesion characteristics post-therapy (Venturi et al., 2024). Thus, RCM provides cellular-level detail, improving the accuracy of melanoma diagnosis compared to dermoscopy alone. It allows for repeated examinations without discomfort or risk to the patient and offers immediate results, facilitating prompt decision-making. RCM aids in the early identification of melanoma, potentially improving patient outcomes (Liu et al., 2024). However, despite all the benefits, RCM requires significant expertise and training to accurately interpret images. While it provides excellent detail, RCM cannot image deeper than the superficial dermis, limiting its use for thicker lesions. The process of capturing and interpreting images can be time-consuming compared to other imaging methods. Moreso, RCM devices are expensive and not widely available in all clinical settings (Liu et al., 2024; Waddell et al., 2018).

According to Venturi and coworkers, RCM is often used in conjunction with other diagnostic tools such as dermoscopy and histopathology to provide a comprehensive assessment of skin lesions. RCM can provide additional details to clarify the diagnosis when dermoscopic findings are ambiguous (Venturi et al., 2024). It allows for noninvasive monitoring of suspicious lesions over time for patients with multiple atypical nevi or a history of melanoma (Liu et al., 2024; Waddell et al., 2018). RCM also enables presurgical assessment of lesion margins to guide excision and ensure complete removal (Venturi et al., 2024). In this context, RCM is a powerful tool in the monitoring and assessment of melanoma, offering high-resolution, noninvasive imaging of skin lesions. Its ability to provide detailed cellular images enhances diagnostic accuracy and aids in the early detection of melanoma (Venturi et al., 2024). While it requires significant expertise and resources, its benefits in improving patient outcomes make it a valuable addition to dermatological practice (Liu et al., 2024; Waddell et al., 2018).

OPTICAL COHERENCE TOMOGRAPHY

OCT is a noninvasive imaging technique widely used in dermatology for the assessment and monitoring of skin lesions, including melanoma (Latriglia et al., 2023). OCT uses light waves to capture cross-sectional images of the skin, providing detailed information about skin structure and pathology. It is akin to an optical ultrasound, providing cross-sectional images of the skin with micrometer resolution. This noninvasive imaging technique is valuable for assessing tumor thickness and extent, critical factors in melanoma staging (Ferrante di Ruffano et al., 2018). OCT helps in distinguishing benign from malignant lesions by evaluating structural differences within the skin. Its use is expanding in routine clinical practice due to its ability to monitor treatment response and detect recurrence. It provides high-resolution images, allowing for the visualization of skin layers and structures at a micrometer scale (Perwein et al., 2022). OCT can image skin layers up to 1–2 mm deep, covering the epidermis, dermis, and part of the subcutaneous tissue. It offers real-time imaging capabilities, providing immediate results for clinical decision-making (Latriglia et al., 2023). Similar to dermatoscopy and RCM, OCT is noninvasive, making it suitable for repeated use without causing patient discomfort or risk (Schuh et al., 2022).

OCT helps identify specific features of melanoma by providing cross-sectional images of the skin. Thus, it offers key diagnostic criteria for epidermal and dermal architecture, tumor invasion, atypical cell structures, and blood vessel changes (Latriglia et al., 2023). The epidermal and dermal architecture as a diagnostic tool focuses on the abnormalities in the structure of the epidermis and dermis, such as thickening or disruption. Tumor invasion reports on the evidence of melanoma cells invading the dermal layers, which can be seen as areas of low reflectivity due to the presence of melanin (Schuh et al., 2022). OCT helps with the visualization of atypical melanocyte clusters or nests, which appear as hyper-reflective areas. It also identifies increased vascularity and abnormal blood vessel patterns, which are often associated with melanoma (Latriglia et al., 2023). OCT is valuable for monitoring patients with suspicious lesions or a history of melanoma. It establishes a baseline image for suspicious lesions, allowing for accurate comparison over time. Regular OCT imaging sessions enable the detection of subtle changes in lesions, which may indicate malignant transformation (Perwein et al., 2022). OCT can assess the effectiveness of treatments, such as surgical excision or topical therapies, by monitoring changes in lesion structure. It provides high-resolution, cross-sectional images that enhance the understanding of lesion morphology and can be used repeatedly for monitoring without harming the patient. Immediate imaging allows for prompt clinical decision-making. OCT helps in the early detection of melanoma by identifying structural abnormalities (Ferrante di Ruffano et al., 2018).

However, OCT requires skilled operators to accurately capture and interpret images. While it provides excellent detail, it cannot image deeper skin structures beyond 1–2 mm. OCT devices are expensive, and the imaging process can be time-consuming, potentially limiting their widespread use (Perwein et al., 2022). OCT is often used alongside other diagnostic tools, such as dermoscopy, RCM, and histopathology, to provide a comprehensive assessment of skin lesions. OCT can help differentiate between benign nevi and malignant melanomas by providing detailed structural information. It facilitates presurgical assessment of lesion margins to ensure complete excision (Ferrante di Ruffano et al., 2018). OCT imaging is particularly useful to detect early changes in monitoring high-risk patients with multiple atypical nevi or a history of melanoma (Schuh et al., 2022). Thus, it is a valuable tool in the monitoring and assessment of melanoma, offering high-resolution, noninvasive imaging of skin lesions. Its ability to provide detailed cross-sectional images enhances diagnostic accuracy and aids in the early detection of melanoma (Perwein et al., 2022). While it requires expertise and resources, the benefits of OCT in improving patient outcomes make it a significant addition to dermatological practice (Schuh et al., 2022).

MULTIPHOTON MICROSCOPY

MPM is an advanced imaging technique used in dermatology to provide high-resolution, three-dimensional images of skin tissue (Basra et al., 2024). MPM is particularly valuable in melanoma monitoring and assessment due to its ability to visualize skin structures at a cellular and subcellular level (Shapiro et al., 2024). It utilizes near-infrared light to excite fluorophores within the skin, generating high-resolution images of cellular and subcellular structures. This technique is particularly advantageous for its depth penetration and minimal photodamage (Soglia et al., 2022). MPM can visualize skin layers and cellular morphology in real time, aiding in the differentiation of melanoma from benign lesions. It also holds potential for assessing the effectiveness of treatments by visualizing dynamic changes in the tumor microenvironment. MPM provides high-resolution images, allowing for detailed visualization of skin structures down to the cellular level. It can generate three-dimensional images, enabling a comprehensive assessment of skin lesions (Basra et al., 2024). MPM is noninvasive and safe for repeated use, which is ideal for monitoring skin changes over time, and can image deeper layers of the skin (up to about 500 micrometers) than some other imaging modalities, reaching the superficial dermis. MPM utilizes two-photon excitation to produce autofluorescence from endogenous molecules (e.g., NADH, FAD) and second harmonic generation from collagen, providing intrinsic contrast without the need for external dyes (Shapiro et al., 2024).

MPM helps identify specific features of melanoma by providing detailed images of skin tissue in melanoma assessment. It is used in key diagnostic provisions that include cellular and subcellular structures, nuclear morphology, melanin distribution, and tissue architecture (Shapiro et al., 2024). Visualization of individual melanocytes, keratinocytes, and other skin cells, allowing for the identification of atypical cells. MPM helps identify specific nuclear morphology features through the assessment of nuclear size, shape, and density, which can indicate malignancy. It also allows the visualization of melanin within melanocytes and keratinocytes, aiding in the differentiation of benign and malignant lesions (Soglia et al., 2022). MPM facilitates the evaluation of overall tissue architecture, including the organization and integrity of the epidermis and dermis. The specific features of melanoma identified by MPM include (1) the presence of large, irregularly shaped melanocytes with prominent nucleoli, (2) melanocytes scattered individually or in clusters throughout the epidermis, (3) irregular and disrupted DEJ with infiltration of atypical cells, and (4) abnormal collagen fiber patterns detected by second harmonic generation imaging (Shapiro et al., 2024; Soglia et al., 2022).

MPM is valuable for monitoring patients at high risk of melanoma and for follow-up of suspicious lesions. It establishes detailed baseline images of suspicious lesions, allowing for accurate comparison over time (Patel et al., 2023). Regular MPM imaging sessions enable the detection of subtle changes in lesions, which may indicate malignant transformation. It can assess the effectiveness of treatments by monitoring changes in lesion structure and cellular morphology post-therapy (Shapiro et al., 2024; Soglia et al., 2022). MPM provides high-resolution, three-dimensional images of skin tissue at a cellular level. It is safe for repeated use, allowing for continuous monitoring of lesions over time. MPM is capable of imaging deeper skin layers than some other noninvasive techniques. It uses endogenous fluorescence, eliminating the need for external contrast agents (Patel et al., 2023; Soglia et al., 2022). Nevertheless, MPM systems are expensive and not widely available in clinical settings. It also requires specialized equipment and significant expertise to operate and interpret images. Moreso, imaging and analysis can be time-consuming compared to other diagnostic methods. While it can image deeper than some methods, it still does not penetrate as deeply as some other modalities like ultrasound or MRI (Shapiro et al., 2024; Soglia et al., 2022).

MPM is often used in conjunction with other diagnostic tools such as dermoscopy, RCM, and histopathology to provide a comprehensive assessment of skin lesions. It is particularly useful for challenging diagnoses, margin assessment, and high-risk patient monitoring (Soglia et al., 2022). When dermoscopic or RCM findings are ambiguous, MPM can provide additional detail to clarify the diagnosis. It is often used in margin assessment to conduct presurgical assessment of lesion margins to guide excision and ensure complete removal. MPM is used in high-risk monitoring, where regular MPM imaging is conducted to detect early changes for high-risk patients with multiple atypical nevi or a history of melanoma (Shapiro et al., 2024; Soglia et al., 2022). Hence, MPM is a powerful tool in the monitoring and assessment of melanoma, offering high-resolution, three-dimensional imaging of skin tissue at a cellular level. Its ability to provide detailed visualization of cellular and subcellular structures enhances diagnostic accuracy and aids in the early detection of melanoma (Basra et al., 2024). While it requires significant expertise and resources, the benefits of MPM in improving patient outcomes make it a valuable addition to dermatological practice (Basra et al., 2024; Patel et al., 2023; Shapiro et al., 2024).

MOLECULAR IMAGING TECHNIQUES

Molecular imaging techniques play a crucial role in the monitoring and assessment of melanoma, offering high-resolution, functional insights that enhance diagnostic accuracy and treatment planning. They are critical tools in providing detailed information at the molecular and cellular levels (van der Hiel et al., 2024). By integrating these advanced imaging modalities into clinical practice, healthcare providers achieve more precise detection, staging, and monitoring of melanoma, ultimately improving patient outcomes. These techniques enhance the ability to detect, diagnose, and monitor the progression and treatment response of melanoma. While there are challenges related to cost, accessibility, and complexity, the benefits of molecular imaging in providing detailed, actionable information make it an invaluable tool in the fight against melanoma (Lee et al., 2024).

Positron Emission Tomography

PET is a powerful imaging technique used in the monitoring and assessment of melanoma, particularly for detecting metastatic disease and evaluating treatment response (van der Hiel et al., 2024). PET scans, often combined with CT or MRI, provide functional imaging by highlighting areas of metabolic activity, which can be indicative of cancerous tissue. It allows for the visualization of metabolic activity within lesions (Lee et al., 2024). Radiotracers, such as fluorodeoxyglucose (FDG), accumulate in highly active melanoma cells due to their high metabolic rate, making PET a powerful tool for detecting metabolic activity, metastatic disease, and evaluating treatment response (Dimitrakopoulou-Strauss, 2019). PET provides whole-body scans, making it particularly useful for detecting metastatic disease. It is often combined with CT (PET/CT) or MRI (PET/MRI) to provide both metabolic and anatomical information, enhancing diagnostic accuracy (Lee et al., 2024; van der Hiel et al., 2024).

PET in melanoma assessment helps identify primary melanoma lesions, especially those that are metabolically active. It is highly effective in detecting metastases to lymph nodes, liver, lungs, bones, and brain. It helps in staging the disease by identifying the extent of spread (Dimitrakopoulou-Strauss, 2019; Lee et al., 2024). PET is used to monitor recurrence in patients with a history of melanoma, detecting new metastatic lesions that may not be visible with other imaging modalities (van der Hiel et al., 2024). PET scans can guide surgical planning by identifying the extent of the disease and aiding in the determination of surgical margins. It helps in targeting radiotherapy by delineating active tumor areas (van der Hiel et al., 2024). PET scans are used to assess the effectiveness of systemic therapies such as chemotherapy and immunotherapy responses. A decrease in metabolic activity on PET indicates a positive response to treatment (Dimitrakopoulou-Strauss, 2019; van der Hiel et al., 2024). PET has high sensitivity for detecting distant metastases, making it invaluable for staging and monitoring advanced melanoma. It can scan the entire body in a single session, providing a comprehensive overview of the disease (Lee et al., 2024). PET offers insights into the metabolic activity of tumors, which can be more informative than structural changes alone. It also detects metabolic changes before anatomical changes become apparent, allowing for earlier intervention (van der Hiel et al., 2024).

Nevertheless, PET involves exposure to ionizing radiation, which can be a concern for some patients, especially with repeated scans. High metabolic activity is not exclusive to cancer cells; infections and inflammation can also show increased uptake, leading to false positives (Dimitrakopoulou-Strauss, 2019). PET scans are expensive and may not be available in all healthcare settings. While PET provides functional information, its spatial resolution is lower compared to CT or MRI, which can limit the precise localization of small lesions (Lee et al., 2024; van der Hiel et al., 2024). PET is integrated into the management of melanoma patients alongside other diagnostic and therapeutic tools. For example, PET/CT or PET/MRI is often performed at the time of initial diagnosis to determine the stage of melanoma and plan appropriate treatment (van der Hiel et al., 2024). Regular PET scans can assess the effectiveness of ongoing treatment and guide adjustments in therapy and are used in post-treatment surveillance to monitor for signs of recurrence, particularly in high-risk patients. PET is also used to guide biopsies and surgeries of suspicious areas and help plan surgical excisions by delineating active tumor margins (Lee et al., 2024).

Hence, PET is a critical tool in the monitoring and assessment of melanoma, providing detailed functional imaging that complements anatomical imaging modalities (Dimitrakopoulou-Strauss, 2019). Its ability to detect metabolic activity makes it particularly useful for staging, detecting metastases, and evaluating treatment response (van der Hiel et al., 2024). While it has limitations, such as radiation exposure and potential for false positives, the benefits of PET in providing comprehensive and early detection of melanoma spread and recurrence make it an invaluable asset in the management of this disease (Lee et al., 2024; van der Hiel et al., 2024).

Photoacoustic Imaging

PAI is an emerging noninvasive imaging technique that combines the high spatial resolution of optical imaging with the deep tissue penetration of ultrasound. This hybrid method is particularly useful in melanoma monitoring and assessment because it provides detailed information about the morphology and function of skin lesions (Fakhoury et al., 2024). PAI can detect melanin and blood vessels within lesions, offering insights into tumor angiogenesis and hypoxia. PAI's ability to provide functional and molecular information complements structural imaging techniques, enhancing overall diagnostic accuracy (von Knorring et al., 2024). PAI offers high spatial resolution comparable to optical imaging while allowing deeper tissue penetration, up to several centimeters. It provides both anatomical details and functional information about tissue properties, such as oxygen saturation and blood volume (Lee et al., 2023). PAI can visualize endogenous chromophores like melanin, hemoglobin, and lipid without the need for external contrast agents, making it particularly suited for melanoma, which is rich in melanin (Fakhoury et al., 2024). PAI helps identify specific features of melanoma by providing high-resolution images of skin tissue. It can visualize melanin concentration in lesions, which is a primary feature of melanoma (Lee et al., 2023). PAI can detect vascular changes such as abnormal blood vessel patterns and increased blood volume, often seen in melanomas. It can also detect differences in oxygen saturation between normal and cancerous tissues and can provide functional insights into the metabolic state of the lesion (von Knorring et al., 2024).

PAI can provide detailed structural information about the shape, size, and depth of lesions. Thus, PAI is valuable for monitoring patients with suspicious lesions or a history of melanoma. It establishes a detailed baseline image of a suspicious lesion, allowing for accurate comparison over time (von Knorring et al., 2024). Regular PAI imaging sessions enable the detection of subtle changes in lesions, which may indicate malignant transformation or response to treatment. PAI can monitor changes in vascularity, oxygen saturation, and lesion morphology to assess the effectiveness of therapies such as surgery, chemotherapy, and immunotherapy. It provides high-resolution images of both the structure and function of skin lesions and is safe for repeated use, making it ideal for continuous monitoring (Lee et al., 2023). PAI is capable of imaging deeper tissues compared to purely optical methods and offers insights into the vascular and metabolic state of lesions. It utilizes natural tissue chromophores, eliminating the need for external contrast agents (von Knorring et al., 2024). However, as an emerging technology, PAI is not yet widely available in clinical practice. It requires specialized equipment and expertise to operate and interpret the images. PAI images can be affected by factors such as tissue heterogeneity and motion artifacts (Fakhoury et al., 2024).

PAI is increasingly being integrated into the management of melanoma alongside other imaging techniques such as dermoscopy, RCM, and PET. It is particularly useful for identifying early-stage melanoma by visualizing melanin distribution and vascular changes. It is used in regular imaging and monitoring of high-risk patients with multiple atypical nevi or a history of melanoma to detect early changes (von Knorring et al., 2024). PAI can help guide biopsies by identifying the most suspicious areas and delineating tumor margins for surgical planning. It is also used for assessment of treatment response, monitoring changes in vascularity and oxygenation post-therapy to evaluate the efficacy of treatments (Lee et al., 2023). In this context, PAI is a promising tool in the monitoring and assessment of melanoma, offering high-resolution, noninvasive imaging that combines anatomical and functional information. Its ability to visualize melanin, blood vessels, and metabolic states provides comprehensive insights into skin lesions, enhancing diagnostic accuracy and aiding in early detection and treatment monitoring. While it is still an emerging technology with some limitations, the potential benefits of PAI in the characterization of melanoma (**Figure 8.2**) make it a valuable addition to dermatological practice, particularly in the management of melanoma (Fakhoury et al., 2024; Lee et al., 2023).

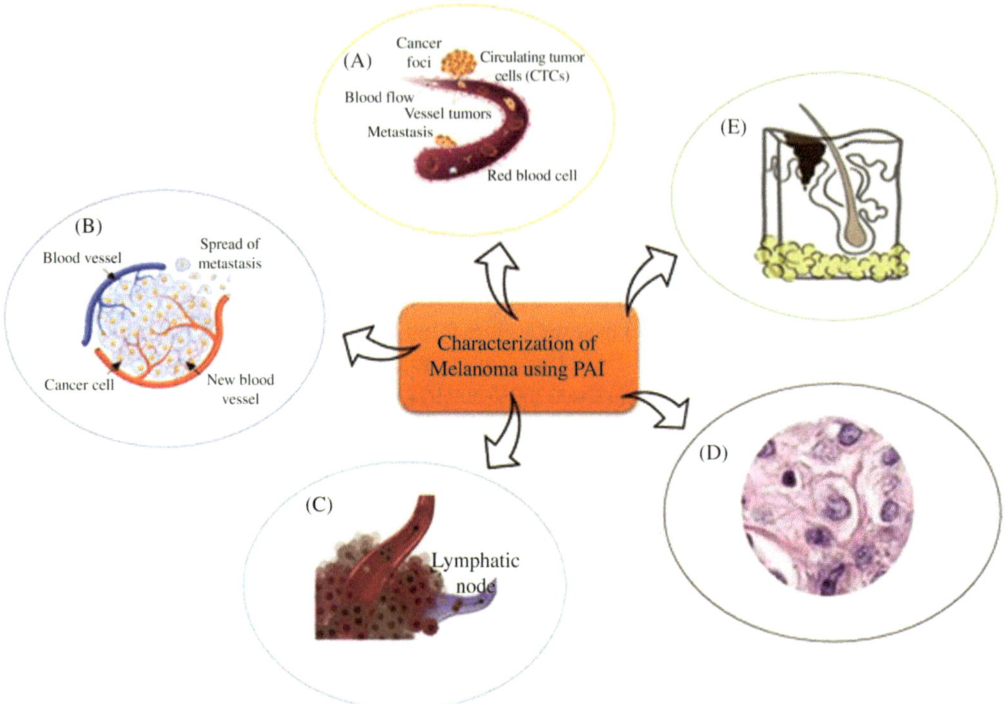

FIGURE 8.2 **Characterization of melanoma using photoacoustic imaging (PAI).** (A) Circulating tumor cell (CTC) detection, (B) Tumor angiogenesis, (C) Lymph node metastasis detection, (D) Virtual histology, and (E) Detection and depth measurement.

ARTIFICIAL INTELLIGENCE AND MACHINE LEARNING

AI and ML are revolutionizing the field of dermatology, particularly in the diagnosis, monitoring, and assessment of melanoma (Wei et al., 2024; Yee et al., 2024). These advanced technologies leverage large datasets of dermatoscopic images and sophisticated algorithms to enhance diagnostic accuracy, predict outcomes, and personalize treatment plans (Anderson et al., 2024). ML models, trained in extensive image libraries assist, clinicians in distinguishing benign from malignant lesions, reducing diagnostic errors, and improving early detection rates. AI algorithms analyze dermoscopic, confocal, and histopathological images to detect melanoma with high accuracy (Schreidah et al., 2024). ML models can predict melanoma progression, treatment response, and patient outcomes based on clinical data. The AI-powered tools assist clinicians in making informed decisions by providing real-time analysis and recommendations (Wei et al., 2024; Yee et al., 2024). AI algorithms, particularly convolutional neural networks (CNNs), are trained on large datasets of dermoscopic images to identify patterns indicative of melanoma. These systems can differentiate between benign and malignant lesions with high sensitivity and specificity (Schreidah et al., 2024; Yee et al., 2024).

AI models can analyze RCM images to detect cellular and subcellular features of melanoma, such as atypical melanocytes and disorganized DEJs (Wei et al., 2024). In histopathological image analysis, AI tools assist pathologists by highlighting areas of concern in histopathological slides, improving the accuracy and speed of melanoma diagnosis (Yee et al., 2024). ML models analyze patient data, including genetic, clinical, and imaging information in predictive modeling and prognostics, to stratify patients based on their risk of melanoma development and progression (Wei et al., 2024). AI predicts how a patient responds to specific treatments, such as immunotherapy or targeted therapy, by analyzing patterns in historical data. AI models use patient data to predict survival rates and disease-free intervals, helping clinicians to develop personalized treatment plans (Schreidah et al., 2024). AI algorithms track changes in skin lesions over time using sequential images, identifying subtle changes that may indicate malignancy. AI tools monitor patients' post-treatment to detect signs of recurrence early, improving the chances of successful intervention (Schreidah et al., 2024). AI algorithms achieve diagnostic accuracies comparable to or exceeding those of expert dermatologists (Yee et al., 2024).

Automated analysis by AI reduces the time required for diagnosis and assessment, allowing for faster clinical decision-making. It provides consistent analysis, minimizing the variability associated with human interpretation (Wei et al., 2024). AI can detect subtle changes in lesions that may be missed by the human eye, enabling earlier diagnosis and intervention. AI and ML enable the development of personalized treatment plans based on individual patient data and predicted outcomes (Yee et al., 2024). Nonetheless, the accuracy of AI models depends on the quality and diversity of the training data. Biased or incomplete datasets can lead to inaccurate predictions (Wei et al., 2024). Some AI models, particularly deep learning algorithms, operate as "black boxes," making it difficult to understand how they arrive at their conclusions (Schreidah et al., 2024). Implementing AI tools in clinical settings requires significant resources, including training for healthcare providers and integration with existing systems. The use of AI in healthcare raises issues related to patient privacy, data security, and regulatory approval (Yee et al., 2024).

AI and ML are being integrated into various aspects of melanoma management, often in conjunction with traditional diagnostic tools. AI-powered systems assist clinicians as decision support systems by providing real-time analysis and diagnostic recommendations based on patient data (Schreidah et al., 2024). In the context of telemedicine, AI enables remote monitoring and assessment of skin lesions, improving access to dermatological care, particularly in underserved areas. It accelerates research by analyzing large datasets to identify new biomarkers and therapeutic targets for melanoma (Yee et al., 2024). Hence, AI and ML are transforming the monitoring and assessment of melanoma by enhancing diagnostic accuracy, predicting outcomes, and personalizing treatment plans. These technologies offer significant benefits, including improved efficiency, consistency, and early detection (Wei et al., 2024; Yee et al., 2024). However, challenges related to data quality, interpretability, and integration into clinical practice must be addressed to fully realize their potential (Wei et al., 2024). As AI and ML continue to evolve, they are poised to play an increasingly important role in the fight against melanoma, improving patient outcomes and advancing the field of dermatology (Schreidah et al., 2024; Wei et al., 2024).

LIMITATIONS AND CHALLENGES

Next-generation imaging technologies for melanoma monitoring and assessment face several limitations and challenges, despite their significant advancements and potential. Understanding these obstacles is crucial for the ongoing development and integration of these tools in clinical practice (Garrison et al., 2023). The implementation of advanced imaging technologies often involves substantial costs related to equipment, maintenance, and training. This financial burden can limit accessibility, particularly in low-resource settings. Ensuring widespread availability of these technologies remains a significant challenge (Stafford et al., 2023). Many next-generation imaging techniques require specialized knowledge and training to operate effectively. This complexity can hinder their adoption in routine clinical practice. For instance, interpreting images from RCM or MPM necessitates expertise that not all healthcare providers possess (Subbiah, 2023). The quality of images produced by advanced imaging technologies can be affected by various factors, including operator skill, patient skin type, and the specific technology used. Variability in image quality can impact diagnostic accuracy and consistency, posing a challenge for reliable melanoma assessment (Wei et al., 2024; Yee et al., 2024).

Integrating next-generation imaging technologies into existing clinical workflows can be challenging. The time required for imaging and analysis might extend patient visit durations, and seamless integration with electronic health records (EHR) systems is often complex and time-consuming

(Wei et al., 2024; Yee et al., 2024). New imaging technologies must undergo rigorous regulatory approval processes to ensure their safety and efficacy. This can be a lengthy and costly process (Subbiah, 2023). Additionally, the validation of these technologies through large-scale clinical trials is essential to establish their reliability and effectiveness in diverse patient populations. While AI and ML hold great promise in enhancing diagnostic accuracy, the "black box" nature of some AI algorithms can be a limitation (Wei et al., 2024). Clinicians may find it challenging to understand and trust AI-generated insights without clear explanations of how conclusions were reached. Ensuring transparency and interpretability of AI models is crucial for their acceptance in clinical practice (Yee et al., 2024). The use of advanced imaging and AI technologies raises ethical and privacy concerns, particularly regarding the handling and storage of sensitive patient data. Ensuring robust data protection measures and addressing ethical considerations are essential to maintain patient trust and compliance with regulations (Subbiah, 2023).

Proving the clinical utility and efficacy of next-generation imaging technologies in improving patient outcomes remains a challenge. While these technologies offer enhanced imaging capabilities, demonstrating that they lead to better clinical decisions and improved survival rates through comprehensive clinical studies is necessary for widespread adoption (Wei et al., 2024). While next-generation imaging technologies offer remarkable potential in revolutionizing melanoma monitoring and assessment, they are not without limitations and challenges (Subbiah, 2023). Addressing these issues requires a multifaceted approach, including reducing costs, enhancing training, improving integration into clinical workflows, ensuring regulatory compliance, and demonstrating clear clinical benefits. By overcoming these obstacles, the healthcare community can fully leverage these advanced tools to improve melanoma diagnosis and patient care (Wei et al., 2024; Yee et al., 2024).

CONCLUSION

Next-generation imaging technologies are poised to revolutionize the field of melanoma detection, monitoring, and assessment. By providing detailed, noninvasive, and highly accurate visualization of skin lesions, these advanced tools significantly enhance the capabilities of healthcare providers in diagnosing and managing melanoma. Technologies such as enhanced dermatoscopy, RCM, OCT, MPM, and molecular imaging techniques like PET and PAI offer unparalleled insights into the structural and functional characteristics of skin lesions. The integration of AI and ML further amplifies the potential of these imaging modalities, enabling precise pattern recognition and predictive analytics that improve early detection and diagnostic accuracy.

These advancements are not only transforming clinical practice but also paving the way for personalized treatment strategies, ultimately leading to better patient outcomes. Next-generation imaging technologies represent a significant advancement in melanoma care. By facilitating earlier detection, more accurate diagnosis, and effective monitoring of treatment responses, these technologies are set to drastically improve melanoma management and patient survival rates. As these technologies continue to evolve and integrate with other medical innovations, their role in combating melanoma will become increasingly vital, heralding a new era of precision medicine in dermatology.

REFERENCES

Anderson, A. D. G., Lo, S. N. and Guitera, P. 2024. Commentary: Real-world post-deployment performance of a novel machine learning-based digital health technology for skin lesion assessment and suggestions for post-market surveillance, *Frontiers in Medicine (Lausanne)*, 11, p. 1345659.

Basra, M., Shapiro, L., Patel, H., Payne, C., Brazen, B. and Biglione, A. 2024. Exploring the utilization of imaging modalities in the diagnosis of basal cell carcinoma: A scoping review, *Cureus*, 16(3), p. e56047.

Bouton, C., Schmeltz, H., Lévèque, C., Gaultier, A., Quereux, G., Dreno, B., Nguyen, J. M. and Rat, C. 2024. Early diagnosis of melanoma: A randomized trial assessing the impact of the transmission of photographs taken with a smartphone from the general practitioner to the dermatologist on the time to dermatological consultation, *BMC Health Services Research*, 24(1), p. 660.

Boutros, A., Croce, E., Ferrari, M., Gili, R., Massaro, G., Marconcini, R., Arecco, L., Tanda, E. T. and Spagnolo, F. 2024. The treatment of advanced melanoma: Current approaches and new challenges, *Critical Reviews in Oncology/Hematology*, 196, p. 104276.

Dimitrakopoulou-Strauss, A. 2019. Monitoring of patients with metastatic melanoma treated with immune checkpoint inhibitors using PET-CT, *Cancer Immunology, Immunotherapy*, 68(5), pp. 813–822.

Fakhoury, J. W., Lara, J. B., Manwar, R., Zafar, M., Xu, Q., Engel, R., Tsoukas, M. M., Daveluy, S., Mehregan, D. and Avanaki, K. 2024. Photoacoustic imaging for cutaneous melanoma assessment: A comprehensive review, *Journal of Biomedical Optics*, 29(1), p. S11518.

Ferrante di Ruffano, L., Dinnes, J., Deeks, J. J., Chuchu, N., Bayliss, S. E., Davenport, C., Takwoingi, Y., Godfrey, K., O'Sullivan, C., Matin, R. N., Tehrani, H., Williams, H. C. and Cochrane Skin Cancer Diagnostic Test Accuracy Group. 2018. Optical coherence tomography for diagnosing skin cancer in adults. *Cochrane Database of Systematic Reviews*, 12(12), p. CD013189.

Garrison, Z. R., Hall, C. M., Fey, R. M., Clister, T., Khan, N., Nichols, R. and Kulkarni, R. P. 2023. Advances in early detection of melanoma and the future of at-home testing, *Life (Basel)*, 13(4), p. 974.

Holmes, G. A., Vassantachart, J. M., Limone, B. A., Zumwalt, M., Hirokane, J. and Jacob, S. E. 2018. Using dermoscopy to identify melanoma and improve diagnostic discrimination, *Federal Practitioner*, 35(4), pp. S39–S45.

Jitian Mihulecea, C. R., Iancu, G. M., Leventer, M. and Rotaru, M. 2023. The many roles of dermoscopy in melanoma detection, *Life (Basel)*, 13(2), p. 477.

Latriglia, F., Ogien, J., Tavernier, C., Fischman, S., Suppa, M., Perrot, J. L. and Dubois, A. 2023. Line-field confocal optical coherence tomography (LC-OCT) for skin imaging in dermatology, *Life (Basel)*, 13(12), p. 2268.

Lee, H., Choi, W., Kim, C., Park, B. and Kim, J. 2023. Review on ultrasound-guided photoacoustic imaging for complementary analyses of biological systems in vivo, *Experimental Biology and Medicine (Maywood)*, 248(9), pp. 762–774.

Lee, K. J., Betz-Stablein, B., Stark, M. S., Janda, M., McInerney-Leo, A. M., Caffery, L. J., Gillespie, N., Yanes, T. and Soyer, H. P. 2022. The future of precision prevention for advanced melanoma, *Frontiers in Medicine (Lausanne)*, 8, p. 818096.

Lee, S. T., Kovaleva, N., Senko, C., Kee, D. and Scott, A. M. 2024. Positron emission tomography/computed tomography transformation of oncology: Melanoma and skin malignancies, *PET Clinics*, 19(2), pp. 231–248.

Liu, H., Jiang, H. and Shan, Q. (2024). Reflectance confocal microscopy versus dermoscopy for the diagnosis of cutaneous melanoma: A head-to-head comparative meta-analysis. *Melanoma Research*, 34(4), pp. 355–365. doi: 10.1097/CMR.0000000000000980.

Manne, S., Heckman, C. J., Frederick, S., Schaefer, A. A., Studts, C. R., Khavjou, O., Honeycutt, A., Berger, A. and Liu, H. 2024. A digital intervention to improve skin self-examination among survivors of melanoma: Protocol for a type-1 hybrid effectiveness-implementation randomized trial, *JMIR Research Protocols*, 13, p. e52689.

McGale, J., Hama, J., Yeh, R., Vercellino, L., Sun, R., Lopci, E., Ammari, S. and Dercle, L. 2023. Artificial intelligence and radiomics: Clinical applications for patients with advanced melanoma treated with immunotherapy, *Diagnostics (Basel)*, 13(19), p. 3065.

Ojukwu, K., Eguchi, M. M., Adamson, A. S., Kerr, K. F., Piepkorn, M. W., Murdoch, S., Barnhill, R. L., Elder, D. E., Knezevich, S. R. and Elmore, J. G. 2024. Immunohistochemistry for diagnosing melanoma in older adults, *JAMA Dermatology*, 160(4), pp. 434–440.

Patel, R. H., Foltz, E. A., Witkowski, A. and Ludzik, J. 2023. Analysis of artificial intelligence-based approaches applied to non-invasive imaging for early detection of melanoma: A systematic review, *Cancers (Basel)*, 15(19), p. 4694.

Perwein, M. K. E., Welzel, J., De Carvalho, N., Pellacani, G. and Schuh, S. 2022. Dynamic optical coherence tomography: A non-invasive imaging tool for the distinction of nevi and melanomas, *Cancers (Basel)*, 15(1), p. 20.

Schreidah, C. M., Gordon, E. R., Adeuyan, O., Chen, C., Lapolla, B. A., Kent, J. A., Reynolds, G. B., Fahmy, L. M., Weng, C., Tatonetti, N. P., Chase, H. S., Pe'er, I. and Geskin, L. J. 2024. Current status of artificial intelligence methods for skin cancer survival analysis: A scoping review, *Frontiers in Medicine (Lausanne)*, 11, p. 1243659.

Schuh, S., Ruini, C., Perwein, M. K. E., Daxenberger, F., Gust, C., Sattler, E. C. and Welzel, J. 2022. Line-field confocal optical coherence tomography: A new tool for the differentiation between nevi and melanomas? *Cancers (Basel)*, 14(5), p. 1140.

Shapiro, L., Basra, M., Patel, H., Payne, C., Brazen, B. and Biglione, A. 2024. Utilization of imaging modalities in the diagnosis of melanoma: A scoping review, *Cureus*, 16(2), p. e54058.

Smith, A. L., Smit, A. K., Laginha, B. I., Singh, N., Gallo, B., Martin, L. and Cust, A. E. 2024. Implementing systematic melanoma risk assessment and risk-tailored surveillance in a skin cancer focussed dermatology clinic: A qualitative study of feasibility and acceptability to patients and clinic staff, *Cancer Medicine*, 13(2), p. e6976.

Soglia, S., Pérez-Anker, J., Lobos Guede, N., Giavedoni, P., Puig, S. and Malvehy, J. 2022. Diagnostics using non-invasive technologies in dermatological oncology, *Cancers (Basel)*, 14(23), p. 5886.

Stafford, H., Buell, J., Chiang, E., Ramesh, U., Migden, M., Nagarajan, P., Amit, M. and Yaniv, D. 2023. Non-melanoma skin cancer detection in the age of advanced technology: A review, *Cancers (Basel)*, 15(12), p. 3094.

Subbiah, V. 2023. The next generation of evidence-based medicine, *Nature Medicine*, 29(1), pp. 49–58.

van der Hiel, B., Aalbersberg, E. A., van den Eertwegh, A. J. M., de Wit-van der Veen, L. J., Stokkel, M. P. M., Lopez-Yurda, M., Boellaard, R., Kapiteijn, E. W., Hospers, G. A. P., Aarts, M. J. B., de Vos, F. Y. F. L., Boers-Sonderen, M. J., van der Veldt, A. A. M., de Groot, J. W. B. and Haanen, J. B. A. G. 2024. The predictive value of FDG PET/CT for determining progression-free survival in advanced stage III-IV BRAF-mutated melanoma patients treated with targeted therapy – what can be learned from progression? *Clinical Nuclear Medicine*, 49(2), pp. 138–145.

Venturi, F., Veronesi, G., Baraldi, C. and Dika, E. (2024). Reflectance confocal microscopy as noninvasive tool for monitoring tirbanibulin efficacy in actinic keratosis. *Photodiagnosis and Photodynamic Therapy*, 48, p. 104235.

von Knorring, T., Blanche, P., Holstad Pedersen, H., Rosenkrantz Hölmich, L., Løth Mårtensson, N., Reichl, C., Karmisholt, K. and Mogensen, M. (2024). Diagnostic accuracy of expeditious bedside evaluation of cutaneous malignant melanoma using photoacoustic imaging. *Journal of the European Academy of Dermatology and Venereology*, doi: 10.1111/jdv.20046.

Waddell, A., Star, P. and Guitera, P. 2018. Advances in the use of reflectance confocal microscopy in melanoma, *Melanoma Management*, 5(1), p. MMT04.

Wei, M. L., Tada, M., So, A. and Torres, R. 2024. Artificial intelligence and skin cancer, *Frontiers in Medicine (Lausanne)*, 11, p. 1331895.

Wolner, Z. J., Yélamos, O., Liopyris, K., Rogers, T., Marchetti, M. A. and Marghoob, A. A. 2017. Enhancing skin cancer diagnosis with dermoscopy, *Dermatologic Clinics*, 35(4), pp. 417–437.

Yee, J., Rosendahl, C. and Aoude, L. G. 2024. The role of artificial intelligence and convolutional neural networks in the management of melanoma: A clinical, pathological, and radiological perspective, *Melanoma Research*, 34(2), pp. 96–104.

9 Patient-Centric Technologies
Empowering Individuals in Melanoma Care

Demetra Demetriou and Zodwa Dlamini
SAMRC Precision Oncology Research Unit (PORU), DSTI/NRF SARChI Chair in Precision Oncology and Cancer Prevention (POCP), Pan African Cancer Research Institute (PACRI), University of Pretoria, Pretoria, South Africa

Mahlatse Kgokolo
University of Pretoria, Pretoria, South Africa

Ashokkumar Deenabandu and Sandra McGuigan
Fortrea Inc., Durham, North Carolina, USA

Kamal S. Saini
Fortrea Inc., Durham, North Carolina, USA
and
Addenbrooke's Hospital, Cambridge University Hospitals NHS Foundation Trust, Cambridge, UK

INTRODUCTION

Skin cancer accounts for one out of every three cancer diagnoses, per Skin Cancer Foundation Statistics. Melanoma is one of the most aggressive forms of skin cancer due to its propensity to spread, including distant metastases, in contrast to non-melanoma skin cancers such as squamous cell carcinoma (SCC) and basal cell carcinoma (BCC) that have relatively good prognoses. The melanocytes are the source of melanoma, a complicated disease with a high degree of genetic diversity and mutational burden (Pacheco et al., 2011). Aside from other uncommon varieties (such as mucosal surfaces, uveal tracts, and leptomeninges), cutaneous melanoma makes up approximately 5% of all cutaneous malignancies and is also a lethal form of skin cancer (Ward and Farma, 2017). Technology has enabled patients to become more involved with their medical journey, tailoring it to their individual preferences and displaying the need for a patient-centric approach. Melanoma patients should receive treatment in medical facilities that guarantee multidisciplinary involvement and a holistic approach. Modern healthcare facilities, particularly those that treat cancer patients, need to change their information technology (IT)/digital infrastructure to strengthen the integrated, patient-centered systems.

The modern clinical encounter now revolves around active patient participation and patient-centered care. Patient-centered care is described as "care that is respectful of and responsive to individual patient preferences, needs, and values, and ensuring that patient values guide all clinical decisions" by the National Academy of Medicine (Corrigan, 2005). With its wide range of data measurement, information management, and process automation capabilities, technology is essential to the healthcare system's ability to appropriately consider patient preferences, requirements, and values into account when making

DOI: 10.1201/9781003511625-9

clinical decisions. The most essential aspect of making such decisions is to ensure that medical care is provided safely and efficiently. The stakes are too high for the best use of every resource available to us to enhance patient safety, with hundreds of thousands of needless deaths and millions of avoidable adverse events occurring annually. Health information technology (HIT) is one of the most significant developments in the healthcare industry that clinicians can use to increase accountability, improve outcomes, and control costs. The improved management of health information using electronic health records that facilitate consistent documentation and better access to patient records and administrative efficiency, in addition to methods that enhance and standardize communication, has been shown to result in significant safety advantages by decreasing medication mistakes, decreasing adverse drug reactions, and enhancing adherence to recommended practices (Alotaibi and Federico, 2017). With this era of evolving digital health comes a lot of challenges (Wachter, 2015). The automation of clinical procedures and the electronic administration of health information are significant steps toward mitigating the risk to patient safety associated with variations in the delivery of healthcare.

Along with enabling patient interaction throughout the continuum of care, IT must also allow for an understanding of and attention to patients' preferences, requirements, and values in addition to preventing adverse events. To encourage patient empowerment and involvement, for instance, there is a rising need for healthcare professionals and patients to communicate better and more efficiently. This has led to the utilization of consumer eHealth tools and patient-centric technologies (Grando et al., 2015; Rozenblum et al., 2015). Patients are empowered to know their treatment plan in advance, enhance the quality of treatment they receive, and the way healthcare practitioners evaluate their performance when they use technologies that encourage them to report their experiences, results, and follow-up activities. Patient-centric technologies enable patients to take a more active role in their care by giving them the power to control their health, collective decision-making, select physicians, and obtain health information (Rozenblum et al., 2015). Patient-centric health records and patient portals, for instance, enable patients to examine, confirm, and act on their health information from convenient locations outside of the conventional provider setting. Using additional tools, patients can interact with other patients who have comparable medical conditions, plan care amongst caregivers, and communicate directly with their care team, thereby expanding and strengthening their network of healthcare providers (Rozenblum et al., 2015).

Additionally, patients can now access mobile health apps that provide personalized education, monitoring, networking, and information based on their convenience and requirements. Secure messaging and telehealth facilitate contact between patients and physicians as well as promote easy interaction between patients with similar conditions. When used in tandem, these resources help foster trust, manage expectations, and improve openness at times of patient vulnerability. Social media and other innovative platforms, including mobile applications, give patients and their families new ways to get involved in their care, self-manage their health issues, learn from others who have similar ailments, communicate better with their healthcare professionals, and even report safety concerns. Additionally, they open new avenues for doctors to interact with patients in ways that suit them best, advancing the trend toward patient-centered care (Hawkins et al., 2016; Rozenblum and Bates, 2013; Rozenblum et al., 2017).

Increasing patient involvement through HIT has proven to encourage patient behavior resulting in better health outcomes, increased satisfaction and efficiency of care delivery, lower costs, and higher standards of patient safety and care quality (Davis Giardina et al., 2014; Wagner et al., 2012). In a study conducted in the medical intensive care unit (ICU) by Dykes and colleagues, it was found that implementing a structured program for patient-centered care and engagement and an IT platform with tools for patient-centric information and safety checklists reduced the adverse events and increased satisfaction among patients and care partners (Dykes et al., 2017).

PATIENT-CENTRIC TECHNOLOGIES

By empowering patients to participate more actively in their care, patient-centric technology has the potential to deliver holistic healthcare and enhance both quality of care delivery and patient safety. Advances in evolving technology will accelerate the shift to patient-centered care, where attempts to prevent unfavorable outcomes are just as important as respecting patients' wants, preferences,

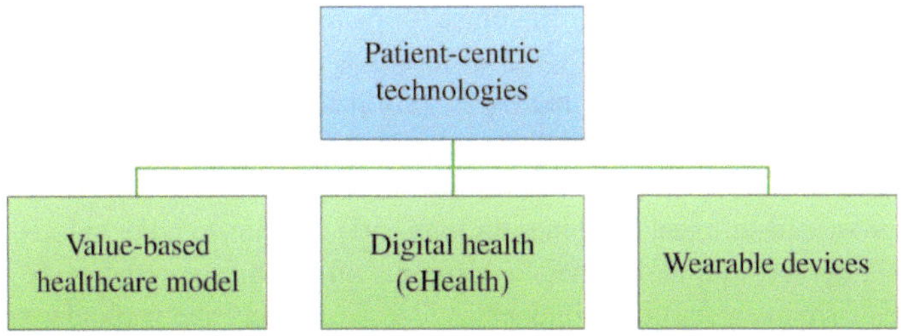

FIGURE 9.1 **Patient-centric technologies.** These technologies include value-based healthcare, digital health, wearables, patient-centric applications, and more.

and values. This is achieved by keeping an emphasis on people rather than systems. Technology can play an unparalleled role in improving the safety, effectiveness, and coordination of healthcare by merging these activities. **Figure 9.1** shows patient-centric technologies.

Value-Based Healthcare Model and Integrated Practice Units

In addition to lowering mortality, the main objectives of optimal care are to improve the quality of life and manage adverse effects over the long term (Porter and Teisberg, 2006). A value-based healthcare (VBHC) model, initially discussed by Porter and Teisberg (2006), strives to improve health outcomes and service quality as assessed against the cost of patient care (Porter and Teisberg, 2006, 2007). Improving the quality of life with minimal disruption of patient routine is one of the key treatment goals for patients with cancer. By gathering and assessing data, patients' demands can be matched with improved and standardized treatment results, lessening the toll that cancer takes on their lives (Johansen and Saunders, 2017). As a result, cancer patients will receive comparable care from various institutes. The implementation of a VBHC model has several advantages for all parties involved, including payers, healthcare providers, and patients (**Figure 9.2**).

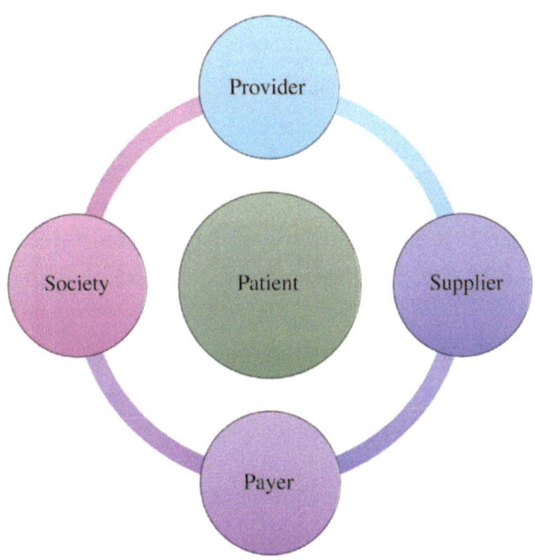

FIGURE 9.2 **Advantages of value-based healthcare in the integrated practice unit's full-cycle system for greater survival rates and efficient treatment.** Patients are in the center of the cycle with key advantages of better overall health, lower cost of care, and allowing the patient to be more engaged with goals. The advantages for the provider include patient-centered care, high efficiency, cost-effective care delivery, multidisciplinary approach, and cooperation with healthcare professionals with optimal healthcare solutions. The advantages for the supplier include cost negotiations, risk-sharing agreements, and innovation. The advantages for the payer include increased coverage of reimbursement, focused investments, improved patient-level outcomes, and limited costs. The advantages for society include wider geographic implementation of care, overall risk reduction, effective use of available resources, evidence-based prevention strategies, and reduced costs to government and healthcare systems.

VBHC models provide improved health outcomes for patients while lowering full-cycle costs, including those connected to hospital stays and medical resource utilization (Johansen and Saunders, 2017; Porter and Teisberg, 2006). In these models, healthcare professionals are crucial in managing and providing patient-centered care, and they are also more likely to involve patients in reaching the suggested objectives (Porter and Teisberg, 2007). Preventive measures and awareness efforts can help patients lower attributable risk factors and improve early clinical outcomes through early diagnosis and/or tailored therapy (Johansen and Saunders, 2017). As a result, the financial constraints on healthcare systems are decreased, and the necessary investments are more sensible, efficient, and targeted at meeting particular needs (**Figure 9.2**).

The cost of cancer treatments is rising in tandem with their increased potency, complexity, and innovation (Johansen and Saunders, 2017). Based on health technology assessment (HTA), alternative reimbursement and price regulatory pathways are being put up to enable access to those therapies at a reasonable cost (Vogler et al., 2018). As a result, by calculating the true worth or benefit of a patient's therapy, it may be possible to reach successful agreements on risk-sharing and price, which would welcome newcomers to the market (Porter and Teisberg, 2007). Given the VBHC model, healthcare systems need to change fast. To improve cancer care and health outcomes, current healthcare facilities—especially those devoted to the disease—must transform into integrated, patient-centered systems where patients participate in the decision-making processes and their input is given weight (Narbutas et al., 2017; Porter and Teisberg, 2007). Consequently, a multidisciplinary, all-encompassing, and holistic plan of action that addresses every stage of the cancer patient's care setting is the focus of integrated practice units (IPUs) (Borras et al., 2014).

The processes for developing high-quality IPUs based on specialized, multidisciplinary cancer care are demonstrated by several case studies (Chiusole et al., 2015; Dummer et al., 2017; Gallicchio et al., 2015; Stordeur et al., 2016). **Table 9.1** summarizes the data retrieved from the best practice paths for patient-centricity and more efficient medical care in melanoma clinics. Multidisciplinary teams, scalability, room for clinical and organizational innovation, increased research, and attention to outcomes measures (e.g., registries, real-world evidence, and aggregated data), as well as firm beliefs about time and expense spending, are all essential components of IPUs. Value creation for patients must be the overarching objective. To accomplish this objective and create an IPU devoted to the treatment of melanoma, **Table 9.2** offers useful strategies for melanoma patients, considering their various aspects of diagnosis and management of melanoma.

TABLE 9.1
Effective Workflows and Essential Elements Guiding the Establishment of a Multidisciplinary, Patient-Focused Organization Founded on Top-Notch Melanoma Clinics

Crucial Elements	Procedure	Objectives and Accomplishments	References
Care continuity	Multidisciplinary teams (e.g., doctors, pharmacists, and nurses); eHealth (digitalization of medical and clinical records).	Data analysis and utilization; uniformity and traceability; and universities and other collaborative networks for research projects Empowerment and engagement of patients (e.g., local patient advocacy groups).	Chiusole et al. (2015) Redondo et al. (2019) Stordeur et al. (2016)
The value to the patients	Identifying the main players and defining the goals, responsibilities, schedules, and operational domains.	Joint protocols and guidelines, standards for process quality and safety, patient selection criteria, and enough facilities.	Gallicchio et al. (2015) Redondo et al. (2019) Stordeur et al. (2016)
Measurement of outcomes	Prompt patient care, quantification of expenses, and risk-adjusted results.	All-inclusive accreditation for superior oncology treatment and model. customization for different cancer types and patient demographics.	Chiusole et al. (2015) Dummer et al. (2017) Redondo et al. (2019)

TABLE 9.2
Effective Strategies to Enhance the Advantages of a Multidisciplinary Approach in the Treatment of Patients with Cutaneous Melanoma: From Diagnosis through End-Stage Management

Dimension	Diagnosis	Treatment	Palliative Care	References
Symptoms	Incorporate general practitioners and other experts to evaluate the influence of disease-related symptoms, and clinical practice should have access to structured psychosocial therapies and psychoeducation that are customized to each patient's circumstances.	Use of PROMs to measure side effects, such as pain, nausea and vomiting, sleeplessness, fatigue, dyspnea, diarrhea, constipation, appetite loss, and anxiety, and to identify areas for improvement in cancer therapy.	Patient participation in the early adoption of supportive care techniques and/or palliative care.	Kasparian (2013) Redondo et al. (2019) Taplin and Rodgers (2010)
Relatives and caretakers	Redesign the environment's structure to accommodate the patient and his or her family (e.g., make appointment scheduling easier, figure out ways to cut down on clinical wait times). Distribute resources (such as workshops, pamphlets, and public websites) that facilitate knowledge sharing and experience sharing among the cancer community.	Acknowledge the influence and viewpoints of patients and their families throughout care (e.g., missing follow-up appointments). Encourage trust and frank and open conversation about the patient's requirements, including family members and friends in treatment choices.	At the end of life, recognize requirements and manage family distress and emotional stability; provide psychosocial support (e.g., group meetings, supportive services) to improve quality of life and lessen regret among patients, family, and caregivers while lowering the risk of psychiatric morbidity.	Redondo et al. (2019) Soukup et al. (2018) Zaider and Kissane (2009)
Comorbidities	Incorporate general practitioners and other specialists to evaluate the influence of additional comorbidity-related symptoms and distinguish them from effects specific to a certain disease.	Make a recommendation regarding a patient's cancer therapy based on more comprehensive medical facts, such as their medical history, current medications and comorbidities, and their treatment preferences.	Analyze the effect of comorbidities on the likelihood of survival, fragility, and complications/ life-threatening issues. Provide support measures that address the consequences and comorbidities' effects as well.	Bebe et al. (2019) Redondo et al. (2019) Soukup et al. (2018)
Advanced melanoma	Encourage community-based skin screening programs to lower the number of cases diagnosed at later stages. Enhance communication between oncologists and geriatricians to ensure best care practices and to assess patient's tolerance to treatment and length of life.	Expand knowledge about the cellular and molecular alterations in advanced melanoma (e.g., clinical trials in the senior population).	Provide round-the-clock, centralized palliative/supportive care in the unit, staffed by physical therapists and specialty nurses.	Gallicchio et al. (2015) Redondo et al. (2019) Russo et al. (2015)

Abbreviation: PROMs, patient-reported outcome measures.

DIGITAL HEALTH

The term "eHealth" refers to the digitalization of healthcare. In 1999, the term "eHealth" was introduced to refer to the application of IT and electronic communication in the healthcare industry (Mitchell, 1999). Digitalized healthcare system offers a wide range of eHealth services due to the innovation and development of an increasing number of technologies aimed to customize and transform healthcare delivery. eHealth generally has a favorable impact on the results of medical care (Wildenbos et al., 2016). The advantages of eHealth services include the most up-to-date patient health status information, enhanced cost-effectiveness, and improved professional communication (Catwell and Sheikh, 2009; Elbert et al., 2014). Healthcare organizations have been assessing and implementing eHealth services to enhance patient care for several years. Because these new services assist to better support treatment procedures, the development of mobile phones and the widespread availability of apps for fitness, wellness, and prevention scenarios have enhanced the importance of eHealth for the healthcare business (Colditz, 1999; Crouter et al., 2003).

Telehealth and technology-based training help reduce disparities by providing healthcare to isolated and rural places that lack adequate infrastructure (Bashshur and Shannon, 2012). The advantages of eHealth and the degree of acceptance of digital intervention in the early diagnosis of cutaneous melanoma have been assessed by several researchers over the past decade (Hall and Murchie, 2014; Loiselle et al., 2013; Murchie et al., 2015). Reduced travel and waiting times, cost-effectiveness, and enhanced access to healthcare services are some of the key advantages of telemedicine and teledermatology (TD) (Loiselle et al., 2013). According to a 2006 study, patients favor telemedicine if it allows them to consult with their doctors more quickly. A qualitative analysis, however, discovered that patients' attitudes toward technology are only favorable when the tool is customized and tailored to the needs and traits of the recipients (Hall and Murchie, 2014). Furthermore, the data that is currently available also indicates that telemedicine benefits healthcare professionals in addition to patients. According to a previous study, general practitioners (GPs) value the use of TD when they need to seek a second opinion or send a patient to a dermatologist (Al-Qirim, 2003).

New approaches to encourage adherence to the required visits/review and increase the number and variety of people conducting skin self-examination may be provided by the recent rise in the use of eHealth melanoma detection tools, which are digital resources that help patients undergo screening frequently outside of the professional context (Alpay et al., 2011). As these digital tools are patient-initiated and patient-centric, with the ability to conduct such consultations outside of clinical settings that are readily accessible and reasonably priced, eHealth technologies for skin surveillance may lessen psychological and practical obstacles in comparison with routine standard of care physical visits. With almost half of the population owning a smartphone and having access to the Internet that allows accessing health information online, eHealth tools for skin screening could more easily fit people's usual habits and create new avenues for melanoma screening adherence (Smith, 2012).

Patients in isolated geographical locations that have limited or no access to experts or those facing physical obstacles that impede their capacity to get care may also benefit from the growing availability of eHealth equipment. With fewer healthcare facilities and an aging population, e-Health technology could be especially helpful for older populations, who are typically more isolated (Fairbrother and Fairbrother, 2010). Even while older persons utilize technology less than younger adults (Glazebrook et al., 2006), research has shown that senior patients who have received device training find it easy to use and express high levels of satisfaction with the way e-Health services are delivered (Dolev et al., 2011). Thus, these techniques can potentially increase the at-risk population's screening rates.

Wearables

Second only to breast cancer in terms of malpractice and misdiagnosis claims, melanoma misdiagnosis significantly lowers a patient's chance of survival (Eftekhari et al., 2019). The insufficiency of the current methods to significantly lower the death rate from skin cancer and improve early verified diagnosis highlights the significance of developing accurate, quantitative, early, and decisive skin cancer diagnostic techniques (McQuade et al., 2018). The chance of getting a second primary melanoma is noticeably higher for those who have survived melanoma (Bradford et al., 2010). Exposure to ultraviolet radiation (UVR) is the most potent risk factor for melanoma (Gilchrest et al., 1999; Kricker et al., 2007; Narayanan et al., 2010). Consequently, to avoid recurrent melanomas in this population, treatments to encourage good sun behavior are required among melanoma survivors. Smartwatches and other wearable technology have gained popularity and offer a fresh approach to clinical monitoring and health intervention. To minimize unintentional sun exposure, emerging wearable solutions include UVR sensors to detect exposure and recommendations to lessen exposure (Vogel et al., 2023).

Rapid and accurate point-of-care (POC) testing for skin cancer is now possible, thanks to the development of biosensors on wearable devices, which have become important clinical instruments (Chatzilakou et al., 2024). These biosensing methods improve accuracy, decrease the need for biopsies, and enable early detection. Smartwatches, hydrogel-coated microneedle patches for biomarker sampling, and microneedle bandage sensors are a few examples of these wearable devices (Al Sulaiman et al., 2019). Melanoma biosensors consist of a physical transduction element and a recognition element positioned in close spatial proximity to each other. Hence, biosensors are analytical tools for the diagnosis of skin cancer that are made up of three main parts: (i) the detector, which senses the biological component unique to skin cancer or the stimulus (biorecognition); (ii) the transducer, which converts the stimulus associated with skin cancer into an output signal (signalization); and (iii) the signal processing system, which measures the output signal (Nagel et al., 1992).

The advancement of wearable biometric monitoring devices (BMDs) has made it possible to remotely monitor patients' health outside of hospitals more frequently and with high resolution. BMDs are wearable sensors embedded in smartphones or wearable equipment that gather physiological, biological, environmental, or behavioral data (Arnerić et al., 2017; Elenko et al., 2015; Topol et al., 2015). The hundreds of data points gathered by BMDs, when combined with the advancements in artificial intelligence (AI), may aid in diagnosis, patient outcome prediction, and assisting healthcare providers in choosing the best course of action for their patients (Fagherazzi and Ravaud, 2019; Hinton, 2018).

Clothing Technology

Clothing is not just a fashion statement but can assist in decreasing melanoma risk through advanced clothing technology. Clothing technology highlights innovations in materials, production techniques, and the integration of smart technologies into clothing and textiles. All clothing provides some protection from the sun, but some materials, known as ultraviolet protection factor (UPF) clothing, are specifically created and tested to provide quantifiable protection. Sunglasses, hats, long sleeves, and other sun-protective apparel are examples of accessories that serve as physical barriers to UVR absorption and are crucial in the prevention of melanoma (Djavid et al., 2021). Avoiding the sun and wearing long sleeves have both been linked to lower chances of sunburns and a decreased risk of developing melanoma (Patel and Chien, 2021).

Different dyes and weave patterns have varying degrees of success when it comes to preventing UVR in clothing. Several studies have shown that colored clothing offers more UV protection. Dark-colored clothing, such as red, black, or navy blue, has consistently demonstrated significantly less UVR transmission than lighter-colored clothing, such as pastels or yellow or white clothes (Davis et al., 1997; Sarkar, 2004). The Skin Cancer Foundation has reported that clothing with bright or dark colors absorbs a greater amount of UV radiation than clothes with lighter colors or no color at all, which is consistent with this conclusion. The ability of various fabric materials to reduce UVR transmittance varies depending on how tightly they are woven. One study found that knitted textiles and linen, two of the most permeable materials, had the lowest UPF levels. Conversely, materials used to make polo shirts and blends of polyester and cotton had outstanding UPF ratings, much exceeding a UPF of 50 (Aguilera et al., 2014). Low fabric porosity has been linked to polyester clothing and polo shirts' success in lowering UVR transmittance, suggesting that clothing with better BSA coverage can provide a stronger barrier against sun exposure and thereby lessen the need for sunscreen application.

Patient-Centric Apps

The use of mobile applications for melanomas is growing in popularity. The mobile app stores offer a plethora of commercially available applications for melanoma (Kassianos et al., 2015; Tellez et al., 2017). These apps serve a variety of functions, from managing medication and side effects to preventing UV exposure. By seeing changes in moles, apps that promote skin self-monitoring aim to aid in the early detection of melanoma. Most studies on these smartphone apps for melanoma self-monitoring have concentrated on their creation or diagnostic precision (Chuchu et al., 2018; Ersser et al., 2019; Freeman et al., 2020; Yas et al., 2017). However, research on the real-world application of these apps outside of well-regulated lab environments is scarce. Numerous apps tailored to dermatology have been created to assist those who have never had skin cancer or those who have already been diagnosed with it in determining whether to seek medical attention for a skin lesion. Additionally, these apps aim to support non-specialist clinicians, like GPs, in determining whether to inform patients that their lesion is benign or to refer them for a specialist assessment (Brewer et al., 2013; Hamilton and Brady, 2012). However, in a recent analysis of the precision with which four smartphone apps assessed the risk of melanoma, it demonstrated a significant difference in usefulness and performance (Wolf et al., 2013). Moreover, there have been no regulatory controls or validation procedures applied to smartphone apps in the United States, the United Kingdom, or any other country that are used for the diagnosis or treatment of cancer, including melanoma. Therefore, there is a chance that these applications could potentially undermine users with incorrect information even while they can enhance patient-clinician communication and assessment between non-specialist clinicians and alert patients regarding possible skin cancer.

Apps used in place of a clinical consultation may provide incorrect or deceptive advice or even postpone the diagnosis of melanoma (Robson et al., 2012). Compared to other cancers, melanoma is especially dangerous because most cases are discovered by the patient rather than their doctor, and it takes longer to see a doctor after a patient first notices a change in their skin or a symptom than it does for all other cancers (Baughan et al., 2009). Despite the challenges, melanoma-detecting apps have the potential to assist with early detection. Mole Monitor, MySkinPal, UMSkinCheck, and SkinVision are some of the melanoma applications used (**Figure 9.3**). Kassianos and colleagues identified 39 apps available at that time of the study in 2015 on app stores for melanoma (Kassianos et al., 2015).

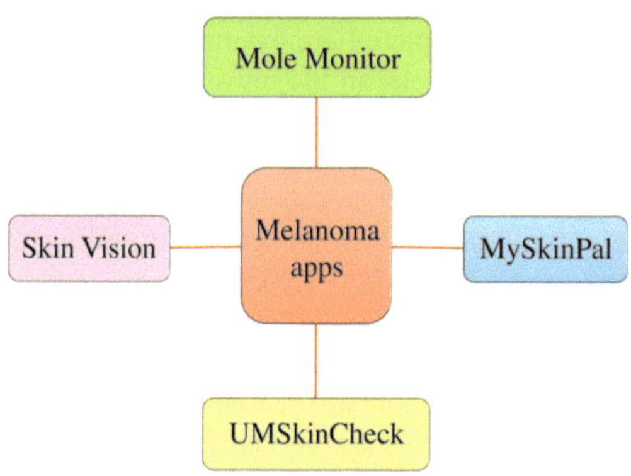

FIGURE 9.3 **Common apps used to look for melanomas.** Although there are many apps available, the common apps used are Mole Monitor, MySkinPal, UMSkinCheck, and SkinVision. These and other apps have the potential to track melanomas and lead to the empowerment of the patient.

Artificial Intelligence in Melanoma

In medicine, AI is being tested extensively in health monitoring, managing medical information, digital medicine, and personalized therapy and has shown promising accuracy in diagnosing disease conditions, especially in dermatology, pathology, and radiology. Machine Learning/Deep Learning algorithms have revolutionized automated assessment in melanoma improving the accuracy even better than the highly skilled dermatologists. Reduced screening costs, more accurate diagnosis of suspicious lesions, and minimizing subjective differences that may prove to be compromising factors in early diagnosis of melanoma are the key advantages of using AI technology. In a systematic review published by Patel and colleagues that evaluated the current status of AI in melanoma, it was shown that in several studies that compared the algorithmic interpretation of images to dermatologists, AI-based algorithms achieved a higher ROC (>80%) in the detection of melanoma (Patel et al., 2023). The use of AI applications in optical coherence tomography and reflectance confocal microscopy has shown promising outcomes in terms of reducing the potential subjective error with improved accuracy and credibility of diagnosis.

Tele-Dermatology

TD is the term for the use of telemedicine in dermatology. TD has historically been divided into two domains: store-and-forward (SaF) TD and real-time (RT) TD (Kaliyadan et al., 2013; Kaliyadan and Ramsey, 2023; Kaliyadan and Venkitakrishnan, 2009). The waiting time for an appointment is decreased when a patient uses SaF TD to connect with a dermatologist through asynchronous consultations. Dermatologists also make extensive use of RT TD. It facilitates communication between the patient and the physician through video channels. Utilizing TD may improve relationships between health domain providers in terms of treatment, monitoring, and the process itself, as well as the perceived quality of services provided. As a result, both the patient and the provider may be more satisfied (Kriwy et al., 2023; Santiago and Lu, 2023). TD and mobile health (mHealth) together can be beneficial to dermatology practices in a synergistic way. TD can deliver treatment straight to the patient's home and shorten travel times or eliminate travel altogether. mHealth can put dermatological care directly in the hands of the public as well as other dermatologists by using specialized apps for smartphones or tablets. The true uniqueness of mHealth integration in TD, which is also evident in dermatology, lies in the ability of people to use applications directly to obtain virtual remote diagnoses and self-care in a way that is distinctly engaging (Giansanti, 2023).

A systematic review of the usage of TD and mHealth in South Africa during the COVID-19 pandemic was proposed by Mbunge and colleagues (Mbunge et al., 2022). The researchers discovered that throughout the epidemic, South Africa embraced a variety of mobile-based digital solutions, such as chatbots, AI, mHealth apps, eHealth and telemedicine, SMS services, and messengers like WhatsApp. These technologies did, however, encounter numerous challenges, such as administrative and budgetary constraints, regulatory and legislative impediments, infrastructure and technology constraints, and cultural limitations. The authors suggested putting effort into community networks, particularly in isolated and rural places, changing mHealth regulations, creating long-term plans for resource mobilization, and connecting reachable global projects that promote this mobile technology (Mbunge et al., 2022). Salmani et al.'s review contained 23 studies, eight of which were from Africa— for example, Ghana, Kenya, Madagascar, Tanzania, and South Africa. This study only looked at mHealth technologies and concentrated on cancer screening. It was determined that users were satisfied with these interventions and that mHealth solutions have a beneficial impact on various elements of cancer screening (Salmani et al., 2020).

LIMITATIONS

Patient-centric technologies face numerous obstacles, from a lack of knowledge among patients and providers to systemic difficulties in implementing the technology. Although technology has enormous potential to enhance patient safety and results, it can only facilitate improved treatment;

it cannot replace the procedures and personnel who provide and receive it. The success of any significant change management project is determined by three factors: people, procedures, and technology. Our recent survey of influential individuals from top US health systems, legislators, and vendors revealed that gaining early support at all levels is more important for the success of HIT in general and innovative predictive analytics technologies in particular (Kakad et al., 2017). Therefore, involving the people who provide and receive care is the next frontier for technology in enhancing patient safety and quality of care.

According to the adoption statistics that are currently available, patients continue to use HIT modalities at low rates (Ahern et al., 2011; Bates and Wells, 2012). Lack of patient awareness, low health literacy, older age, lower socioeconomic status, insufficient computer skills, and unfulfilled technical support needs are some of the factors that may hinder patients from adopting HIT (Rozenblum et al., 2015). A portion of these difficulties are associated with organizational strategies—or the absence of them—that encourage providers and patients to adopt patient-centric technologies like personal health records. By focusing on particular audiences and tracking their uptake, organizations should prioritize strategic investments in this area (Wells et al., 2015). Patient-centric mobile health applications (mHealth apps) present another difficulty. Despite a significant increase in the quantity of mHealth applications and smartphones availability, research indicates that many of these apps lack safety and security, and only a small number of them cater to the needs of patients who could benefit the most (Singh et al., 2016). Lastly, there are situations in which patient-centric HIT may bring up moral and privacy concerns for the patient; one such instance is when a patient is incapable of making decisions for themselves and their proxy decision-makers use the tools on their behalf (Brown et al., 2016). Nonetheless, as their potential is better recognized and utilized by providers, patients, and policymakers, HIT solutions that facilitate patient participation are anticipated to gain significance.

Melanoma screening is important for early diagnosis. As with any screening technique, a thorough examination of the accuracy and effectiveness of each instrument or application is necessary. Part of this evaluation should also look at any potential detrimental effects of using the tool, such as creating a false sense of security with a favorable or unfavorable result. Even while e-Health apps have the potential to improve melanoma detection, most of them lack essential characteristics and are being produced and evaluated on an as-needed basis. Since there aren't many certified tests, it would be very beneficial to broaden the scope of relevant melanoma screening (Tyagi et al., 2012). The use of eHealth devices has the potential to degrade cooperative relationships between doctors and patients (Armstrong et al., 2009) since information is provided in a constrained manner that could cause diagnoses to be misunderstood. In place of clinical visits, eHealth tools may be utilized, and patients may overestimate their accuracy. Patients who exhibit this kind of overconfidence may forget to see a doctor, which could have been crucial in identifying melanoma early enough for treatment (Tyagi et al., 2012).

CONCLUSION

Not only is patient-centered healthcare essential, but it is also critical to acknowledge the urgent need for efficient melanoma screening and preventive methods. Karimkhani and colleagues have pointed out that melanoma continues to be a major factor in the mortality rates from skin cancer worldwide (Karimkhani et al., 2017). The adverse outcomes associated with melanoma can be significantly reduced by early identification and behavioral adjustments, although the increase in screening rate is still difficult to achieve. Low acceptance rates limit the effectiveness of screening procedures, which are limited in number even though they include sophisticated diagnostic tools. This emphasizes the need for novel strategies to boost screening rates, especially in high-risk demographics. Enhancing screening acceptance and engagement by the integration of eHealth tools into widely used platforms, including mobile apps and the Internet, presents a promising opportunity.

These initiatives can efficiently spread knowledge, raise awareness, and motivate proactive health-seeking behaviors by making use of the widespread use of digital technology, particularly among populations at risk for dangerous habits like excessive tanning. Effectively, the development of digital health solutions specific to melanoma prevention and screening is critical in addition to patient-centered treatment. With the widespread use of smart mobile phones with high-resolution cameras and easy access to the Internet, the use of digital technology together with patient empowerment will play a critical role in improving patient outcomes in melanoma by promoting early detection and prompt multidisciplinary intervention, thereby reducing global morbidity and mortality.

REFERENCES

Aguilera, J., De Gálvez, M. V., Sánchez-Roldán, C. and Herrera-Ceballos, E. 2014. New advances in protection against solar ultraviolet radiation in textiles for summer clothing, *Photochememistry and Photobiology*, 90, pp. 1199–1206.

Ahern, D. K., Woods, S. S., Lightowler, M. C., Finley, S. W. and Houston, T. K. 2011. Promise of and potential for patient-facing technologies to enable meaningful use, *American Journal of Preventive Medicine*, 40, pp. S162–S172.

Al Sulaiman, D., Chang, J. Y. H., Bennett, N. R., Topouzi, H., Higgins, C. A., Irvine, D. J. and Ladame, S. 2019. Hydrogel-coated microneedle arrays for minimally invasive sampling and sensing of specific circulating nucleic acids from skin interstitial fluid, *ACS Nano*, 13, pp. 9620–9628.

Alotaibi, Y. K. and Federico, F. 2017. The impact of health information technology on patient safety, *Saudi Medical Journal*, 38, pp. 1173–1180.

Alpay, L., Van Der Boog, P. and Dumaij, A. 2011. An empowerment-based approach to developing innovative e-health tools for self-management, *Health Informatics Journal*, 17, pp. 247–255.

Al-Qirim, N. A. 2003. Teledermatology: The case of adoption and diffusion of telemedicine health Waikato in New Zealand, *Telemedicine Journal and e-Health*, 9, pp. 167–177.

Armstrong, A. W., Watson, A. J., Makredes, M., Frangos, J. E., Kimball, A. B. and Kvedar, J. C. 2009. Text-message reminders to improve sunscreen use: A randomized, controlled trial using electronic monitoring, *Archives of Dermatology*, 145, pp. 1230–1236.

Arnerić, S. P., Cedarbaum, J. M., Khozin, S., Papapetropoulos, S., Hill, D. L., Ropacki, M., Rhodes, J., Dacks, P. A., Hudson, L. D., Gordon, M. F., Kern, V. D., Romero, K., Vradenburg, G., Au, R., Karlin, D. R., Facheris, M. F., Fitzer-Attas, C. J., Vitolo, O. V., Wang, J., Miller, B. M. and Kaye, J. A. 2017. Biometric monitoring devices for assessing end points in clinical trials: Developing an ecosystem, *Nature Reviews Drug Discovery*, 16, pp. 736–736.

Bashshur, R. L. and Shannon, G. W. 2012. Telemedicine as a Modality of Health Care Delivery and Its Implications. *Encyclopedia of Cyber Behavior*. IGI Global.

Bates, D. W. and Wells, S. 2012. Personal health records and health care utilization, *JAMA*, 308, pp. 2034–2036.

Baughan, P., O'neill, B. and Fletcher, E. 2009. Auditing the diagnosis of cancer in primary care: The experience in Scotland, *British Journal of Cancer*, 101(Suppl 2), pp. S87–S91.

Bebe, F. N., Hu, S., Brown, T. L. and Tulp, O. L. 2019. Role, extent, and impact of comorbidity on prognosis and survival in advanced metastatic melanoma: A review, *Journal of Clinical and Aesthetic Dermatology*, 12, p. 16.

Borras, J. M., Albreht, T., Audisio, R., Briers, E., Casali, P., Esperou, H., Grube, B., Hamoir, M., Henning, G. and Kelly, J. 2014. Policy statement on multidisciplinary cancer care, *European Journal of Cancer*, 50, pp. 475–480.

Bradford, P. T., Freedman, D. M., Goldstein, A. M. and Tucker, M. A. 2010. Increased risk of second primary cancers after a diagnosis of melanoma, *Archives of Dermatology*, 146, pp. 265–272.

Brewer, A. C., Endly, D. C., Henley, J., Amir, M., Sampson, B. P., Moreau, J. F. and Dellavalle, R. P. 2013. Mobile applications in dermatology, *JAMA Dermatology*, 149, pp. 1300–1304.

Brown, S. M., Aboumatar, H. J., Francis, L., Halamka, J., Rozenblum, R., Rubin, E., Sarnoff Lee, B., Sugarman, J., Turner, K. and Vorwaller, M. 2016. Balancing digital information-sharing and patient privacy when engaging families in the intensive care unit, *Journal of the American Medical Informatics Association*, 23, pp. 995–1000.

Catwell, L. and Sheikh, A. 2009. Evaluating eHealth interventions: The need for continuous systemic evaluation, *PLOS MED*, 6, p. e1000126.

Chatzilakou, E., Hu, Y., Jiang, N. and Yetisen, A. K. 2024. Biosensors for melanoma skin cancer diagnostics, *Biosensors and Bioelectronics*, 250, p. 116045.

Chiusole, D., Cioffredi, P., Basso, U., Bortolami, A., Crivellari, G., Gennaro, G., Spina, R. and Opocher, G. 2015. OECI accreditation at Veneto Institute of Oncology IOV-IRCCS, general framework and multidisciplinary approach, *Tumori Journal*, 101, pp. S38–S41.

Chuchu, N., Takwoingi, Y., Dinnes, J., Matin, R. N., Bassett, O., Moreau, J. F., Bayliss, S. E., Davenport, C., Godfrey, K., O'connell, S., Jain, A., Walter, F. M., Deeks, J. J. and Williams, H. C. 2018. Smartphone applications for triaging adults with skin lesions that are suspicious for melanoma, *The Cochrane Database of Systematic Reviews*, 12, p. Cd013192.

Colditz, G. A. 1999. Economic costs of obesity and inactivity, *Medicine and Science in Sports and Exercise*, 31, pp. S663–S667.

Corrigan, J. M. 2005. *Crossing the Quality Chasm – Building a Better Delivery System: A New Engineering/Health Care Partnership* (Institute of Medicine & National Academy of Engineering). Washington, DC: The National Academies Press. https://nap.nationalacademies.org/read/11378/chapter/8#94

Crouter, S. E., Schneider, P. L., Karabulut, M. and Bassett, D. R., Jr. 2003. Validity of 10 electronic pedometers for measuring steps, distance, and energy cost, *Medicine and Science in Sports Exercise*, 35, pp. 1455–1460.

Davis Giardina, T., Menon, S., Parrish, D. E., Sittig, D. F. and Singh, H. 2014. Patient access to medical records and healthcare outcomes: A systematic review, *Journal of the American Medical Informatics Association*, 21, pp. 737–741.

Davis, S., Capjack, L., Kerr, N. and Fedosejevs, R. 1997. Clothing as protection from ultraviolet radiation: Which fabric is most effective? *International Journal of Dermatology*, 36, pp. 374–379.

Djavid, A. R., Stonesifer, C., Fullerton, B. T., Wang, S. W., Tartaro, M. A., Kwinta, B. D., Grimes, J. M., Geskin, L. J. and Saenger, Y. M. 2021. Etiologies of melanoma development and prevention measures: A review of the current evidence, *Cancers (Basel)*, 13, p. 4914.

Dolev, J. C., O'sullivan, P. and Berger, T. 2011. The eDerm online curriculum: A randomized study of effective skin cancer teaching to medical students, *Journal of the American Academy of Dermatology*, 65, pp. e165–e171.

Dummer, R., Ramelyte, E., Levesque, M., Goldinger, S. M. and Braun, R. P. 2017. Critical aspects to achieve a high-quality melanoma clinic, *Current Opinion in Oncology*, 29, pp. 145–150.

Dykes, P. C., Rozenblum, R., Dalal, A., Massaro, A., Chang, F., Clements, M., Collins, S., Donze, J., Fagan, M. and Gazarian, P. 2017. Prospective evaluation of a multifaceted intervention to improve outcomes in intensive care: The promoting respect and ongoing safety through patient engagement communication and technology study, *Critical Care Medicine*, 45, pp. e806–e813.

Eftekhari, A., Ahmadian, E., Salatin, S., Sharifi, S., Dizaj, S. M., Khalilov, R. and Hasanzadeh, M. 2019. Current analytical approaches in diagnosis of melanoma, *TrAC Trends in Analytical Chemistry*, 116, pp. 122–135.

Elbert, N. J., Van Os-Medendorp, H., Van Renselaar, W., Ekeland, A. G., Hakkaart-Van Roijen, L., Raat, H., Nijsten, T. E. and Pasmans, S. G. 2014. Effectiveness and cost-effectiveness of eHealth interventions in somatic diseases: A systematic review of systematic reviews and meta-analyses, *Journal of Medical Internet Research*, 16, p. e110.

Elenko, E., Underwood, L. and Zohar, D. 2015. Defining digital medicine, *Nature Biotechnology*, 33, pp. 456–461.

Ersser, S. J., Effah, A., Dyson, J., Kellar, I., Thomas, S., Mcnichol, E., Caperon, E., Hewitt, C. and Muinonen-Martin, A. J. 2019. Effectiveness of interventions to support the early detection of skin cancer through skin self-examination: A systematic review and meta-analysis, *British Journal of Dermatology*, 180, pp. 1339–1347.

Fagherazzi, G. and Ravaud, P. 2019. Digital diabetes: Perspectives for diabetes prevention, management and research, *Diabetes & Metabolism*, 45, pp. 322–329.

Fairbrother, K. and Fairbrother, E. 2010. Smack-a-mole game teaches skin cancer awareness and raises funds for the Dermatology Nurses' Association, *Journal of the Dermatology Nurses' Association*, 2, pp. 218–221.

Freeman, K., Dinnes, J., Chuchu, N., Takwoingi, Y., Bayliss, S. E., Matin, R. N., Jain, A., Walter, F. M., Williams, H. C. and Deeks, J. J. 2020. Algorithm based smartphone apps to assess risk of skin cancer in adults: Systematic review of diagnostic accuracy studies, *BMJ*, 368, p. m127.

Gallicchio, R., Scapicchio, D., Musto, P. and Storto, G. 2015. Achievement of European standards by CROB-IRCCS, *Tumori Journal*, 101, pp. S47–S50.

Giansanti, D. 2023. Advancing dermatological care: A comprehensive narrative review of tele-dermatology and mHealth for bridging gaps and expanding opportunities beyond the COVID-19 pandemic, *Healthcare*, 11, p. 1911.

Gilchrest, B. A., Eller, M. S., Geller, A. C. and Yaar, M. 1999. The pathogenesis of melanoma induced by ultraviolet radiation, *New England Journal of Medicine*, 340, pp. 1341–1348.

Glazebrook, C., Garrud, P., Avery, A., Coupland, C. and Williams, H. 2006. Impact of a multimedia intervention “skinsafe” on patients’ knowledge and protective behaviors, *Preventive Medicine*, 42, pp. 449–454.
Grando, M., Rozenblum, R. and Bates, D. 2015. *Information Technology for Patient Empowerment in Healthcare*. de Gruyter.
Hall, S. and Murchie, P. 2014. Can we use technology to encourage self-monitoring by people treated for melanoma? A qualitative exploration of the perceptions of potential recipients, *Supportive Care in Cancer*, 22, pp. 1663–1671.
Hamilton, A. D. and Brady, R. R. W. 2012. Medical professional involvement in smartphone ‘apps’ in dermatology, *British Journal of Dermatology*, 167, pp. 220–221.
Hawkins, J. B., Brownstein, J. S., Tuli, G., Runels, T., Broecker, K., Nsoesie, E. O., Mciver, D. J., Rozenblum, R., Wright, A. and Bourgeois, F. T. 2016. Measuring patient-perceived quality of care in US hospitals using Twitter, *BMJ Quality & Safety*, 25, pp. 404–413.
Hinton, G. 2018. Deep learning—A technology with the potential to transform health care, *JAMA*, 320, pp. 1101–1102.
Johansen, N. J. and Saunders, C. M. 2017. Value-based care in the worldwide battle against cancer, *Cureus,* 9, p. e1039.
Kakad, M., Rozenblum, R. and Bates, D. W. 2017. *Getting buy-in for predictive analytics in health care.* Harvard Business Review.
Kaliyadan, F. and Ramsey, M. L. 2023. *Teledermatology*. Treasure Island (FL): StatPearls Publishing.
Kaliyadan, F. and Venkitakrishnan, S. 2009. Teledermatology: Clinical case profiles and practical issues, *Indian Journal of Dermatology, Venereology and Leprology*, 75, pp. 32–35.
Kaliyadan, F., Amin, T. T., Kuruvilla, J. and Ali, W. H. A. B. 2013. Mobile teledermatology–patient satisfaction, diagnostic and management concordance, and factors affecting patient refusal to participate in Saudi Arabia, *Journal of Telemedicine and Telecare*, 19, pp. 315–319.
Karimkhani, C., Green, A. C., Nijsten, T., Weinstock, M. A., Dellavalle, R. P., Naghavi, M. and Fitzmaurice, C. 2017. The global burden of melanoma: Results from the Global Burden of Disease Study 2015, *Br J Dermatol*, 177, pp. 134–140.
Kasparian, N. A. 2013. Psychological stress and melanoma: Are we meeting our patients’ psychological needs? *Clinics in Dermatology*, 31, pp. 41–46.
Kassianos, A. P., Emery, J. D., Murchie, P. and Walter, F. M. 2015. Smartphone applications for melanoma detection by community, patient and generalist clinician users: A review, *Br J Dermatol*, 172, pp. 1507–1518.
Kricker, A., Armstrong, B. K., Goumas, C., Litchfield, M., Begg, C. B., Hummer, A. J., Marrett, L. D., Theis, B., Millikan, R. C., Thomas, N., Culver, H. A., Gallagher, R. P., Dwyer, T., Rebbeck, T. R., Kanetsky, P. A., Busam, K., From, L., Mujumdar, U., Zanetti, R. and Berwick, M. 2007. Ambient UV, personal sun exposure and risk of multiple primary melanomas, *Cancer Causes Control*, 18, pp. 295–304.
Kriwy, P., Nötzold, A., Seitz, A.-T. and Berger, R. 2023. Akzeptanz der Teledermatologie: Ergebnisse einer Befragung sächsischer Haus- und HautärztInnen, *Gesundheitswesen*, 85, pp. 1149–1156.
Loiselle, C. G., Peters, O., Haase, K. R., Girouard, L., Körner, A., Wiljer, D. and Fitch, M. 2013. Virtual navigation in colorectal cancer and melanoma: An exploration of patients’ views, *Supportive Care in Cancer*, 21, pp. 2289–2296.
Mbunge, E., Batani, J., Gaobotse, G. and Muchemwa, B. 2022. Virtual healthcare services and digital health technologies deployed during coronavirus disease 2019 (COVID-19) pandemic in South Africa: A systematic review, *Global Health Journal*, 6, pp. 102–113.
McQuade, J. L., Daniel, C. R., Hess, K. R., Mak, C., Wang, D. Y., Rai, R. R., Park, J. J., Haydu, L. E., Spencer, C., Wongchenko, M., et al. 2018. Association of body-mass index and outcomes in patients with metastatic melanoma treated with targeted therapy, immunotherapy, or chemotherapy: A retrospective, multicohort analysis, *Lancet Oncology*, 19, pp. 310–322.
Mitchell, J. 1999. *From Telehealth to e-Health: The Unstoppable Rise of e-Health.* Department of Communications, Information Technology and the Arts.
Murchie, P., Allan, J. L., Brant, W., Dennis, M., Hall, S., Masthoff, J., Walter, F. M. and Johnston, M. 2015. Total skin self-examination at home for people treated for cutaneous melanoma: Development and pilot of a digital intervention, *BMJ Open*, 5, p. e007993.
Nagel, B., Dellweg, H. and Gierasch, L. M. 1992. Glossary for chemists of terms used in biotechnology (IUPAC Recommendations 1992), *Pure and Applied Chemistry*, 64, pp. 143–168.
Narayanan, D. L., Saladi, R. N. and Fox, J. L. 2010. Ultraviolet radiation and skin cancer, *Int J Dermatol*, 49, pp. 978–986.

Narbutas, Š., York, K., Stein, B. D., Magsanoc-Alikpala, K., Majima, Y., Kalo, Z., Almasi, T. and Inotai, A. 2017. Overview on patient centricity in cancer care, *Frontiers in Pharmacology*, 8, p. 698.

Pacheco, I., Buzea, C. and Tron, V. 2011. Towards new therapeutic approaches for malignant melanoma, *Expert Reviews in Molecular Medicine*, 13, p. e33.

Patel, R. H., Foltz, E. A., Witkowski, A. and Ludzik, J. 2023. Analysis of artificial intelligence-based approaches applied to non-invasive imaging for early detection of melanoma: A systematic review, *Cancers*, 15, p. 4694.

Patel, S. P. and Chien, A. L. 2021. Sun protective clothing and sun avoidance: The most critical components of photoprotection in patients with melanoma, *Dermatolic Surgery*, 47, pp. 333–337.

Porter, M. E. and Teisberg, E. O. 2006. Redefining *health care*: Creating *value-based competition on results*. Harvard Business Press.

Porter, M. E. and Teisberg, E. O. 2007. How physicians can change the future of health care, *JAMA*, 297, pp. 1103–1111.

Redondo, P., Ribeiro, M., Lopes, M., Borges, M. and Gonçalves, F. R. 2019. Holistic view of patients with melanoma of the skin: How can health systems create value and achieve better clinical outcomes? *Ecancermedicalscience*, 13, p. 959.

Robson, Y., Blackford, S. and Roberts, D. 2012. Caution in melanoma risk analysis with smartphone application technology, *British Journal of Dermatology*, 167, pp. 703–704.

Rozenblum, R. and Bates, D. W. 2013. Patient-centred healthcare, social media and the internet: the perfect storm? *BMJ Quality & Safety*, 22(3), pp. 183–186.

Rozenblum, R., Greaves, F. and Bates, D. W. 2017. The role of social media around patient experience and engagement, *BMJ Quality & Safety*, 26, pp. 845–848.

Rozenblum, R., Miller, P., Pearson, D., Marielli, A., Grando, M. and Bates, D. 2015. Patient-Centered Healthcare, Patient Engagement and Health Information Technology: The Perfect Storm. *Information Technology for Patient Empowerment in Healthcare*. 1st ed. Berlin: Walter de Gruyter, 3–22.

Russo, A. E., Ferrau, F., Antonelli, G., Priolo, D., Mccubrey, J. A. and Libra, M. 2015. Malignant melanoma in elderly patients: Biological, surgical and medical issues, *Expert Review of Anticancer Therapy*, 15, pp. 101–108.

Salmani, H., Ahmadi, M. and Shahrokhi, N. 2020. The impact of mobile health on cancer screening: A systematic review, *Cancer Informatics*, 19, p. 1176935120954191.

Santiago, S. and Lu, J. 2023. Patient satisfaction in teledermatology: An updated review, *Current Dermatology Reports*, 12, pp. 23–26.

Sarkar, A. K. 2004. An evaluation of UV protection imparted by cotton fabrics dyed with natural colorants, *BMC Dermatology*, 4, p. 15.

Singh, K., Drouin, K., Newmark, L. P., Lee, J., Faxvaag, A., Rozenblum, R., Pabo, E. A., Landman, A., Klinger, E. and Bates, D. W. 2016. Many mobile health apps target high-need, high-cost populations, but gaps remain, *Health Affairs*, 35, pp. 2310–2318.

Smith, A. 2012. *46% of American Adults Are Smartphone Owners*. Pew Internet & American Life Project.

Soukup, T., Lamb, B. W., Arora, S., Darzi, A., Sevdalis, N. and Green, J. S. A. 2018. Successful strategies in implementing a multidisciplinary team working in the care of patients with cancer: An overview and synthesis of the available literature, *Journal of Multidisciplinary Healthcare*, 11, pp. 49–61.

Stordeur, S., Vrijens, F. and Leroy, R. 2016. Reference centres for adults with rare and complex cancers—Policy recommendations to improve the organisation of care in Belgium, *Revue d'Épidémiologie et de Santé Publique*, 64, pp. 1–6.

Taplin, S. H. and Rodgers, A. B. 2010. Toward improving the quality of cancer care: Addressing the interfaces of primary and oncology-related subspecialty care, *Journal of the National Cancer Institute Monographs*, 2010, pp. 3–10.

Tellez, W. A., Nieto-Gutierrez, W. and Taype-Rondan, A. 2017. Sunscreen mobile apps: A content analysis, *European Research in Telemedicine/La Recherche Européenne en Télémédecine*, 6, pp. 157–163.

Topol, E. J., Steinhubl, S. R. and Torkamani, A. 2015. Digital medical tools and sensors, *JAMA*, 313, pp. 353–354.

Tyagi, A., Miller, K. and Cockburn, M. 2012. e-Health tools for targeting and improving melanoma screening: A review, *Journal of Skin Cancer*, 2012, p. 437502.

Vogel, R. I., Luo, X., Brown, K., Jewett, P., Dona, A. C., Nagler, R. H., Ahmed, R. L., Martinson, B. C. and Lazovich, D. 2023. A UVR-sensor wearable device intervention to reduce sun exposure in melanoma survivors: Results from a randomized controlled trial, *PLOS ONE*, 18, p. e0281480.

Vogler, S., Paris, V. and Panteli, D. 2018. European Observatory Policy Briefs. In: Richardson, E., Palm, W. and Mossialos, E. (eds.) *Ensuring Access to Medicines: How to Redesign Pricing, Reimbursement and Procurement?* Copenhagen (Denmark): European Observatory on Health Systems and Policies©

World Health Organization. 2018. Acting as the host organization for, and secretariat of, the European Observatory on Health Systems and Policies.

Wachter, R. M. 2015. *The Digital Doctor: Hope, Hype, and Harm at the Dawn of Medicine's Computer Age*. New York: McGraw-Hill Education.

Wagner, P. J., Dias, J., Howard, S., Kintziger, K. W., Hudson, M. F., Seol, Y.-H. and Sodomka, P. 2012. Personal health records and hypertension control: A randomized trial, *Journal of the American Medical Informatics Association*, 19, pp. 626–634.

Ward, W. H. and Farma, J. M (Eds.). 2017. *Cutaneous melanoma: Etiology and therapy* [Internet]. Brisbane (AU): Codon Publications. https://pubmed.ncbi.nlm.nih.gov/29461771/

Wells, S., Rozenblum, R., Park, A., Dunn, M. and Bates, D. W. 2015. Organizational strategies for promoting patient and provider uptake of personal health records, *Journal of the American Medical Informatics Association*, 22, pp. 213–222.

Wildenbos, G. A., Peute, L. W. and Jaspers, M. W. 2016. Impact of patient-centered eHealth applications on patient outcomes: A review on the mediating influence of human factor issues, *Yearbook of Medical Informatics*, 113–119.

Wolf, J. A., Moreau, J. F., Akilov, O., Patton, T., English, J. C., Ho, J. and Ferris, L. K. 2013. Diagnostic inaccuracy of smartphone applications for melanoma detection, *JAMA Dermatology*, 149, pp. 422–426.

Yas, Q. M., Zaidan, A. A., Zaidan, B. B., Hashim, M. and Lim, C. K. 2017. A systematic review on smartphone skin cancer apps: Coherent taxonomy, motivations, open challenges and recommendations, and new research direction, *Journal of Circuits, Systems and Computers*, 27, p. 1830003.

Zaider, T. and Kissane, D. 2009. The assessment and management of family distress during palliative care, *Current Opinion in Supportive and Palliative Care*, 3, pp. 67–71.

10 Unveiling Synergistic Future Horizons in Melanoma Combination Therapies

Talent Chipiti and Zodwa Dlamini
SAMRC/UP Precision Oncology Research Unit, DSTI/NRF SARChI Chair in Precision Oncology (POCP) and Cancer Prevention, Pan African Cancer Research Institute (PACRI), University of Pretoria, Pretoria, South Africa

Zukile Mbita
University of Limpopo, Sovenga, South Africa

Elisa Marie Ledet
Tulane Cancer Center's Prostate Cancer Biorepository, Tulane Cancer Center, Tulane University, New Orleans, Louisiana, USA

INTRODUCTION

Melanoma is a significant global health concern, leading to high mortality rates each year. In South Africa, the number of new cases is increasing annually, with a mortality rate of around 20%. The high mortality rate is mainly due to melanoma's ability to spread to other parts of the body and its resistance to traditional treatments, posing a considerable challenge for healthcare providers worldwide (World Health Organization, 2023). Skin cancer is a major concern in South Africa, particularly for individuals with lighter natural skin tones, who face a higher risk. Minimizing exposure to ultraviolet (UV) rays can decrease the chances of developing skin cancer (South African National Cancer Registry, 2023).

Basal cell carcinoma and squamous cell carcinoma are the two most common types of skin cancer. Melanoma, the third most prevalent type of skin cancer, is particularly dangerous due to its tendency to metastasize to other parts of the body, including vital organs, leading to higher mortality rates. Basal cell carcinoma typically grows slowly and can damage surrounding tissue, potentially causing cosmetic disfigurement if not treated early, but it is unlikely to spread to distant areas or result in death. On the other hand, while squamous cell carcinoma of the skin is usually not life-threatening, it can grow significantly or spread to other parts of the body if left untreated, leading to serious complications (Centers for Disease Control and Prevention [CDC], 2022; Mayo Clinic, 2021; McDaniel et al., 2022).

Combination therapies represent a promising strategy for treating melanoma, aiming to enhance treatment effectiveness while reducing side effects. This overview explores combination therapies for melanoma globally, with a particular focus on Africa and South Africa. Historically, Africa has faced limited access to advanced treatments, but recent efforts are improving accessibility and building local capacity. In South Africa, a burgeoning research landscape is driving the development of tailored combination approaches, including the integration of immunotherapy with targeted therapies, chemotherapy, and radiation. For instance, the combination of pembrolizumab (an immunotherapy drug) with dabrafenib and trametinib (targeted therapies) is used to treat advanced melanoma (Ferrucci et al., 2020).

Globally, landmark trials have demonstrated that combining immunotherapy and targeted therapy is effective and broadens treatment options (Robert et al., 2016). Ongoing research aims to

DOI: 10.1201/9781003511625-10

optimize treatment sequencing, identify biomarkers, and explore novel combinations to combat resistance (Larkin et al., 2019). Collaborative efforts are crucial for progress and ensuring equitable access to cutting-edge therapies worldwide. Synergistic approaches are essential in managing melanoma, offering enhanced effectiveness while minimizing side effects. By combining multiple modalities, these approaches target cancer cells through various pathways, such as inhibiting the MAPK/ERK pathway, blocking immune checkpoints, and targeting specific genetic mutations (e.g., BRAF and MEK inhibitors) (Kohler et al., 2015). This multipronged attack helps overcome resistance and reduce the risk of recurrence, allowing for personalized treatment strategies that leverage genomic profiling and immune monitoring (Sullivan, 2020).

Research initiatives are directed toward developing combination therapies that are specifically suited to the genetic and environmental factors influencing melanoma in South African patients. These combination therapies, which often include immunotherapy and targeted therapy, have shown promise in improving patient outcomes by leveraging synergistic effects to enhance therapeutic efficacy while minimizing adverse side effects (South African National Cancer Registry, 2023).

Overview of the Evolving Field of Combination Therapies for Melanoma Treatment

Melanoma, a highly aggressive form of skin cancer, poses significant challenges to patients and clinicians alike, necessitating innovative treatment strategies to improve outcomes. The exploration of combination therapies, which harness synergistic interactions between different therapeutic modalities, holds promise for enhancing efficacy and mitigating resistance mechanisms (Farhana, 2023).

Combination therapies have emerged as a promising strategy in melanoma treatment, offering the potential to enhance efficacy while minimizing adverse effects (Sosman et al., 2012). This chapter explores the evolving landscape of combination therapies for melanoma on a global scale, with a specific focus on Africa and South Africa. We examine recent advancements in the field, including the integration of immunotherapy, targeted therapy, and traditional treatments, to provide a comprehensive understanding of the current state and prospects.

In Africa, access to advanced melanoma treatments has historically been limited, exacerbated by healthcare infrastructure challenges and disparities in resource allocation (Marsden et al., 2017). However, recent efforts have been sought to bridge this gap, with initiatives aimed at improving access to novel therapies and building local capacity for melanoma management. For instance, organizations like the African Organization for Research and Training in Cancer (AORTIC) have been instrumental in advocating for improved cancer care infrastructure and education across the continent (AORTIC, 2022).

In South Africa, a burgeoning melanoma research landscape has contributed to the development of innovative combination approaches tailored to the unique genetic and environmental factors prevalent in the region (Arnold et al., 2022).

Melanoma is a significant health concern in South Africa, especially among the white population, where incidence rates are considerably higher compared to other racial groups. According to recent statistics, melanoma accounts for a substantial portion of the country's cancer burden, with an estimated annual incidence rate of about 4.7 per 100,000 individuals. This rate is notably higher in men (6.4 per 100,000) than in women (3.1 per 100,000), reflecting global trends where men are generally at a higher risk of developing melanoma (Ferlay et al., 2020; National Cancer Registry, 2019).

In South Africa, specialized melanoma treatment centers are pivotal in managing and treating this aggressive form of skin cancer. Some of the leading centers include:

1. *Groote Schuur Hospital in Cape Town*: This tertiary referral hospital is renowned for its comprehensive cancer care services, including advanced melanoma treatment. It offers a range of therapies, including surgical oncology, radiation therapy, and medical oncology.
2. *Chris Hani Baragwanath Academic Hospital in Johannesburg*: As one of the largest hospitals in the world, it provides extensive oncology services and has a dedicated team for skin cancer, including melanoma.

3. *Netcare Milpark Hospital in Johannesburg*: Known for its state-of-the-art oncology unit, this hospital offers cutting-edge treatments, including immunotherapy and targeted therapies for melanoma.
4. *Tygerberg Hospital in Cape Town*: This academic hospital is affiliated with Stellenbosch University and provides specialized oncology services, including treatment for melanoma.
5. *WITS Donald Gordon Medical Centre in Johannesburg*: This private hospital is associated with the University of the Witwatersrand and offers comprehensive cancer care, including advanced treatments for melanoma.

These facilities are equipped with state-of-the-art technology and staffed by multidisciplinary teams who create personalized treatment plans for melanoma patients. The emphasis on early detection and innovative treatments, such as immunotherapy and targeted therapy, is crucial for improving patient outcomes.

The demographic distribution of melanoma in South Africa shows that it mainly affects individuals of European descent, with a higher occurrence in older age groups. Due to its geographical location, the higher levels of UV radiation in the country contribute to the increased risk. Public health initiatives that focus on awareness and early detection are crucial in addressing the growing incidence of melanoma in South Africa (Coory et al., 2013; Norval and Kelfkens, 2020).

Collaborative efforts between academic institutions, healthcare providers, and industry partners have led to the initiation of clinical trials exploring novel combination regimens and establishing specialized melanoma treatment centers (Eggermont et al., 2019).

Globally, groundbreaking clinical trials such as CheckMate 067 and COMBI-d have showcased the remarkable efficacy of combining immunotherapy, which boosts the body's natural defenses to fight cancer, with targeted therapy regimens that specifically target the cancer cells. These trials have demonstrated significant improvements in both overall survival and progression-free survival (PFS) rates for patients with melanoma. This groundbreaking approach offers new hope for patients battling this challenging disease, providing more effective treatment options and potentially extending and improving their quality of life (Larkin et al., 2015; Robert et al., 2015a). Additionally, the advent of novel agents targeting key signaling pathways and immune checkpoints has expanded the armamentarium of available treatment options (Dummer et al., 2018).

Importance of Synergistic Approaches in Enhancing Treatment Efficacy and Minimizing Side Effects

Synergistic approaches in cancer management, particularly in the context of melanoma treatment, hold significant importance in enhancing treatment efficacy while minimizing side effects. Melanoma, a highly aggressive form of skin cancer, presents unique challenges due to its tendency for rapid metastasis and resistance to traditional treatments. Synergistic approaches offer a multifaceted strategy to combat these challenges by leveraging the complementary mechanisms of different therapeutic modalities.

***Enhanced Efficacy*:** Combining multiple treatment modalities, such as immunotherapy, targeted therapy, chemotherapy, and radiation therapy, can target melanoma cells through multiple pathways simultaneously. This multi-pronged approach increases the likelihood of eradicating cancer cells effectively, reducing the risk of disease recurrence and metastasis (Hodi et al., 2014).

***Overcoming Resistance*:** Melanoma, a type of skin cancer, often acquires resistance to treatments aimed at single targets due to a variety of factors, including genetic mutations and strategies that allow the cancer to evade the immune system. To address this, researchers and clinicians have been exploring synergistic treatment approaches, which involve targeting multiple pathways involved in tumor growth and progression simultaneously. By doing so, they aim to increase the likelihood of achieving a durable response to treatment, which is of great importance in managing advanced melanoma (Hugo et al., 2015).

***Minimizing Side Effects*:** Combination therapies can allow for lower doses of individual drugs, reducing the risk of toxic side effects associated with high-dose monotherapy. By using different mechanisms of action, synergistic combinations can exploit tumor-specific vulnerabilities while sparing normal tissues, leading to improved tolerability and quality of life for patients (Spain et al., 2016).

***Targeting Heterogeneity*:** Melanomas exhibit significant intra-tumoral and inter-tumoral heterogeneity, with distinct subpopulations of cancer cells harboring different genetic mutations and immune profiles. Synergistic approaches can target multiple subpopulations simultaneously, addressing the diverse nature of the disease and reducing the likelihood of treatment resistance (Luke et al., 2017).

***Immunomodulation*:** When immunotherapy agents are combined with other treatment modalities, such as targeted therapy or chemotherapy, it has been observed that it can lead to enhanced antitumor immune responses. For instance, targeted therapies have the potential to sensitize tumor cells to immune-mediated killing, thus making them more vulnerable to the body's immune system. On the other hand, chemotherapy can play a role in modulating the tumor microenvironment (TME), creating conditions that are more conducive to immune cell infiltration. This combined approach can potentially bolster the body's natural defenses against cancerous cells (Gide et al., 2019).

***Personalized Medicine*:** Synergistic approaches allow for personalized treatment strategies tailored to the unique molecular and immunological characteristics of each patient's tumor. By integrating genomic profiling, biomarker analysis, and immune monitoring, clinicians can identify optimal combination regimens that maximize therapeutic efficacy while minimizing the risk of toxicity (Snyder et al., 2014).

Synergistic approaches in melanoma treatment offer a promising avenue for improving patient outcomes by enhancing treatment efficacy and minimizing side effects. As our understanding of the molecular and immune landscape of melanoma continues to evolve, the development of novel combination therapies holds the potential to revolutionize the standard of care for this challenging disease.

CURRENT LANDSCAPE OF MELANOMA TREATMENT

Melanoma, the most aggressive form of skin cancer, has undergone significant advancements in treatment in recent decades. This section will provide a detailed overview of treatment options, including surgery, chemotherapy, immunotherapy, and targeted therapy, as well as the associated limitations and challenges. It will also highlight the importance of combination therapy and potential combination therapies.

EXISTING TREATMENT MODALITIES, THEIR LIMITATIONS, AND CHALLENGES ASSOCIATED WITH MONOTHERAPY APPROACHES

Melanoma, a serious form of skin cancer, has several monotherapy treatment options, each with its own set of benefits and challenges as highlighted in **Figure 10.1**. These therapies include surgery, chemotherapy, immunotherapy, targeted therapy, and radiation therapy, each playing a crucial role depending on the stage and characteristics of the cancer.

Surgery, often the primary treatment for early-stage melanoma, can be highly effective in removing localized tumors but becomes less viable as the disease progresses to advanced stages (Balch et al., 2009). Chemotherapy, though sometimes beneficial, frequently results in severe side effects and demonstrates limited efficacy in treating advanced melanoma (Chapman et al., 1999). Immunotherapy has significantly advanced melanoma treatment by boosting the body's immune response to cancer cells; however, it is effective only in a subset of patients and can lead to immune-related adverse effects. Targeted therapy, aimed at specific genetic mutations in melanoma cells, shows promise but often encounters issues with resistance and subsequent relapse. Radiation therapy, useful for palliative care or treating inoperable tumors, is limited by the potential damage it can cause to surrounding healthy tissues. Each monotherapy approach faces significant limitations, underscoring the necessity for combined treatment strategies to enhance patient outcomes (Mitchell et al., 2020; Robert et al., 2015b).

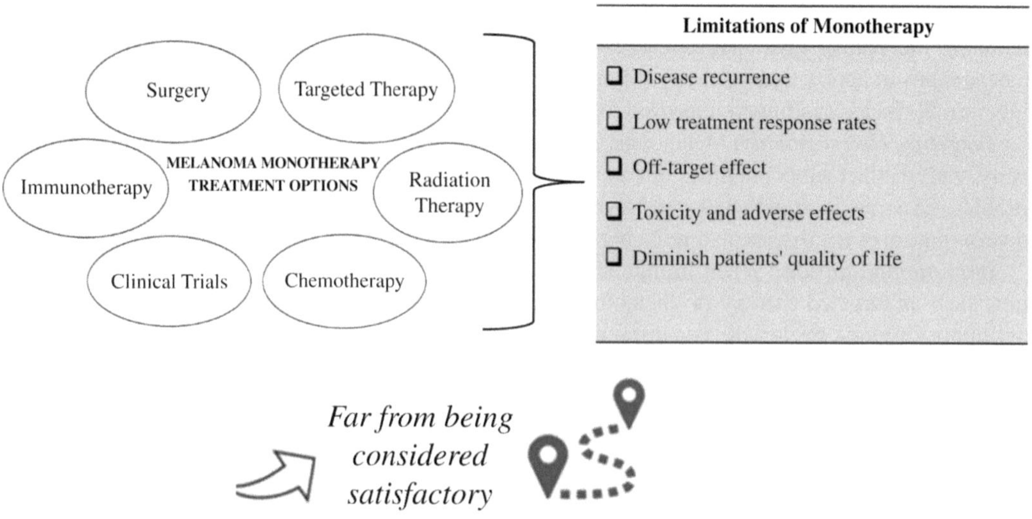

FIGURE 10.1 **An illustration of the current monotherapy treatment modalities available for melanoma, including surgery, chemotherapy, immunotherapy, targeted therapy, and radiation therapy outcomes.** Each has its benefits and challenges. While surgery is effective for early-stage melanoma, it becomes less viable in advanced stages. Chemotherapy has limited efficacy and severe side effects. Immunotherapy is effective in some patients but can lead to immune-related adverse effects. Targeted therapy shows promise but encounters issues with resistance and relapse. Radiation therapy is useful for palliative care but can damage surrounding healthy tissues. Combined treatment strategies are necessary to improve patient outcomes.

Surgery

Surgery is the primary treatment for early-stage melanoma and involves the excision of the tumor with a margin of healthy tissue to ensure complete removal. For localized melanomas, this method is often curative. Sentinel lymph node biopsy is performed to determine if the cancer has spread to regional lymph nodes, guiding further treatment decisions (Balch et al., 2009). In cases where melanoma has metastasized, surgical resection of metastatic sites may be considered, although this is less common. While surgery is effective for early-stage melanoma, its role diminishes significantly in metastatic disease. Surgical excision is not feasible for widespread metastatic melanoma, and recurrence is a major concern even after successful initial surgery (Balch et al., 2009).

Chemotherapy

Historically, chemotherapy was a mainstay for treating advanced melanoma. Agents such as dacarbazine (DTIC) and temozolomide were commonly used. However, response rates to chemotherapy are generally low, and the benefits are limited, often accompanied by significant side effects (Chapman et al., 1999). Consequently, chemotherapy has been largely supplanted by more effective treatments like immunotherapy and targeted therapy. The primary limitation of chemotherapy is its low efficacy in melanoma, with response rates typically below 20% (Chapman et al., 1999). Moreover, chemotherapeutic agents do not specifically target melanoma cells, leading to considerable toxicity and adverse effects, which can diminish patients' quality of life. Resistance to chemotherapy also develops quickly, limiting its long-term effectiveness.

Immunotherapy

Immunotherapy presents a new method for treating melanoma by utilizing the body's immune system to effectively target and eliminate cancer cells. There are various types of immunotherapies available for melanoma treatment.

Immunotherapy for melanoma includes checkpoint inhibitors (CPIs) like pembrolizumab, nivolumab, and atezolizumab, which target proteins on immune cells to enhance the immune response against melanoma cells. Additionally, therapies like IL-2, tumor-infiltrating lymphocyte (TIL) therapy, oncolytic virus therapy, BCG vaccine, and imiquimod cream are also used to treat melanoma. These treatments can cause side effects such as fatigue, skin rash, and flu-like symptoms (Mitchell et al., 2020; Swetter et al., 2024).

The development of immunotherapy has brought about a revolutionary shift in the approach to treating melanoma. Specifically, CPIs like ipilimumab (anti-CTLA-4), nivolumab, and pembrolizumab (both anti-PD-1) work by augmenting the immune system's capacity to identify and eliminate cancer cells. This mechanism marks a significant advancement in the fight against melanoma, offering new hope for patients (Hodi et al., 2010; Robert et al., 2015b). The use of these agents has led to notable improvements in the survival rates of patients with advanced melanoma. Another form of immunotherapy, known as adoptive cell transfer (ACT), involves the infusion of autologous TILs after *ex vivo* expansion. This method has shown promising results in the treatment of advanced melanoma (Rosenberg et al., 2008). Despite the breakthroughs achieved with immunotherapy, several challenges persist. Not all patients respond to CPIs, with response rates varying between 20–40% for anti-PD-1 therapies and around 10–15% for anti-CTLA-4 monotherapy (Hodi et al., 2010; Robert et al., 2015b). Moreover, immune-related adverse events (irAEs) can be severe, including colitis, hepatitis, and endocrinopathies, necessitating careful management and sometimes discontinuation of therapy (Postow et al., 2018).

Targeted Therapy

Targeted therapy focuses on specific genetic mutations within melanoma cells. The most notable targets are mutations in the BRAF gene, present in approximately 50% of melanomas. BRAF inhibitors (vemurafenib and dabrafenib) and MEK inhibitors (trametinib and cobimetinib) have shown efficacy in treating BRAF-mutant melanoma by disrupting the MAPK/ERK signaling pathway, which is crucial for cell proliferation and survival (Flaherty et al., 2010). These treatments often lead to rapid tumor regression and improved survival. Targeted therapies, particularly those aimed at BRAF mutations, often lead to the rapid development of resistance. The initial response is typically dramatic, but the duration of response is usually limited, with most patients experiencing disease progression within 6–12 months (Long et al., 2014). Combination therapies with BRAF and MEK inhibitors have improved outcomes but do not completely overcome resistance. Additionally, these therapies can have significant side effects, such as rash, diarrhea, and hepatotoxicity.

The treatment landscape for melanoma has transformed remarkably with the introduction of immunotherapy and targeted therapy, offering new hope for patients with advanced disease. However, each modality has its limitations and challenges, particularly when used as monotherapy. Ongoing research aims to optimize these treatments, explore combination strategies, and develop new therapeutic approaches to improve outcomes and manage resistance and adverse effects. The integration of multidisciplinary care and personalized treatment plans based on genetic profiling and immune status is essential to advancing melanoma management.

Synergistic Potential of Combination Therapies in Melanoma Treatment

The synergy between different treatment modalities holds considerable promise in melanoma treatment. Preclinical studies have provided compelling evidence of enhanced efficacy and reduced toxicity with combination approaches. For instance, studies in mouse models of melanoma have demonstrated improved tumor control when combining BRAF inhibitors with anti-PD-1 antibodies compared to monotherapy (Shin et al., 2020). Similarly, the combination of MEK inhibitors with CTLA-4 blockade has been shown to alter the TME favorably for immune cell infiltration and activity (Ebert et al., 2016).

Clinical trials have further validated the potential of combination therapies in melanoma treatment. For example, the CheckMate 067 trial investigated the combination of nivolumab and ipilimumab versus either agent alone in advanced melanoma, showing improved survival outcomes with the combination approach (Larkin et al., 2019). Furthermore, the COMBI-i trial evaluated the combination of dabrafenib, trametinib, and spartalizumab in patients with advanced BRAF-mutant melanoma, demonstrating higher response rates and longer PFS compared to standard targeted therapy alone (Atkins et al., 2023).

Overall, the synergistic potential of combination therapies in melanoma treatment offers a promising avenue for improving patient outcomes. Both preclinical and clinical studies have underscored the enhanced efficacy and reduced toxicity associated with these approaches. Moving forward, continued research and clinical investigation are essential to further elucidate the optimal combinations, dosing regimens, and patient selection criteria to maximize the benefits of combination therapies in melanoma treatment.

EXPLORATION OF SYNERGISTIC INTERACTIONS BETWEEN DIFFERENT TREATMENT MODALITIES

Combination therapies in melanoma typically involve the use of multiple agents that target different pathways or mechanisms of tumor growth and survival. The rationale behind this approach is to enhance therapeutic effects while minimizing the chances of resistance, a common problem in monotherapy. Combination therapies utilize the principle that different treatment modalities can target distinct pathways and mechanisms involved in melanoma progression. For instance, combining immunotherapy with targeted therapy can simultaneously disrupt tumor cell signaling and enhance the immune system's ability to recognize and destroy cancer cells (Rager et al., 2022). The rationale behind such combinations includes:

- *Targeting Multiple Pathways*: Cancer cells are renowned for their adaptability and their ability to evade therapeutic interventions. One of the reasons behind this resilience lies in their reliance on multiple signaling pathways for survival and proliferation. These pathways, which control various cellular processes, such as growth, proliferation, and apoptosis, are often disrupted in cancer cells (Sharma et al., 2019; Xia et al., 2014).

  When a single pathway is targeted with a therapeutic agent, cancer cells can sometimes escape the treatment by activating alternative pathways to maintain their survival. This phenomenon, known as compensatory signaling, undermines the efficacy of monotherapy and contributes to treatment resistance. To tackle this challenge, combination therapies in cancer treatment aim to disrupt multiple signaling pathways simultaneously. By targeting different pathways with complementary mechanisms of action, these combination approaches can effectively block the various routes that cancer cells may use to survive and proliferate (Lopez and Banerji, 2017). This strategy prevents the cells from compensating for the inhibition of one pathway by activating another, thereby enhancing the overall efficacy of the treatment. For instance, combination therapy may entail the simultaneous inhibition of both the MAPK pathway (with BRAF inhibitors) and the PI3K/AKT pathway (with PI3K inhibitors) in melanoma cells (Aasen et al., 2019).

  By targeting these two key pathways, which are commonly disrupted in melanoma, the combination therapy can exert a more potent and sustained antitumor effect compared to targeting either pathway alone. This approach not only increases the likelihood of inducing tumor cell death but also reduces the chance of treatment resistance development. By depriving cancer cells of multiple survival pathways, combination therapies represent a promising strategy to overcome resistance mechanisms and improve patient outcomes in cancer treatment (Rager et al., 2022).

- *Overcoming Resistance*: Tumors frequently develop resistance to monotherapies. Combination therapies can address this by targeting multiple resistance mechanisms simultaneously

(Ferrucci et al., 2020). Cancer cells can adapt to single-drug therapies through various mechanisms, leading to treatment failure. Combination therapies target multiple resistance mechanisms, reducing the likelihood of resistance development and enhancing therapeutic efficacy.

- *Genetic Mutations and Pathway Activation*: Tumors can acquire mutations that make certain drugs less effective. For example, in the case of melanoma, secondary mutations in the MAPK pathway can reduce the efficacy of BRAF inhibitors. Combining BRAF inhibitors with MEK inhibitors can effectively target both the primary driver mutation and the downstream signaling pathway, thereby reducing the likelihood of resistance (Long et al., 2014).
- *Tumor Microenvironment Modulation*: The TME is pivotal in cancer progression and resistance, encompassing various cell types, signaling molecules, and extracellular matrix components that shield tumor cells from therapeutic agents. Disrupting these protective mechanisms involves combining therapies that target the tumor cells with those that modify the microenvironment. For example, combining CPIs with anti-angiogenic agents can enhance immune cell infiltration and improve antitumor activity (Motz and Coukos, 2011).
- *Phenotypic Plasticity*: It's important to keep in mind that cancer cells can undergo changes that help them survive treatment. For example, they can undergo epithelial-to-mesenchymal transition (EMT), which makes them more resistant to certain therapies and more invasive. To address this, it's beneficial to target multiple pathways involved in EMT and cell survival. An effective approach is to combine inhibitors of the PI3K/AKT pathway with those targeting the MAPK pathway, as this can prevent cancer cells from altering their characteristics to evade treatment (Engelman and Cantley, 2006).
- *Combination with Immunotherapy*: Immunotherapies, such as CPIs, have significantly transformed cancer treatment by leveraging the body's immune system to combat cancer. However, their effectiveness can be hindered by the presence of immunosuppressive cells and factors within the TME. Combining immunotherapies with targeted therapies can enhance the immune response by increasing the visibility of tumor cells to the immune system and reducing immunosuppressive signals. For example, combining PD-1 inhibitors with vascular endothelial growth factor (VEGF) inhibitors has demonstrated improved outcomes in various cancers, including melanoma and renal cell carcinoma (Motzer et al., 2019).
- *Addressing Multiple Resistance Mechanisms*: Combination therapies can thwart cancer cells from developing escape routes by simultaneously targeting various resistance mechanisms. For instance, the combination of BRAF and MEK inhibitors in melanoma not only aims at the primary oncogenic pathway but also counteracts compensatory signaling through other pathways, resulting in more enduring treatment responses (Robert et al., 2016).

Combination therapies constitute a potent strategy for surmounting the multifaceted nature of tumor resistance. By concurrently addressing multiple resistance mechanisms, these therapies have the potential to augment treatment efficacy, diminish the likelihood of resistance development, and ameliorate patient outcomes in melanoma and other cancers.

- *Enhanced Immune Response*: Immunotherapies, such as PD-1/PD-L1 inhibitors, can be significantly enhanced by treatments that improve the immune system's ability to recognize cancer cells or alter the TME to promote immune activity. Combining CPIs with targeted therapies is a promising strategy in this regard.
  - *Increased Tumor Antigen Expression*: One of the ways combination therapies enhance the immune response is by increasing the expression of tumor antigens. Targeted therapies, such as BRAF and MEK inhibitors, can lead to changes in the tumor cells that make

them more recognizable to the immune system. This increased antigen expression allows immune cells, particularly T cells, to identify and attack the cancer cells more effectively. For example, a study by Ribas et al. (2017a) demonstrated that combining the BRAF inhibitor vemurafenib with the PD-1 inhibitor pembrolizumab increased the expression of melanoma antigens, thereby improving the efficacy of the immune response.

- *Immune Cell Infiltration*: Another critical mechanism is the enhancement of immune cell infiltration into the tumor. Targeted therapies can modulate the TME, making it more conducive to immune cell infiltration. This change allows immune cells, such as cytotoxic T lymphocytes (CTLs), to penetrate the tumor more effectively and exert their antitumor effects. Ribas et al. (2017b) showed that the combination of targeted therapies with CPIs led to a significant increase in the infiltration of immune cells into melanoma tumors. This increased infiltration is crucial for a robust and sustained immune response against the cancer cells.
- *Modification of the Tumor Microenvironment*: Targeted therapies can also modify the TME to be more favorable for immune activity. For instance, these therapies can reduce the presence of immunosuppressive cells, such as regulatory T cells (Tregs) and myeloid-derived suppressor cells (MDSCs), which typically inhibit the immune response. By diminishing these immunosuppressive elements, the combination of targeted therapies with immunotherapies can create a more supportive environment for immune cell function. This modification enhances the overall efficacy of the immune response against the tumor.
- *Clinical Evidence*: Clinical evidence supports the enhanced efficacy of combining CPIs with targeted therapies. In a study involving patients with BRAF-mutant melanoma, the combination of the BRAF inhibitor dabrafenib, the MEK inhibitor trametinib, and the PD-1 inhibitor pembrolizumab showed improved PFS and overall response rates (ORRs) compared to monotherapy (Ribas et al., 2017a). These findings highlight the potential of combination therapies to provide superior clinical outcomes by enhancing the immune response.

- *Reduced Toxicity*: One of the critical challenges in combination therapies is managing increased toxicity. To address this, researchers are exploring various strategies, such as adjusting dosages and sequencing treatments. For example, the use of lower doses of targeted therapies in combination with immunotherapy has been shown to reduce side effects while maintaining therapeutic efficacy. Sequential administration, where targeted therapy is given initially to reduce tumor burden followed by immunotherapy, can also help in managing toxicity (Ribas et al., 2019). Additionally, the development of biomarkers to predict response and toxicity can help tailor combination therapies to individual patients, potentially improving outcomes and reducing adverse effects. Ongoing research aims to identify such biomarkers and refine treatment protocols to maximize the benefits of combination therapies while minimizing risks (Boutros et al., 2024). The synergistic potential of combination therapies in melanoma treatment represents a significant advancement in oncology. By combining different modalities, such as targeted therapy and immunotherapy, clinicians can achieve improved efficacy and potentially overcome the limitations of monotherapy. Preclinical and clinical studies have demonstrated the benefits of these approaches, although increased toxicity remains a challenge. Future research and clinical trials will continue to optimize these strategies, aiming to provide durable responses and improved quality of life for melanoma patients.

Targeted Therapy and Immunotherapy

Combination therapies represent a cutting-edge approach in the treatment landscape of melanoma, offering a multifaceted strategy to improve patient outcomes. These combinations leverage the synergistic potential of various treatment modalities, including immunotherapy, targeted therapy,

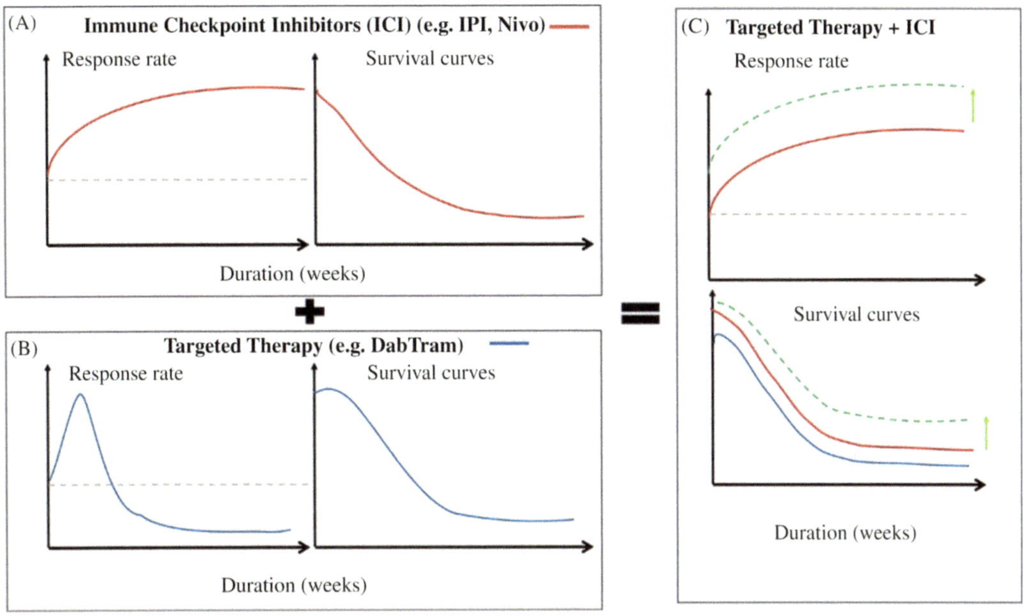

FIGURE 10.2 **This figure displays the typical response kinetics of patients and their survival rates when using monotherapy compared to combination therapy.** This can be seen in the form of Kaplan–Meier curves. Targeted therapy (B), such as MAPKi, initially shows better early survival advantages; however, these advantages diminish over time. Conversely, adding an immune checkpoint inhibitor (ICI) (A) like IPI or Nivo, which has a slower onset of response, extends the initial rapid response induced by MAPKi. As a result, the Kaplan–Meier curves are characterized by less steep initial slopes but longer and higher plateauing tails. In (C), it can be observed that the combination of ICI and targeted therapy can result in both superior response and survival rates as compared to individual monotherapy. *Abbreviations*: Dab, dabrafenib; DabTram, dabrafenib+trametinib; IPI, ipilimumab; MAPKi, mitogen-activated pathway kinase inhibitors; Nivo, nivolumab.

chemotherapy, and other emerging approaches, as can be witnessed in the illustration in **Figure 10.2**. By concurrently targeting multiple pathways involved in melanoma progression and immune evasion, combination therapies aim to enhance therapeutic efficacy while mitigating the development of resistance and minimizing treatment-related toxicity (Long et al., 2014).

Targeted therapies, such as BRAF and MEK inhibitors, directly interfere with specific molecules involved in melanoma cell growth. BRAF inhibitors (e.g., vemurafenib and dabrafenib) target the mutated BRAF protein, which is found in about 50% of melanomas and drives cell proliferation. MEK inhibitors (e.g., trametinib and cobimetinib) inhibit the downstream MEK protein in the same pathway, providing a more comprehensive blockade of the signaling pathway. While these therapies have shown significant efficacy in reducing tumor size, their benefits are often temporary due to the development of resistance mechanisms within the cancer cells (Long et al., 2014).

Immunotherapies, particularly CPIs such as PD-1 inhibitors (nivolumab and pembrolizumab) and CTLA-4 inhibitors (ipilimumab), enhance the body's immune response against melanoma cells by blocking proteins that inhibit immune activation. This allows the immune system to better recognize and destroy cancer cells (Hodi et al., 2010; Robert et al., 2015b).

The combination of targeted therapy with immunotherapy has shown promising synergistic potential. For example, the rapid tumor regression induced by targeted therapy can reduce the immunosuppressive TME, potentially making the tumor more susceptible to immune attack as illustrated in **Figure 10.3**. Conversely, the immune activation provided by immunotherapy can help in recognizing and destroying residual cancer cells that might escape targeted therapy, thus potentially preventing or delaying resistance (Shin et al., 2020).

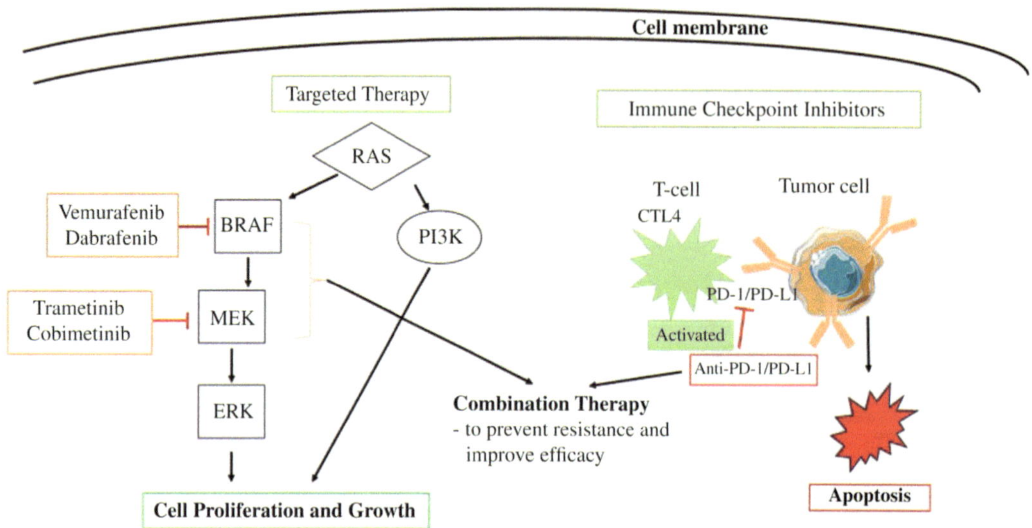

FIGURE 10.3 An illustration of the molecular pathways involved in melanoma development and progression, along with the key targets of current monotherapies and potential combination therapies. The combination of BRAF and MEK inhibitors, such as Dabrafenib and Trametinib, works synergistically to inhibit both BRAF and MEK, preventing resistance and improving efficacy. When ICIs, exemplified by Nivolumab and Ipilimumab, are combined with targeted therapy, they enhance the immune response against melanoma by targeting PD-1 and CTLA-4. Furthermore, combining targeted therapy with ICIs, like BRAF/MEK inhibitors with PD-1/PD-L1 inhibitors, aims to address both tumor cell proliferation and the immune environment, providing a comprehensive approach to treatment.

Chemotherapy and Immunotherapy

The use of traditional chemotherapy in treating melanoma has lessened with the rise of targeted and immune-based therapies. However, there is growing interest in combining chemotherapy with immunotherapy. Chemotherapy drugs can cause immunogenic cell death, leading to the release of tumor antigens and boosting the body's antitumor immune response. This potential synergy with immunotherapy is gaining attention, especially in cases where other treatments may not be suitable (Larkin et al., 2019; Sordo-Bahamonde et al., 2023).

The combination of chemotherapy with immunotherapy takes advantage of the immunogenic cell death triggered by chemotherapy drugs to enhance the body's immune response against tumors. Although traditional chemotherapy has become less common in managing melanoma, its ability to induce immunogenic cell death suggests a new way to work alongside immunotherapies (Emens and Middleton, 2015). Chemotherapy drugs like dacarbazine (DTIC), temozolomide, and platinum-based drugs can induce immunogenic cell death, promoting the release of tumor antigens and activating dendritic cells and CTLs to enhance the antitumor immune response. Furthermore, chemotherapy-induced immunogenic cell death can make tumor cells more vulnerable to immune-mediated destruction by upregulating immune checkpoint molecules (Ugurel et al., 2013).

The use of ICIs combined with standard chemotherapy has produced encouraging outcomes in various types of cancer. This is particularly evident in the case of difficult-to-treat tumors, with minimal overlapping side effects between the drugs. The addition of chemotherapy to PD-1 blockade with pembrolizumab has significantly enhanced patient outcomes in lung cancer. It has halved the risk of death compared to chemotherapy alone in both non-squamous and squamous non-small cell lung cancer (NSCLC) (Socinski et al., 2018). Additionally, the combination of chemotherapy with the anti-PD-L1 antibody atezolizumab or the anti-PD-1 antibody nivolumab plus ipilimumab has also demonstrated survival advantages in NSCLC patients (Paz-Ares et al., 2018). Notably, neoadjuvant nivolumab combined with chemotherapy has shown significant improvements in event-free survival and pathological complete response rates in NSCLC patients who are eligible for surgical removal of the tumor (Sordo-Bahamonde et al., 2023).

The goal of combining chemotherapy with immunotherapy is to capitalize on these immunomodulatory effects. Immunotherapies such as CPIs (e.g., anti-PD-1/PD-L1 antibodies and anti-CTLA-4 antibodies) and adoptive cell therapies enhance the body's immune response against cancer cells. When used in combination with chemotherapy, immunotherapies can further stimulate the immune system, leading to synergistic antitumor effects. While less common than combining targeted therapies with immunotherapy, some studies have shown promising results in combining chemotherapy with immunotherapy, particularly in cases where other therapies are not suitable. The combined effects of chemotherapy-induced immunogenic cell death and immunotherapy-mediated immune activation could provide new treatment options for melanoma patients.

More research is required to determine the best combinations, sequences, and dosing regimens for chemotherapy and immunotherapy in melanoma treatment. Ongoing clinical trials are also evaluating the safety and efficacy of these combination approaches in different patient populations (**Table 10.1**). As our understanding of the complex interplay between chemotherapy and immunotherapy continues to evolve, this dual-modality strategy holds promise for improving outcomes in melanoma patients.

TABLE 10.1
A Comprehensive Catalogue of Ongoing Clinical Trials Aimed at Assessing the Combinations, Sequences, and Dosing Regimens of Chemotherapy and Immunotherapy in the Context of Melanoma Treatment

Trial Name	Description	Status	References
CheckMate 067	Evaluates the combination of nivolumab (an anti-PD-1 therapy) and ipilimumab (an anti-CTLA-4 therapy) versus monotherapy in untreated advanced melanoma.	Ongoing	Larkin et al. (2019).
KEYNOTE-022	Investigates pembrolizumab (anti-PD-1) in combination with dabrafenib and trametinib (BRAF/MEK inhibitors) in advanced melanoma patients.	Ongoing	Ribas et al. (2019)
COMBI-i	Examines spartalizumab (anti-PD-1) with dabrafenib and trametinib in patients with BRAF V600 mutation-positive advanced melanoma.	Ongoing	Dummer et al. (2020)
NCT04000486	Evaluates the safety and efficacy of combining pembrolizumab with chemotherapy in metastatic melanoma patients.	Ongoing	Garbe et al. (2020)
NCT03470922	Investigates nivolumab combined with chemotherapy (temozolomide) in patients with stage IV melanoma.	Ongoing	Ascierto et al. (2019)
TRIM	Studies tremelimumab (anti-CTLA-4) with durvalumab (anti-PD-L1) and chemotherapy in advanced melanoma patients.	Ongoing	Jansen et al. (2020)
NCT03568375	Evaluates the combination of ipilimumab, nivolumab, and dacarbazine in metastatic melanoma.	Ongoing	Eggermont et al. (2018)

Many chemo-immunotherapy combinations have shown promise in treating various cancers, but only a few have been successful. Utilizing advanced technologies such as spatial transcriptomics and single-cell sequencing could help enhance our understanding of the TME and improve treatment strategies. Improving preclinical models and identifying new biomarkers are crucial for advancing chemo-immunotherapy. The increasing availability of ICIs and a wide range of chemo-immunotherapy combinations offer hope for innovative cancer therapy strategies shortly (Sordo-Bahamonde et al., 2023).

EXAMINATION OF PRECLINICAL AND CLINICAL STUDIES DEMONSTRATING ENHANCED EFFICACY AND REDUCED TOXICITY WITH COMBINATION APPROACHES IN MELANOMA TREATMENT

Preclinical Studies

Preclinical studies provide the initial proof-of-concept for combination therapies. For instance, in mouse models of melanoma, the combination of BRAF inhibitors and anti-PD-1 antibodies has shown improved tumor control compared to either agent alone. These studies indicate that the initial tumor shrinkage by targeted therapy can enhance the effectiveness of subsequent immunotherapy by increasing the infiltration of immune cells into the tumor (Shin et al., 2020).

Another preclinical study demonstrated that MEK inhibitors could enhance the antitumor activity of CTLA-4 blockade by altering the TME to be more favorable for immune cell infiltration and activity (Ebert et al., 2016). These findings support the rationale for combining targeted therapies with immunotherapies to achieve a more robust antitumor response. The combination of MAPK inhibitors (MAPKi) with CPIs has been proposed to enhance antitumor immunity for treating metastatic melanoma, based on promising preclinical studies showing synergistic effects from their combined or sequential use (Haist et al., 2023). Haist et al. (2023) conducted initial studies demonstrating that combining anti-PD-1 or PD-L1 monoclonal antibodies (mAb) with BRAF inhibitors (BRAFi) resulted in slowed tumor growth, increased the number and activity of TIL, and prolonged survival in a PTEN−/− melanoma mouse model. The study also observed positive changes in the TME, including higher intratumoral CTLs and elevated levels of proinflammatory cytokines (Haist et al., 2023).

Molecularly targeted tyrosine kinase inhibitors (TKIs) have shown efficacy in treating metastatic melanoma. However, extended use of these agents as monotherapy can lead to resistance. Resistance has been linked to epithelial-mesenchymal transition and upregulation of oncogenic proteins. Combining TKIs with immunotherapies targeting key proteins in the RAS/RAF/MAPK or PI3K/AKT pathways can delay resistance onset and improve survival in metastatic melanoma (Table 10.2) (Rager et al., 2022).

TABLE 10.2
Preclinical Combination Therapies for Melanoma

Drug 1	Target	Drug 2	Target	Type of Study	References
Compd A	RAF	Trametinib	MEK	Preclinical	Atefi et al. (2015)
Trametinib/PD901	MEK	PHGDH siRNA	NRAS	Preclinical	Nguyen et al. (2020)
Trametinib	MEK	GSK2334470	PDPK1	Preclinical	Cai et al. (2022)
Trametinib	MEK	XMD9-92	ERK5	Preclinical	Adam et al. (2020)
Trametinib	MEK	CCG-222740	MRTF	Preclinical	Appleton et al. (2021)
LY2801653	cMET	Trametinib	MEK1/2	Preclinical	Cheng et al. (2017)
ASN007	ERK1/2	Copanlisib	ERK1/2	Preclinical	Portelinha et al. (2021)
Everolimus	mTOR	XAV939	Wnt	Preclinical	Etnyre et al. (2014)
Cobimetinib	MEK	CD147 inhibitor	PI3K	Preclinical	Landras et al. (2022)
Abemaciclib	CDK4/6	Merestinib	cMET	Preclinical	Ohara et al. (2021)

In a similar vein, early treatment with BRAF inhibitors (BRAFi) in patients with metastatic melanoma has demonstrated favorable changes in the TME, supporting the efficacy of triple combination therapy (Spain et al., 2016). Subsequent studies have highlighted the enhanced antitumor effects of combining BRAF inhibitor dabrafenib, MEK inhibitor trametinib, and a PD-1 blocking monoclonal antibody compared to monotherapy in a BRAFV600E melanoma model. This combination resulted in increased tumor antigen expression, elevated MHC class I levels, greater TIL influx, and enhanced antitumor activity as indicated by heightened expression of IFN-γ (Boutros et al., 2024; Ribas et al., 2017a).

Further research has demonstrated that combining BRAFi with CPI can enhance the effectiveness of adoptive T-cell transfer and antibody-mediated CCL2 neutralization in addressing immunomodulatory cell infiltration in tumors (Lau et al., 2021; Quirk et al., 2015). These synergistic effects of MAPKi with anti-PD-1/PD-L1 mAb were observed in both BRAF-mutated and wild-type melanoma models, indicating that MEKi influences T-cell function through paradoxical ERK activation (Ascierto et al., 2024; Shin et al., 2020).

Ascierto et al. (2024) found that the triple combination of BRAF/MEKi plus anti-PD-1 inhibitors depended on CTL recruitment in a BRAFV600E/PTEN−/− melanoma model. Short-term BRAF/MEK inhibition increased tumor immune cell infiltration but decreased over time, highlighting the importance of optimal treatment timing (Ascierto et al., 2024). A recent study confirmed the benefits of combining MAPKi and CPI, noting even better tumor control with a quadruple combination including DT and CPI therapy in a BRAFV600E-mutant melanoma model (Haist et al., 2023). However, combining anti-CTLA-4 mAb with BRAFi (vemurafenib) reduced TIL levels, questioning their synergy (Quirk et al., 2015).

Sequential treatment strategies, although less researched, aim to avoid cross-resistance by combining complementary mechanisms, allowing one therapy to enhance the response to the other while reducing toxicity. For instance, commencing with anti-PD-1/PD-L1 mAb treatment before MAPKi has been proven to enhance antitumor immunity and survival compared to using anti-PD-L1 treatment alone (Wang et al., 2021). This sequential approach also led to sustained intracranial tumor responses, addressing the issue of intracranial resistance that often arises with continuous MAPKi administration (Wang et al., 2021). Intermittent dosing or short-term cessation of MAPKi can reverse tumor resistance, providing a strategy for overcoming resistance to continuous BRAF/MEK inhibitor therapy (Haugh et al., 2021; Zhong et al., 2022).

Preclinical studies have shown that combining targeted therapies with immunotherapies in melanoma treatment can enhance antitumor responses. This can be achieved by altering the TME and increasing immune cell infiltration and activity. Studies in mouse models have demonstrated the synergistic effects of combining BRAF inhibitors with anti-PD-1/PD-L1 antibodies, resulting in slowed tumor growth and improved survival. Additionally, the timing and sequence of treatment play crucial roles in optimizing therapeutic efficacy and overcoming resistance. Overall, these findings provide valuable insights into the development of more effective combination therapies for melanoma patients.

Clinical Studies

Several clinical trials have demonstrated the enhanced efficacy of combination therapies in melanoma. The COMBI-i trials, a phase III study, evaluated the combination of dabrafenib (BRAF inhibitor), trametinib (MEK inhibitor), and spartalizumab (anti-PD-1 antibody) in patients with advanced BRAF-mutant melanoma. The results showed a higher ORR and longer PFS compared to standard targeted therapy alone, indicating a significant benefit from the combination approach (Ferrucci et al., 2020).

In the CheckMate 067 trial, researchers investigated the efficacy of combining nivolumab, a PD-1 inhibitor, and ipilimumab, a CTLA-4 inhibitor, compared to each agent alone in the treatment of advanced melanoma. The results demonstrated that the combination therapy led to significantly improved survival outcomes, including a higher ORR and longer PFS compared to the individual agents. However, it's important to note that this combination also resulted in an increase in treatment-related adverse events, highlighting the critical need for careful monitoring and management of potential toxicities (Larkin et al., 2019).

The phase I clinical trial, which marked the initial stage of research, aimed to investigate the potential benefits of combining a CPI (IPI) with a single-agent MAPKi (vemurafenib) in treating patients with BRAF-mutated metastatic malignant melanoma. Unfortunately, the trial had to be discontinued due to the emergence of serious adverse effects, specifically liver toxicity and skin rashes (NCT01400451) (Ribas et al., 2013). Given the adverse toxicity profiles and lower response rates associated with single-agent BRAF inhibitors, recent research has given priority to combining BRAF and MEK inhibitors instead of using single-agent BRAF inhibitors. This strategic shift is driven by the aim to maximize efficacy while minimizing adverse effects. Moreover, there is an observed higher incidence of adverse events related to vemurafenib compared to dabrafenib, emphasizing the importance of thoroughly considering drug-specific adverse events when designing combination therapies. This approach could lead to improved treatment outcomes and enhanced patient safety in the context of BRAF inhibitor-based therapies (Amin et al., 2016).

Another phase I study (NCT01767454) found that combining DT with IPI had a better safety profile regarding hepatotoxicity (Puzanov et al., 2014) but led to severe immune-associated colitis, most commonly associated with IPI treatment (Minor et al., 2015).

Owing to the unfavorable toxicity profile of IPI combinations, subsequently conducted trials predominantly prioritized the investigation of MAPKi combinations with PD-1/PD-L1 inhibitors, which exhibited a more manageable toxicity profile. Nevertheless, the consideration of tolerability remained paramount for triple combination regimens (Haist et al., 2023).

Numerous double and triple clinical combination regimens have been tested, and this process is ongoing. The aim is to combine single treatments to improve effectiveness while also using data from preclinical trials. Most combinations of targeted cancer therapies have shown effectiveness in preclinical models of metastatic melanoma. The choices for clinical trials were guided by the established toxicity profiles of these combinations. Key proteins in the RAS/RAF/MAPK or PI3K/AKT pathways were also targeted, and this is highlighted in **Table 10.3** (Rager et al., 2022).

TABLE 10.3
Clinical Phase Trial: Drug Combination Therapies for Melanoma

Drug 1 (Target)	Drug 2 (Target)	Drug 3 (Target)	Phase	References
MK-2206 (AKT)	Carboplatin/Paclitaxel, Docetaxel, or Erlotinib		I	Molife et al. (2014)
Pazopanib (VEGFR/ PDGFR/c-KIT)	Paclitaxel (Antineoplastic)		II	Fruehauf et al. (2018)
Vemurafenib (BRAF)	Cobimetinib (MEK)	Atezolizumab (PD-L1)	III	Gutzmer et al. (2020)
Dabrafenib (BRAF)	Trametinib (MEK)	Pembrolizumab (PD-1)	I/II	Rager et al. (2022)
Dasatinib (KIT)	Dacarbazine		1	Algazi et al. (2012)
Binimetinib (MEK)	Ribociclib (CDK4/6)		Ib/II	Schuler et al. (2022)
Sorafenib (KIT)	Carboplatin	Paclitaxel	I/II	Jilaveanu et al. (2009)
Apatinib (VEGFR)	Camrelizumab/SHR-1210 (PD-1)		II/III	Liang et al. (2019)
Axitinib (VEGFR)	Toripalimab (PD-1)		Ib	Sheng et al. (2019)
Tivantinib (cMET)	Sorafenib (VEGFR/PDGFR/RAF)		I	Puzanov et al. (2015)
Bevacizumab (VEGFR)	Paclitaxel (Antineoplastic)	Carboplatin (Antineoplastic)	II	Yan et al. (2021)
Lenvatinib (VEGFR)	Pembrolizumab (PD-1)		Ib/II	Rager et al. (2022)
Dabrafenib (BRAF)	Trametinib (MEK)	Spartalizumab (PD-1)	III	Dummer et al. (2022)
Pimasertib (MEK1/2)	Voxtalisib (pan-PI3K)		Ib	Schram et al. (2018)
Bevacizumab (VEGFR)	Ipilimumab (CTLA-4)		I	Hodi et al. (2014)

Sullivan and colleagues noted comparable response rates but observed that the triple combination of atezolizumab, vemurafenib, and cobimetinib resulted in more enduring responses and longer median PFS compared to treatment with vemurafenib and cobimetinib alone (Sullivan et al., 2019). Analysis of biomarkers suggested that the run-in period of vemurafenib and cobimetinib induced favorable changes in the TME, which supported the subsequent IMspire 150 phase III trial (NCT02908672). This trial confirmed a significantly prolonged PFS in the triple combination arm (Gutzmer et al., 2020; Haist et al., 2023).

The FDA has given the green light for the use of this combination in treating metastatic melanoma. Even though both groups had similar median overall survival and ORRs, the triple combination therapy was well-tolerated overall. However, it's worth noting that there were slightly more serious treatment-related adverse events associated with this therapy compared to the other options (Gutzmer et al., 2020). The combination of pembrolizumab plus DT was compared to DT only in advanced BRAF-mutant melanoma patients in the phase I/II KEYNOTE 022 trial (NCT02130466). Although the triple therapy improved median PFS, it did not reach pre-specified significance criteria. The ORR was weaker, attributed to adverse prognostic features among patients. However, the addition of pembrolizumab increased the rate of complete response and duration of response. More people in the group that received the triple combination treatment experienced serious side effects, which led to more of them stopping the treatment (Haist et al., 2023).

The COMBI-i trial assessed spartalizumab plus DT, demonstrating high efficacy but not meeting its primary endpoint, with a higher occurrence of serious treatment-related adverse events in the triple combination arm (Dummer et al., 2018). Collectively, these trials indicate a modest additional benefit of triple combination regimens compared to MAPKi combinations, albeit with an unfavorable toxicity profile. It's important to note that none of these trials included an IPI plus Nivo comparator arm, which is currently considered standard of care; thus caution is advised in the widespread first-line use of triple combination regimens for BRAFV600 mutant melanoma patients. Nevertheless, subgroup analyses suggest that patients with a high disease burden may experience greater benefits, and further biomarker-driven analyses may help pinpoint these populations more accurately (Dummer et al., 2018).

The immunomodulatory properties of MAPKi to enhance the efficacy of other immunotherapies, such as ACT and CAR-T-cell therapy, suggest potential avenues for MAPKi as immunotherapy adjuvants. Short-term administration of vemurafenib before adoptive transfers of autologous TIL has been suggested as a safe and feasible option (Borch et al., 2021; Haist et al., 2023).

The highlighted clinical trials in melanoma have highlighted the enhanced efficacy of combination therapies involving MAPKi and immunotherapy agents. These combinations have shown improved ORRs and PFS compared to standard targeted therapy alone. Careful management of adverse effects is crucial, as some trials have demonstrated increased toxicity. Further studies are needed to identify populations that would benefit most from these treatments. The immunomodulatory properties of MAPKi suggest the potential for enhancing the efficacy of other immunotherapies, offering additional avenues for treatment.

FUTURE HORIZONS AND PROSPECTS

The future of melanoma treatment is poised to benefit significantly from ongoing research and innovations in combination therapy. As the field evolves, several emerging trends and novel approaches are expected to enhance treatment efficacy and overcome current limitations, particularly concerning resistance mechanisms.

Researchers are working to optimize treatment sequencing, identify predictive biomarkers, and explore novel combination strategies to improve outcomes and address resistance mechanisms (Hodi et al., 2018). Collaboration among academia, industry, and healthcare stakeholders is crucial for advancing progress in melanoma treatment and ensuring global access to cutting-edge therapies (Luke et al., 2017).

Researchers are continuously identifying new molecular targets that can be exploited for melanoma therapy. For instance, recent studies have focused on targeting the PI3K/AKT/mTOR pathway, which is often dysregulated in melanoma and associated with resistance to BRAF and MEK inhibitors. Combining inhibitors of this pathway with existing therapies could potentially enhance treatment responses and delay resistance (Ribas et al., 2019). Additionally, epigenetic modifications are being explored as therapeutic targets. Drugs that inhibit histone deacetylases (HDACs) or bromodomain and extraterminal (BET) proteins can modify the expression of genes involved in melanoma progression and immune evasion, thereby providing new avenues for combination therapy (Sweis et al., 2016).

Innovative drug combinations are also at the forefront of melanoma research. Combining ICIs with oncolytic viruses, for instance, is a promising strategy. Oncolytic viruses selectively infect and kill cancer cells while simultaneously stimulating an antitumor immune response. When used in combination with CPIs, these viruses can enhance the immune-mediated destruction of melanoma cells (Ribas et al., 2017a). Another exciting area is the combination of adoptive cell therapy (ACT) with CPIs. ACT involves the infusion of autologous TILs that are expanded *ex vivo*. When combined with checkpoint blockade, this approach can significantly enhance the antitumor activity of TILs and improve clinical outcomes (Rosenberg et al., 2008).

Optimizing the sequencing and scheduling of combination therapies is critical to maximizing their efficacy. Studies have shown that the sequence in which therapies are administered can significantly impact their effectiveness. For example, starting with targeted therapy to reduce tumor burden followed by immunotherapy may improve overall survival compared to concurrent administration (Boutros et al., 2024).

Furthermore, intermittent dosing schedules, as opposed to continuous treatment, are being investigated to mitigate toxicity and manage resistance. This approach allows periods of drug withdrawal, during which the tumor's drug resistance mechanisms may be reset, potentially restoring the tumor's sensitivity to treatment (Zhong et al., 2022).

CONSIDERATION OF PERSONALIZED MEDICINE APPROACHES AND PRECISION ONCOLOGY IN MELANOMA TREATMENT

Personalized medicine involves tailoring treatment based on the individual characteristics of each patient's tumor. This approach leverages genomic profiling and other biomarkers to select the most appropriate therapies. For instance, the identification of specific genetic mutations, such as BRAF V600E, guides the use of targeted therapies (Hodis et al., 2012).

The integration of next-generation sequencing (NGS) into clinical practice allows for a comprehensive analysis of tumor genomes, helping to identify actionable mutations and predict responses to therapy. This precision oncology approach enables the design of customized treatment regimens that are more effective and less toxic (Krauthammer et al., 2015).

Identifying biomarkers that predict response to therapy is crucial for optimizing treatment strategies. For example, PD-L1 expression levels can indicate the likelihood of response to PD-1/PD-L1 inhibitors. Additionally, tumor mutational burden (TMB) has emerged as a potential biomarker for immunotherapy, with higher TMB associated with better responses to CPIs (Snyder et al., 2014).

Research is also focused on identifying biomarkers of resistance. Understanding the mechanisms underlying resistance to targeted and immunotherapy can help in developing strategies to overcome it. For instance, secondary mutations in the MAPK pathway are a common resistance mechanism to BRAF inhibitors, and identifying these mutations can guide the use of second-line therapies (Nazarian et al., 2010).

Collaboration among academia, industry, and healthcare stakeholders is essential for advancing melanoma treatment. Academic research provides the foundational knowledge and early-stage discoveries, while industry partners bring the resources and expertise needed for drug development and clinical trials. Healthcare providers ensure that new treatments are effectively translated into clinical practice.

Moreover, global collaboration is necessary to ensure equitable access to cutting-edge therapies. This involves not only sharing scientific knowledge but also addressing disparities in healthcare infrastructure and access to new treatments. Collaborative efforts such as international clinical trials and global health initiatives are crucial for making advanced melanoma treatments available worldwide (Luke et al., 2017).

The future of melanoma treatment lies in the continued exploration of combination therapies, the identification of novel therapeutic targets, and the integration of personalized medicine approaches. By leveraging these strategies, researchers and clinicians aim to improve treatment outcomes, manage resistance, and reduce toxicity. Collaborative efforts across the globe will be essential in ensuring that these advancements benefit all melanoma patients, regardless of their geographic location.

CHALLENGES AND CONSIDERATIONS IN MELANOMA COMBINATION THERAPIES

The integration of combination therapies in the treatment of melanoma not only holds great promise but also presents several challenges and considerations. Understanding and addressing these challenges is critical to optimizing treatment outcomes and improving patient care.

One of the primary challenges in implementing combination therapies for melanoma is the complexity of the treatment regimens. Combining multiple therapeutic agents can result in complicated dosing schedules and increased potential for drug-drug interactions, which can be difficult to manage clinically (Gide et al., 2018). This complexity often requires more intensive monitoring and management to ensure patient adherence and to mitigate adverse effects.

Combination therapies, while potentially more effective, can also lead to increased toxicity compared to monotherapy. For example, combining ICIs with targeted therapies can amplify irAEs, which can be severe and sometimes life-threatening (Larkin et al., 2015). Managing these toxicities requires a delicate balance between maintaining the efficacy of the treatment and ensuring patient safety.

Tumor resistance remains a significant barrier to the success of combination therapies. Melanoma cells can develop resistance to therapies through various mechanisms, such as genetic mutations, adaptive responses, and alterations in the TME (Nazarian et al., 2010). Identifying and overcoming these resistance mechanisms is crucial for the long-term efficacy of combination treatments.

The cost of combination therapies can be prohibitively high, limiting accessibility for many patients, especially in low- and middle-income countries. The financial burden of these treatments can be significant, encompassing not only the cost of the drugs themselves but also the associated healthcare services required for administration and monitoring (Kohler et al., 2015). This economic barrier can prevent widespread adoption and equitable access to advanced melanoma treatments.

One strategy to overcome the challenges of combination therapies is the use of personalized medicine approaches. By tailoring treatments based on individual patient characteristics, such as genetic profiles and biomarker expression, clinicians can optimize therapy selection and dosing, potentially reducing toxicity and improving efficacy (Krauthammer et al., 2015). Ongoing research into predictive biomarkers is essential to identify patients who are most likely to benefit from specific combination therapies.

Implementing sequential or adaptive therapy approaches can help manage toxicity and resistance. Sequential therapy involves administering treatments one after another, rather than simultaneously, to minimize overlapping toxicities and allow for better management of side effects (Boutros et al., 2024). Adaptive therapy, on the other hand, adjusts the treatment regimen based on the tumor's response, potentially delaying the development of resistance by varying the therapeutic pressure on the tumor (Gatenby et al., 2009).

Enhanced supportive care strategies are critical for managing the increased toxicity associated with combination therapies. This includes proactive monitoring for adverse effects, prompt intervention when side effects occur, and comprehensive patient education to ensure adherence and manage expectations (Postow et al., 2015). Multidisciplinary care teams, including oncologists, nurses, and pharmacists, play a vital role in providing the necessary support to patients undergoing combination therapy.

Collaboration among stakeholders, including researchers, pharmaceutical companies, healthcare providers, and policymakers, is essential to address the cost and accessibility barriers. Efforts to negotiate pricing, increase funding for melanoma research, and implement global access programs can help ensure that advanced combination therapies are available to patients regardless of their geographic location or economic status (Luke et al., 2017).

While combination therapies offer a promising approach to treating melanoma, their implementation is fraught with challenges related to complexity, toxicity, resistance, and cost. Addressing these challenges requires a multifaceted strategy, including personalized medicine, sequential and adaptive therapy approaches, improved supportive care, and collaborative efforts to enhance access. By tackling these hurdles, the melanoma treatment landscape can be significantly improved, leading to better patient outcomes and prolonged survival.

CONCLUSION

The field of melanoma treatment has advanced significantly with the introduction of combination therapies that integrate immunotherapy, targeted therapy, and chemotherapy. These combinations have the potential to greatly improve patient outcomes by addressing the complex nature of this aggressive cancer. By leveraging the complementary mechanisms of different treatments, combination therapies can effectively target melanoma cells. For example, combining BRAF inhibitors with MEK inhibitors has shown significant efficacy in targeting the MAPK/ERK pathway, which is crucial for the proliferation and survival of melanoma cells. Similarly, combining CPIs such as nivolumab and pembrolizumab with traditional therapies can enhance the immune system's ability to recognize and eliminate melanoma cells, leading to improved overall survival rates. These specific combination therapies show promise in the treatment of melanoma, offering new hope for patients with this disease.

In addition, combination therapies have the potential to mitigate the adverse effects associated with high-dose monotherapies by simultaneously targeting multiple subpopulations of melanoma cells and addressing the diverse genetic mutations and immune profiles within the tumor. This approach reduces the likelihood of treatment resistance and recurrence, resulting in a more robust and enduring response. However, the accessibility of advanced melanoma treatments in Africa remains a significant challenge due to limited healthcare infrastructure, high costs, and a shortage of specialized medical personnel, leading to disparities in the availability and effectiveness of these treatments across the continent.

To fully realize the potential of synergistic combination therapies in melanoma treatment, it is essential to focus on enhanced research initiatives, expanded clinical trials, integration of personalized medicine, capacity building, and education, as well as policy and advocacy efforts. These actions can accelerate the development of effective combination therapies and ensure that advancements benefit all patients globally. In South Africa, the current challenges in developing tailored combination approaches include limited access to cutting-edge therapies, insufficient research funding, and the need for more comprehensive genetic and immunological profiling of the patient population to inform personalized treatment plans.

By addressing these key areas, the medical community can make significant progress in improving melanoma treatment outcomes. Synergistic combination therapies hold the promise of revolutionizing the standard of care for melanoma, ultimately leading to improved survival rates and quality of life for patients. Continued research, collaboration, and clinical innovation are imperative to advancing this promising field and achieving the goal of more effective and personalized melanoma treatment.

REFERENCES

Aasen, S. N., Parajuli, H., Hoang, T., Feng, Z., Stokke, K., Wang, J., Roy, K., Bjerkvig, R., Knappskog, S. and Thorsen, F. 2019. Effective treatment of metastatic melanoma by combining MAPK and PI3K signaling pathway inhibitors, *International Journal of Molecular Sciences*, 20(17), p. 4235. https://doi.org/10.3390/ijms20174235

Adam, C., Fusi, L., Weiss, N., Goller, S. G., Meder, K., Frings, V. G., Kneitz, H., Goebeler, M., Houben, R., Schrama, D., et al. 2020. Efficient suppression of NRAS-driven melanoma by co-inhibition of ERK1/2 and ERK5 MAPK pathways, *Journal of Investigative Dermatology*, 140, pp. 2455–2465.e10. https://doi.org/10.1016/j.jid.2020.03.972.

Algazi, A. P., Weber, J. S., Andrews, S. C., Urbas, P., Munster, P. N., DeConti, R. C., Hwang, J., Sondak, V. K., Messina, J. L., McCalmont, T., et al. 2012. Phase I clinical trial of the Src inhibitor dasatinib with dacarbazine in metastatic melanoma, *British Journal of Cancer*, 106, pp. 85–91. https://doi.org/10.1038/bjc.2011.514.

Amin, A., Lawson, D. H., Salama, A. K., Koon, H. B., Guthrie, T., Jr., Thomas, S. S., O'Day, S. J., Shaheen, M. F., Zhang, B., Francis, S., et al. 2016. Phase II study of vemurafenib followed by ipilimumab in patients with previously untreated BRAF-mutated metastatic melanoma, *Journal for ImmunoTherapy of Cancer*, 4, p. 44. https://doi.org/10.1186/s40425-016-0148-7

AORTIC. (2022). African Organization for Research and Training in Cancer. Retrieved from https://www.aortic-africa.org/

Appleton, K. M., Palsuledesai, C. C., Misek, S. A., Blake, M., Zagorski, J., Gallo, K. A., Dexheimer, T. S. and Neubig, R. R. 2021. Inhibition of the myocardin-related transcription factor pathway increases efficacy of trametinib in NRAS-mutant melanoma cell lines, *Cancers*, 13, p. 2012. https://doi.org/10.3390/cancers13092012.

Ascierto, P. A., et al. 2019. Efficacy and safety of nivolumab alone or combined with ipilimumab in patients with melanoma brain metastases: A pooled analysis, *Journal of Clinical Oncology*, 37(35), pp. 2930–2941.

Ascierto, P. A., Casula, M., Bulgarelli, J., Pisano, M., Piccinini, C., Piccin, L., Cossu, A., Mandalà, M., Ferrucci, P. F., Guidoboni, M., Rutkowski, P., Ferraresi, V., Arance, A., Guida, M., Maiello, E., Gogas, H., Richtig, E., Fierro, M. T., Lebbe, C. and Helgadottir, H. 2024. Sequential immunotherapy and targeted therapy for metastatic BRAF V600 mutated melanoma: 4-year survival and biomarkers evaluation from the phase II SECOMBIT trial, *Nature Communications*, 15(1), p. 146. https://doi.org/10.1038/s41467-023-44475-6

Arnold, M., Singh, D., Laversanne, M., Vignat, J., Vaccarella, S., Meheus, F., Cust, A. E., de Vries, E., Whiteman, D. C. and Bray, F. (2022). Global burden of cutaneous melanoma in 2020 and projections to 2040. *JAMA Dermatology*, 158(5), pp. 495–503. https://doi.org/10.1001/jamadermatol.2022.0160

Atefi, M., Titz, B., Avramis, E., Ng, C., Wong, D. J., Lassen, A., Cerniglia, M., Escuin-Ordinas, H., Foulad, D., Comin-Anduix, B., et al. 2015. Combination of pan-RAF and MEK inhibitors in NRAS mutant melanoma, *Molecular Cancer*, 14, p. 27. https://doi.org/10.1186/s12943-015-0293-5.

Atkins, M. B., Lee, S. J., Chmielowski, B., Tarhini, A. A., Cohen, G. I., Truong, T.-G., Moon, H. H., Davar, D., O'Rourke, M., Stephenson, J. J., et al. 2023. Combination dabrafenib and trametinib versus combination nivolumab and ipilimumab for patients with advanced BRAF-mutant melanoma: The DREAMseq Trial—ECOG-ACRIN EA6134, *Journal of Clinical Oncology*, 41(2), pp. 186–197. https://doi.org/10.1200/JCO.22.01763

Balch, C. M., Gershenwald, J. E., Soong, S. J., Thompson, J. F., Atkins, M. B., Byrd, D. R., Buzaid, A. C., Cochran, A. J., Coit, D. G., Ding, S., Eggermont, A. M., Flaherty, K. T., Gimotty, P. A., Kirkwood, J. M., McMasters, K. M., Mihm, M. C. Jr, Morton, D. L., Ross, M. I., Sober, A. J. and Sondak, V. K. 2009. Final version of 2009 AJCC melanoma staging and classification, *Journal of Clinical Oncology*, 27(36), pp. 6199–6206.

Borch, T. H., Harbst, K., Rana, A. H., Andersen, R., Martinenaite, E., Kongsted, P., Pedersen, M., Nielsen, M., Kjeldsen, J. W., Kverneland, A. H., Lauss, M., Hölmich, L. R., Hendel, H., Met, Ö., Jönsson, G., Donia, M. and Svane, I. M. 2021. Clinical efficacy of T-cell therapy after short-term BRAF-inhibitor priming in patients with checkpoint inhibitor-resistant metastatic melanoma, *Journal for Immunotherapy of Cancer*, 9, p. e002703. https://doi.org/10.1136/jitc-2021-002703

Boutros, A., Croce, E., Ferrari, M., Gili, R., Massaro, G., Marconcini, R., Arecco, L., Tanda, E. T. and Spagnolo, F. 2024. The treatment of advanced melanoma: Current approaches and new challenges, *Critical Reviews in Oncology/Hematology*, 196, p. 104276.

Cai, W., Nguyen, M. Q., Wilski, N. A., Purwin, T. J., Vernon, M., Tiago, M. and Aplin, A. E. 2022. A genome-wide screen identifies PDPK1 as a target to enhance the efficacy of MEK1/2 inhibitors in NRAS mutant melanoma, *Cancer Research*, 82, pp. 2625–2639. https://doi.org/10.1158/0008-5472.CAN-21-3217.

Centers for Disease Control and Prevention (CDC). (2022). Skin Cancer. Available from https://www.cdc.gov/cancer/skin/

Chapman, P. B., Einhorn, L. H., Meyers, M. L., Saxman, S., Destro, A. N., Panageas, K. S., Begg, C. B., Agarwala, S. S., Schuchter, L. M., Ernstoff, M. S., Houghton, A. N. and Kirkwood, J. M. 1999. Phase III multicenter randomized trial of the Dartmouth regimen versus dacarbazine in patients with metastatic melanoma, *Journal of Clinical Oncology*, 17(9), pp. 2745–2751.

Cheng, H., Chua, V., Liao, C., Purwin, T. J., Terai, M., Kageyama, K., Davies, M. A., Sato, T. and Aplin, A. E. 2017. Co-targeting HGF/cMET signaling with MEK inhibitors in metastatic uveal melanoma, *Molecular Cancer Therapeutics*, 16, pp. 516–528. https://doi.org/10.1158/1535-7163.MCT-16-0552.

Coory, M., Baade, P., Aitken, J., Smithers, M., McLeod, G. R. and Ring, I. 2013. Trends for in situ and invasive melanoma in Queensland, Australia, 1982–2002, *Cancer Causes & Control*, 17(1), pp. 21–27.

Courtney, K. D., Corcoran, R. B., Engelman, J. A. (2010). The PI3K pathway as drug target in human cancer, *Journal of Clinical Oncology*, 28(6), pp. 1075–1083. https://doi.org/10.1200/JCO.2009.25.3641.

Dummer, R., et al. 2020. Overall survival in patients with BRAF-mutant melanoma receiving encorafenib plus binimetinib versus vemurafenib or encorafenib (COLUMBUS): A multicentre, open-label, randomised, phase 3 trial, *Lancet Oncology*, 21(5), pp. 616–626.

Dummer, R., Ascierto, P. A., Gogas, H. J., Arance, A., Mandala, M., Liszkay, G., Garbe, C., Schadendorf, D., Krajsova, I., Gutzmer, R., Chiarion-Sileni, V., Dutriaux, C., de Groot, J. W. B., Yamazaki, N., Loquai, C., Moutouh-de Parseval, L. A., Pickard, M. D., Sandor, V., Robert, C. and Flaherty, K. T. 2018. Encorafenib plus binimetinib versus vemurafenib or encorafenib in patients with BRAF-mutant melanoma (COLUMBUS): A multicentre, open-label, randomised phase 3 trial, *Lancet. Oncology*, 19(5), pp. 603–615. https://doi.org/10.1016/S1470-2045(18)30142-6

Dummer, R., Long, G. V., Robert, C., Tawbi, H. A., Flaherty, K. T., Ascierto, P. A., Nathan, P. D., Rutkowski, P., Leonov, O., Dutriaux, C., et al. 2022. Randomized phase III trial evaluating spartalizumab plus dabrafenib and trametinib for BRAF V600-mutant unresectable or metastatic melanoma, *Journal of Clinical Oncology*, 40, pp. 1428–1438. https://doi.org/10.1200/JCO.21.01601.

Ebert, P. J., Cheung, J., Yang, Y., McNamara, E., Hong, R., Moskalenko, M., … and Klijn, C. 2016. MAP kinase inhibition promotes T cell and anti-tumor activity in combination with PD-L1 checkpoint blockade, *Immunity*, 44(3), pp. 609–621.

Eggermont, A. M. M., et al. 2018. Adjuvant pembrolizumab versus placebo in resected stage III melanoma, *NEJM*, 378(19), pp. 1789–1801.

Eggermont, A. M. M., Chiarion-Sileni, V., Grob, J. J., Dummer, R., Wolchok, J. D., Schmidt, H., Hamid, O., Robert, C., Ascierto, P. A., Richards, J. M., Lebbe, C., Ferraresi, V., Smylie, M., Weber, J. S., Maio, M., Hosein, F., de Pril, V., Kicinski, M., Suciu, S. and Testori, A. 2019. Adjuvant ipilimumab versus placebo after complete resection of stage III melanoma: Long-term follow-up results of the European Organisation for Research and Treatment of Cancer 18071 double-blind phase 3 randomised trial, *European Journal of Cancer*, 119, pp. 1–10.

Emens, L. A. and Middleton, G. 2015. The interplay of immunotherapy and chemotherapy: Harnessing potential synergies, *Cancer Immunology Research*, 3(5), pp. 436–443. https://doi.org/10.1158/2326-6066.CIR-15-0064

Etnyre, D., Stone, A. L., Fong, J. T., Jacobs, R. J., Uppada, S. B., Botting, G. M., Rajanna, S., Moravec, D. N., Shambannagari, M. R., Crees, Z., et al. 2014. Targeting c-met in melanoma: Mechanism of resistance and efficacy of novel combinatorial inhibitor therapy, *Cancer Biology & Therapy*, 15, pp. 1129–1141. https://doi.org/10.4161/cbt.29451.

Farhana, A. 2023. Enhancing skin cancer immunotheranostics and precision medicine through functionalized nanomodulators and nanosensors: Recent development and prospects, *International Journal of Molecular Sciences*, 24(4), p. 3493. https://doi.org/10.3390/ijms24043493

Ferlay, J., Colombet, M., Soerjomataram, I., Mathers, C., Parkin, D. M., Piñeros, M., … and Bray, F. 2020. Estimating the global cancer incidence and mortality in 2018: GLOBOCAN sources and methods, *International Journal of Cancer*, 144(8), pp. 1941–1953.

Ferrucci, P. F., Di Giacomo, A. M., Del Vecchio, M., Atkinson, V., Schmidt, H., Schachter, J., Queirolo, P., Long, G. V., Stephens, R., Svane, I. M., Lotem, M., Abu-Amna, M., Gasal, E., Ghori, R., Diede, S. J., Croydon, E. S., Ribas, A., Ascierto, P. A., and KEYNOTE-022 International Team. 2020. KEYNOTE-022 part 3: A randomized, double-blind, phase 2 study of pembrolizumab, dabrafenib, and trametinib in *BRAF*-mutant melanoma, *Journal for Immunotherapy of Cancer*, 8(2), p. e001806. https://doi.org/10.1136/jitc-2020-001806

Flaherty, K. T., Puzanov, I., Kim, K. B., Ribas, A., McArthur, G. A., Sosman, J. A., O'Dwyer, P. J., Lee, R. J., Grippo, J. F., Nolop, K. and Chapman, P. B. 2010. Inhibition of mutated, activated BRAF in metastatic melanoma, *New England Journal of Medicine*, 363(9), pp. 809–819. https://doi.org/10.1056/NEJMoa1002011

Fruehauf, J. P., El-Masry, M., Osann, K., Parmakhtiar, B., Yamamoto, M. and Jakowatz, J. G. 2018. Phase II study of pazopanib in combination with paclitaxel in patients with metastatic melanoma, *Cancer Chemotherapy and Pharmacology*, 82, pp. 353–360. https://doi.org/10.1007/s00280-018-3624-6.

Garbe, C., et al. 2020. Systematic review of medical treatment in melanoma: Current status and future prospects, *Lancet Oncology*, 21(9), pp. e343–e354.

Gatenby, R. A., Silva, A. S., Gillies, R. J. and Frieden, B. R. 2009. Adaptive therapy, *Cancer Research*, 69(11), pp. 4894–4903.

Gide, T. N., Wilmott, J. S., Scolyer, R. A. and Long, G. V. 2018. Primary and acquired resistance to immune checkpoint inhibitors in metastatic melanoma, *Clinical Cancer Research*, 25(6), pp. 1572–1578.

Gide, T. N., Silva, I. P., Quek, C., Ahmed, T., Menzies, A. M., Carlino, M. S., … and Wilmott, J. S. 2019. Close proximity of immune and tumor cells underlies response to anti-PD-1 based therapies in metastatic melanoma patients, *OncoImmunology*, 9(1). https://doi.org/10.1080/2162402X.2019.1659093

Gutzmer, R., Stroyakovskiy, D., Gogas, H. Robert, C., Lewis, K., Protsenko, S., Pereira, R. P., Eigentler, T., Rutkowski, P., Demidov, L. et al. 2020. Atezolizumab, vemurafenib, and cobimetinib as first-line treatment for unresectable advanced BRAF(V600) mutation-positive melanoma (IMspire150): Primary analysis of the randomised, double-blind, placebo-controlled, phase 3 trial, *Lancet*, 395, pp. 1835–1844. https://doi.org/10.1016/S0140-6736(20)30934-X

Haist, M., Stege, H., Kuske, M. et al. 2023. Combination of immune-checkpoint inhibitors and targeted therapies for melanoma therapy: The more, the better? *Cancer and Metastasis Reviews*, 42, pp. 481–505. https://doi.org/10.1007/s10555-023-10097-z

Haugh, A. M., Salama, A. K. S. and Johnson, D. B. 2021. Advanced melanoma: Resistance mechanisms to current therapies, *Hematology/oncology Clinics of North America*, 35(1), pp. 111–128. https://doi.org/10.1016/j.hoc.2020.09.005

Hodi, F. S., Chiarion-Sileni, V., Gonzalez, R., Grob, J. J., Rutkowski, P., Cowey, C. L., … and Larkin, J. 2018. Nivolumab plus ipilimumab or nivolumab alone versus ipilimumab alone in advanced melanoma (CheckMate 067): 4-year outcomes of a multicentre, randomised, phase 3 trial, *Lancet Oncology*, 19(11), pp. 1480–1492.

Hodi, F. S., Lawrence, D., Lezcano, C., Wu, X., Zhou, J., Sasada, T., Zeng, W., Giobbie-Hurder, A., Atkins, M. B., Ibrahim, N., et al. 2014. Bevacizumab plus ipilimumab in patients with metastatic melanoma, *Cancer Immunology Research*, 2, pp. 632–642. https://doi.org/10.1158/2326-6066.CIR-14-0053.

Hodi, F. S., Lee, S., McDermott, D. F., Rao, U. N. M., Butterfield, L. H., Tarhini, A. A., … and Atkins, M. B. 2014. Ipilimumab plus sargramostim vs ipilimumab alone for treatment of metastatic melanoma: A randomized clinical trial, *JAMA*, 315(8), pp. 787–796.

Hodi, F. S., O'Day, S. J., McDermott, D. F., Weber, R. W., Sosman, J. A., Haanen, J. B., … and Urba, W. J. 2010. Improved survival with ipilimumab in patients with metastatic melanoma, *New England Journal of Medicine*, 363(8), pp. 711–723.

Hodis, E., Watson, I. R., Kryukov, G. V., Arold, S. T., Imielinski, M., Theurillat, J. P., Nickerson, E., Auclair, D., Li, L., Place, C., Dicara, D., Ramos, A. H., Lawrence, M. S., Cibulskis, K., Sivachenko, A., Voet, D., Saksena, G., Stransky, N., Onofrio, R. C., Winckler, W., … and Chin, L. 2012. A landscape of driver mutations in melanoma, *Cell*, 150(2), pp. 251–263. https://doi.org/10.1016/j.cell.2012.06.024

Hugo, W., Shi, H., Sun, L., Piva, M., Song, C., Kong, X., … and Lu, Y. 2015. Non-genomic and immune evolution of melanoma acquiring MAPKi resistance, *Cell*, 162(6), pp. 1271–1285.

Jansen, Y., et al. 2020. Pembrolizumab plus ipilimumab or placebo in advanced melanoma: Final results of the phase III KEYNOTE-252/ECHO-301 trial, *Journal of Clinical Oncology*, 38(15_suppl), p. 10000.

Jilaveanu, L., Zito, C., Lee, S. J., Nathanson, K. L., Camp, R. L., Rimm, D. L., Flaherty, K. T. and Kluger, H. M. 2009. Expression of sorafenib targets in melanoma patients treated with carboplatin, paclitaxel and sorafenib, *Clinical Cancer Research*, 15, pp. 1076–1085. https://doi.org/10.1158/1078-0432.CCR-08-2280.

Kohler, B. A., Sherman, R. L., Howlader, N., Jemal, A., Ryerson, A. B., Henry, K. A., … and Cronin, K. A. 2015. Annual report to the nation on the status of cancer, 1975–2011, featuring incidence of breast cancer subtypes by race/ethnicity, poverty, and state, *Journal of the National Cancer Institute*, 107(6), p. djv048.

Krauthammer, M., Kong, Y., Ha, B. H., Evans, P., Bacchiocchi, A., McCusker, J. P., … and Schlessinger, J. 2015. Exome sequencing identifies recurrent mutations in NF1 and RASopathy genes in sun-exposed melanomas, *Nature Genetics*, 47(9), pp. 996–1002.

Landras, A., Reger de Moura, C., Villoutreix, B. O., Battistella, M., Sadoux, A., Dumaz, N., Menashi, S., Fernandez-Recio, J., Lebbe, C. and Mourah, S. 2022. Novel treatment strategy for NRAS-mutated melanoma through a selective inhibitor of CD147/VEGFR-2 interaction, *Oncogene*, 41, pp. 2254–2264. https://doi.org/10.1038/s41388-022-02244-7.

Larkin, J., Chiarion-Sileni, V., Gonzalez, R., Grob, J. J., Cowey, C. L., Lao, C. D., … and Dummer, R. 2015. Combined nivolumab and ipilimumab or monotherapy in untreated melanoma, *New England Journal of Medicine*, 373(1), pp. 23–34.

Larkin, J., Chiarion-Sileni, V., Gonzalez, R., Grob, J. J., Rutkowski, P., Lao, C. D., … and Jansen, P. 2019. Five-year survival with combined nivolumab and ipilimumab in advanced melanoma, *New England Journal of Medicine*, 381(16), pp. 1535–1546.

Lau, P. K. H., Cullinane, C., Jackson, S., Walker, R., Smith, L. K., Slater, A., Kirby, L., Patel, R. P., von Scheidt, B., Slaney, C. Y., McArthur, G. A. and Sheppard, K. E. 2021. Enhancing adoptive cell transfer with combination BRAF-MEK and CDK4/6 inhibitors in melanoma, *Cancers*, 13(24), p. 6342. https://doi.org/10.3390/cancers13246342

Liang, L., Wen, Y., Hu, R., Wang, L., Xia, Y., Hu, C., Qiao, Y., Geng, X., Chen, T., Fei, J., et al. 2019. Safety and efficacy of PD-1 blockade-activated multiple antigen-specific cellular therapy alone or in combination with apatinib in patients with advanced solid tumors: A pooled analysis of two prospective trials, *Cancer Immunology, Immunotherapy*, 68, pp. 1467–1477. https://doi.org/10.1007/s00262-019-02375-z.

Long, G. V., Stroyakovskiy, D., Gogas, H., Levchenko, E., De Braud, F., Larkin, J., … and Dummer, R. 2014. Combined BRAF and MEK inhibition versus BRAF inhibition alone in melanoma, *New England Journal of Medicine*, 371(20), pp. 1877–1888.

Lopez, J. S. and Banerji, U. 2017. Combine and conquer: Challenges for targeted therapy combinations in early phase trials, *Nature Reviews. Clinical Oncology*, 14(1), pp. 57–66. https://doi.org/10.1038/nrclinonc.2016.96

Luke, J. J., Flaherty, K. T., Ribas, A. and Long, G. V. 2017. Targeted agents and immunotherapies: Optimizing outcomes in melanoma, *Nature Reviews Clinical Oncology*, 14(8), pp. 463–482.

Mayo Clinic. (2021). Squamous Cell Carcinoma of the Skin. Available from https://www.mayoclinic.org/diseases-conditions/squamous-cell-carcinoma/symptoms-causes/syc-20352480

McDaniel, B., Badri, T. and Steele, R. B. 2022. *Basal Cell Carcinoma.* In StatPearls. StatPearls Publishing. Available from https://www.ncbi.nlm.nih.gov/books/NBK482439/

Minor, D. R., Puzanov, I., Callahan, M. K., Hug, B. A. and Hoos, A. 2015. Severe gastrointestinal toxicity with administration of trametinib in combination with dabrafenib and ipilimumab, *Pigment Cell & Melanoma Research*, 28, pp. 611–612. https://doi.org/10.1111/pcmr.12383

Mitchell, T. C., Karakousis, G. and Schuchter, L. 2020. Chapter 66: Melanoma. In: Niederhuber J. E., Armitage J. O., Doroshow J. H., Kastan M. B., Tepper J. E. (eds.) *Abeloff's Clinical Oncology.* 6th ed. Philadelphia, PA: Elsevier.

Molife, L. R., Yan, L., Vitfell-Rasmussen, J., Zernhelt, A. M., Sullivan, D. M., Cassier, P. A., Chen, E., Biondo, A., Tetteh, E., Siu, L. L., et al. 2014. Phase 1 trial of the oral AKT inhibitor MK-2206 plus carboplatin/paclitaxel, docetaxel, or erlotinib in patients with advanced solid tumors, *J. Hematol. Oncol*, 7, p. 1. https://doi.org/10.1186/1756-8722-7-1.

Motz, G. T., & Coukos, G. (2011). The parallel lives of angiogenesis and immunosuppression: Cancer and other tales. *Nature Reviews Immunology*, 11(4), pp. 253–266. https://doi.org/10.1038/nri2971

Motzer, R. J., Penkov, K., Haanen, J., Rini, B., Albiges, L., Campbell, M. T., Venugopal, B., Kollmannsberger, C., Negrier, S., Uemura, M., et al. 2019. Avelumab plus Axitinib versus Sunitinib for Advanced Renal-Cell Carcinoma, *New England Journal of Medicine*, 380(12), pp. 1103–1115. https://doi.org/10.1056/NEJMoa1816047

National Cancer Registry. (2019). *Cancer in South Africa 2016.* National Cancer Registry, South African National Department of Health.

Swetter, S. M., Johnson, D., Albertini, M. R., Barker, C. A., Bateni, S., Baumgartner, J., Bhatia, S., Bichakjian, C., Boland, G., Chandra, S., et al. 2024. NCCN Guidelines® Insights: Melanoma: Cutaneous, Version 2.2024. *Journal of the National Comprehensive Cancer Network : JNCCN*, 22(5), pp. 290–298. https://doi.org/10.6004/jnccn.2024.0036

Nazarian, R., Shi, H., Wang, Q., Kong, X., Koya, R. C., Lee, H., Chen, Z., Lee, M. K., Attar, N., Sazegar, H., Chodon, T., Nelson, S. F., McArthur, G., Sosman, J. A., Ribas, A. and Lo, R. S. 2010. Melanomas acquire resistance to B-RAF(V600E) inhibition by RTK or N-RAS upregulation, *Nature*, 468(7326), pp. 973–977.

Nguyen, M. Q., Teh, J. L. F., Purwin, T. J., Chervoneva, I., Davies, M. A., Nathanson, K. L., Cheng, P. F., Levesque, M. P., Dummer, R. and Aplin, A. E. 2020. Targeting PHGDH upregulation reduces glutathione levels and resensitizes resistant NRAS-mutant melanoma to MAPK kinase inhibition, *Journal of Investigative Dermatology*, 140, pp. 2242–2252.e47. https://doi.org/10.1016/j.jid.2020.02.047.

Norval, M. and Kelfkens, G. 2020. The effects of ultraviolet radiation on human health in South Africa, *Photochemical & Photobiological Sciences*, 19(2), pp. 201–207.

Ohara, M., Saito, K., Kageyama, K., Terai, M., Cheng, H., Aplin, A. E. and Sato, T. 2021. Dual targeting of CDK4/6 and cMET in metastatic uveal melanoma, *Cancers*, 13, p. 1104. https://doi.org/10.3390/cancers13051104.

Paz-Ares, L., Luft, A., Vicente, D., Tafreshi, A., Gumus, M., Mazieres, J., Hermes, B., Cay, S. F., Csoszi, T., Fulop, A., et al. 2018. Pembrolizumab plus chemotherapy for squamous non-small-cell lung cancer, *New England Journal of Medicine*, 379, pp. 2040–2051. https://doi.org/10.1056/NEJMoa1810865.

Portelinha, A., Thompson, S., Smith, R. A., Da Silva Ferreira, M., Asgari, Z., Knezevic, A., Seshan, V., de Stanchina, E., Gupta, S., Denis, L., et al. 2021. ASN007 is a selective ERK1/2 inhibitor with preferential activity against RAS and RAF-mutant tumors, *Cell Reports. Medicine*, 2, p. 100350. https://doi.org/10.1016/j.xcrm.2021.100350.

Postow, M. A., Callahan, M. K. and Wolchok, J. D. 2015. Immune checkpoint blockade in cancer therapy, *Journal of Clinical Oncology*, 33(17), pp. 1974–1982.

Postow, M. A., Sidlow, R. and Hellmann, M. D. 2018. Immune-related adverse events associated with immune checkpoint blockade, *New England Journal of Medicine*, 378(2), pp. 158–168.

Puzanov, I., Callahan, M. K., Linette, G. P., Patel, S. P., Luke, J. J., Sosman, J. A., Wolchok, J. D., Hamid, O., Minor, D. R. and Orford, K. W. 2014. Phase 1 study of the BRAF inhibitor dabrafenib (D) with or without the MEK inhibitor trametinib (T) in combination with ipilimumab (Ipi) for V600E/K mutation-positive unresectable or metastatic melanoma (MM), *Journal of Clinical Oncology*, 32, pp. 2511–2511. https://doi.org/10.1200/jco.2014.32.15_suppl.2511

Puzanov, I., Sosman, J., Santoro, A., Saif, M. W., Goff, L., Dy, G. K., Zucali, P., Means-Powell, J. A., Ma, W. W., Simonelli, M., et al. 2015. Phase 1 trial of tivantinib in combination with sorafenib in adult patients with advanced solid tumors, *Investigational New Drugs*, 33, pp. 159–168. https://doi.org/10.1007/s10637-014-0167-5.

Quirk, S. K., Shure, A. K. and Agrawal, D. K. 2015. Immune-mediated adverse events of anticytotoxic T lymphocyte-associated antigen 4 antibody therapy in metastatic melanoma, *Translational Research: The Journal of Laboratory and Clinical Medicine*, 166(5), pp. 412–424. https://doi.org/10.1016/j.trsl.2015.06.005

Rager, T., Eckburg, A., Patel, M., Qiu, R., Gantiwala, S., Dovalovsky, K., Fan, K., Lam, K., Roesler, C., Rastogi, A., Gautam, S., Dube, N., Morgan, B., Nasifuzzaman, S. M., Ramaswami, D., Gnanasekar, V., Smith, J., Merchant, A. and Puri, N. 2022. Treatment of metastatic melanoma with a combination of immunotherapies and molecularly targeted therapies, *Cancers*, 14(15), p. 3779. https://doi.org/10.3390/cancers14153779

Ribas, A., Puzanov, I., Dummer, R., Schadendorf, D., Hamid, O., Robert, C., Hodi, F. S., Schachter, J., Pavlick, A. C., Lewis, K. D., et al. 2015. Pembrolizumab versus investigator-choice chemotherapy for ipilimumab-refractory melanoma (KEYNOTE-002): A randomised, controlled, phase 2 trial. *Lancet. Oncology, 16*(8), 908–918. https://doi.org/10.1016/S1470-2045(15)00083-2

Ribas, A., Dummer, R., Puzanov, I., VanderWalde, A., Andtbacka, R. H. I., Michielin, O., Olszanski, A. J., Malvehy, J., Cebon, J., Fernandez, E., Kirkwood, J. M., Gajewski, T. F., Chen, L., Gorski, K. S., Anderson, A. A., Diede, S. J., Lassman, M. E., Gansert, J., Hodi, F. S. and Long, G. V. 2017b. Oncolytic virotherapy promotes intratumoral T cell infiltration and improves anti-PD-1 immunotherapy, *Cell*, 170(6), pp. 1109–1119.e10. https://doi.org/10.1016/j.cell.2017.08.027

Ribas, A., Hodi, F. S., Callahan, M., Konto, C. and Wolchok, J. 2013. Hepatotoxicity with combination of vemurafenib and ipilimumab, *New England Journal of Medicine*, 368, pp. 1365–1366. https://doi.org/10.1056/NEJMc1302338

Ribas, A., Lawrence, D., Atkinson, V., Agarwal, S., Miller, W. H., Carlino, M. S. and Ascierto, P. A. 2017a. Combined BRAF and MEK inhibition with PD-1 blockade immunotherapy in BRAF-mutant melanoma, *Nature Medicine*, 23(7), pp. 936–944.

Ribas, A., Lawrence, D., Atkinson, V., Agarwala, S. S., Miller, W. H., Snider, J., … and Schadendorf, D. 2019. Combined BRAF and MEK inhibition with PD-1 blockade immunotherapy in BRAF-mutant melanoma, *Nature Medicine*, 25(6), pp. 936–940.

Robert, C., Karaszewska, B., Schachter, J., Rutkowski, P., Mackiewicz, A., Stroiakovski, D., Lichinitser, M., Dummer, R., Grange, F., Mortier, L., Chiarion-Sileni, V., Drucis, K., Krajsova, I., Hauschild, A., Lorigan, P., Wolter, P., Long, G. V., Flaherty, K., Nathan, P., Ribas, A. and Schadendorf, D. 2015a. Improved overall survival in melanoma with combined dabrafenib and trametinib, *New England Journal of Medicine*, 372(1), pp. 30–39. https://doi.org/10.1056/NEJMoa1412690

Robert, C., Schachter, J., Long, G. V., Arance, A., Grob, J. J., Mortier, L. and Lebbé, C. 2015b. Pembrolizumab versus ipilimumab in advanced melanoma, *New England Journal of Medicine*, 372(26), pp. 2521–2532.

Robert, L., Ribas, A. and Hu-Lieskovan, S. 2016. Combining targeted therapy with immunotherapy. Can 1+1 equal more than 2? *Seminars in Immunology*, 28(1), pp. 73–80. https://doi.org/10.1016/j.smim.2016.01.001

Rosenberg, S. A., Restifo, N. P., Yang, J. C., Morgan, R. A. and Dudley, M. E. 2008. Adoptive cell transfer: A clinical path to effective cancer immunotherapy, *Nature Reviews Cancer*, 8(4), pp. 299–308.

Schram, A. M., Gandhi, L., Mita, M. M., Damstrup, L., Campana, F., Hidalgo, M., Grande, E., Hyman, D. M. and Heist, R. S. 2018. A phase Ib dose-escalation and expansion study of the oral MEK inhibitor pimasertib and PI3K/MTOR inhibitor voxtalisib in patients with advanced solid tumours, *British Journal of Cancer*, 119, pp. 1471–1476. https://doi.org/10.1038/s41416-018-0322-4.

Schuler, M., Zimmer, L., Kim, K. B., Sosman, J. A., Ascierto, P. A., Postow, M. A., De Vos, F., van Herpen, C. M. L., Carlino, M. S., Johnson, D. B., et al. 2022. Phase Ib/II trial of ribociclib in combination with binimetinib in patients with NRAS-mutant melanoma, *Clinical Cancer Research*, 28, pp. 3002–3010. https://doi.org/10.1158/1078-0432.CCR-21-3872.

Sharma, A., Boise, L. H. and Shanmugam, M. 2019. Cancer metabolism and the evasion of apoptotic cell death, *Cancers*, 11(8), p. 1144. https://doi.org/10.3390/cancers11081144

Sheng, X., Yan, X., Chi, Z., Si, L., Cui, C., Tang, B., Li, S., Mao, L., Lian, B., Wang, X., et al. 2019. Axitinib in combination with toripalimab, a humanized immunoglobulin G4 monoclonal antibody against programmed cell death-1, in patients with metastatic mucosal melanoma: An open-label phase IB trial, *Journal of Clinical Oncology*, 37, pp. 2987–2999. https://doi.org/10.1200/JCO.19.00210.

Shin, M. H., Kim, J., Lim, S. A., Kim, J. and Lee, K. M. 2020. Current insights into combination therapies with MAPK inhibitors and immune checkpoint blockade, *International Journal of Molecular Sciences*, 21(7), p. 2531. https://doi.org/10.3390/ijms21072531

Snyder, A., Makarov, V., Merghoub, T., Yuan, J., Zaretsky, J. M., Desrichard, A., ... and Sznol, M. 2014. Genetic basis for clinical response to CTLA-4 blockade in melanoma, *New England Journal of Medicine*, 371(23), pp. 2189–2199.

Socinski, M. A., Jotte, R. M., Cappuzzo, F., Orlandi, F., Stroyakovskiy, D., Nogami, N., Rodriguez-Abreu, D., Moro-Sibilot, D., Thomas, C. A., Barlesi, F., et al. 2018. Atezolizumab for first-line treatment of metastatic nonsquamous NSCLC, *New England Journal of Medicine*, 378, pp. 2288–2301. https://doi.org/10.1056/NEJMoa1716948.

Sordo-Bahamonde, C., Lorenzo-Herrero, S., Gonzalez-Rodriguez, A. P., Martínez-Pérez, A., Rodrigo, J. P., García-Pedrero, J. M. and Gonzalez, S. 2023. Chemo-immunotherapy: A new trend in cancer treatment, *Cancers*, 15(11), p. 2912. https://doi.org/10.3390/cancers15112912

Sosman, J. A., Kim, K. B., Schuchter, L., Gonzalez, R., Pavlick, A. C., Weber, J. S., ... and Hodi, F. S. 2012. Survival in BRAF V600–mutant advanced melanoma treated with vemurafenib, *New England Journal of Medicine*, 366(8), pp. 707–714.

South African National Cancer Registry. 2023. Melanoma of the Skin. Retrieved from https://www.cansa.org.za/files/2023/03/NCR_2020_Cancer_Stats_Melanoma_of_the_Skin.pdf

Spain, L., Julve, M. and Larkin, J. 2016. Combination dabrafenib and trametinib in the management of advanced melanoma with BRAFV600 mutations, *Expert Opinion on Pharmacotherapy*, 17(7), pp. 1031–1038. https://doi.org/10.1517/14656566.2016.1168805

Sullivan R. J. 2020. Adjuvant nivolumab plus ipilimumab for resected stage IV melanoma, *Lancet (London, England)*, 395(10236), pp. 1524–1525. https://doi.org/10.1016/S0140-6736(20)31044-8

Sullivan, R. J., Hamid, O., Gonzalez, R., Infante, J. R., Patel, M. R., Hodi, F. S., Lewis, K. D., Tawbi, H. A., Hernandez, G., Wongchenko, M. J., et al. 2019. Atezolizumab plus cobimetinib and vemurafenib in BRAF-mutated melanoma patients, *Nature Medicine*, 25, pp. 929–935. https://doi.org/10.1038/s41591-019-0474-7

Sweis, R. F., Spranger, S., Bao, R., Paner, G. P., Stadler, W. M., Steinberg, G., ... and Gajewski, T. F. 2016. Molecular drivers of the non-T-cell-inflamed tumor microenvironment in urothelial bladder cancer, *Cancer Immunology Research*, 4(7), pp. 563–568.

Ugurel, S., Paschen, A. and Becker, J. 2013. Dacarbazine in melanoma: From a chemotherapeutic drug to an immunomodulating agent, *Journal of Investigative Dermatology*, 133, pp. 289–292. https://doi.org/10.1038/jid.2012.341.

Wang, Y., Liu, S., Yang, Z., Algazi, A. P., Lomeli, S. H., Wang, Y., Othus, M., Hong, A., Wang, X., Randolph, C. E., Jones, A. M., Bosenberg, M. W., Byrum, S. D., Tackett, A. J., Lopez, H., Yates, C., Solit, D. B., Ribas, A., Piva, M. and Moriceau, G. 2021. Anti-PD-1/L1 lead-in before MAPK inhibitor combination maximizes antitumor immunity and efficacy, *Cancer Cell*, 39(10), pp. 1375–1387.e6. https://doi.org/10.1016/j.ccell.2021.07.023

World Health Organization. (2023). Global Cancer Observatory: Melanoma of Skin. Retrieved from https://gco.iarc.fr/today/data/factsheets/cancers/16-Melanoma-of-skin-fact-sheet.pdf

Xia, Y., Zhang, Y. L., Yu, C., Chang, T. and Fan, H. Y. 2014. YAP/TEAD co-activator regulated pluripotency and chemoresistance in ovarian cancer initiated cells, *PLOS ONE*, 9(11), p. e109575. https://doi.org/10.1371/journal.pone.0109575

Yan, X., Sheng, X., Chi, Z., Si, L., Cui, C., Kong, Y., Tang, B., Mao, L., Wang, X., Lian, B., et al. 2021. Randomized phase II study of bevacizumab in combination with carboplatin plus paclitaxel in patients with previously untreated advanced mucosal melanoma, *Journal of Clinical Oncology*, 39, pp. 881–889. https://doi.org/10.1200/JCO.20.00902.

Zhong, J., Yan, W., Wang, C., Liu, W., Lin, X., Zou, Z., Sun, W. and Chen, Y. 2022. BRAF inhibitor resistance in melanoma: Mechanisms and alternative therapeutic strategies, *Current Treatment Options in Oncology*, 23(11), pp. 1503–1521. https://doi.org/10.1007/s11864-022-01006-7

11 Collaborative Solutions for Future Challenges in Melanoma

A Technological Roadmap

Nkhensani Chauke-Malinga, Mohammed Alaouna, Thabiso Victor Miya, and Zodwa Dlamini
SAMRC/UP Precision Oncology Research Unit, DSTI/NRF SARChI Chair in Precision Oncology (POCP) and Cancer Prevention, Pan African Cancer Research Institute (PACRI), University of Pretoria, Pretoria, South Africa

Thendo Netshiongolwe and Daniel Sambili
Department of Plastic and Reconstructive Surgery, Faculty of Health Sciences, Steve Biko Academic Hospital, University of Pretoria, Pretoria, South Africa

Richard C. Wu
Division of Medical Oncology, The Ohio State University James Comprehensive Cancer Center, Columbus, Ohio, USA

INTRODUCTION

Low- and middle-income countries (LMICs) suffer from a dual burden of disease: the persistent rise in infectious disease-related morbidity and death is accompanied by a sharp increase in non-communicable chronic diseases, such as cancer. The absolute number of cancer patients receiving a diagnosis each year in LMICs is increasing quickly, despite a slight shift in age-standardized cancer rates (Goss et al., 2014; Mallath et al., 2014). Roughly, 75% of cancer deaths will happen in LMICs by 2030, and 1 in 8 persons will receive a cancer diagnosis at some point in their lives (*Cancer*, 2021). The LMICs will account for the majority of the increase in the global cancer burden over the next 50 years (400% in low-income countries, 168% in middle-income countries, and 53% in high-income countries) (Soerjomataram and Bray, 2021) as a result of increased urbanization, rising life expectancy, rising population, and changing lifestyles (Pramesh et al., 2022). LMICs have greater mortality: incidence ratios than high-income countries, although having age-standardized cancer incidence rates that are lower (Goss et al., 2014; Mallath et al., 2014). In LMICs, efforts in cancer prevention should focus on lowering exposure to common modifiable risk factors including alcohol, tobacco, and obesity, enhancing care access, and improving the prognosis of people who are diagnosed

DOI: 10.1201/9781003511625-11

with the disease (Gelband et al., 2016). While the majority of current efforts are directed toward building and expanding treatment facilities, comparatively less focus is placed on producing recommendations that are specific to a given nation for successful palliative care, early detection, prevention, access, and survivability with a focus on value and quality (Pramesh et al., 2022).

In Africa, the incidence rates of melanoma in particular vary across different regions. For instance, a study from South Africa reported that the incidence of melanoma in the Caucasian population was similar to that found in European countries (Norval and Wright, 2017). However, melanoma is less common in Asia and Africa compared to Europe and North America (Han et al., 2017). In South Africa, melanoma poses a significant health burden, with relatively low incidence rates but notable disparities between different population groups (Gordon et al., 2016). The incidence of melanoma in South Africa is reported to be 2.7 per 100,000, with a significantly higher occurrence in the white population (23.2 per 100,000) (Wet et al., 2020). Additionally, research has suggested that the incidence rate of malignant melanoma in the mucosa of the head and neck is higher in Asian and African countries compared to Western countries (Liu et al., 2020). Furthermore, the epidemiological landscape of melanoma in Africa presents unique challenges. Data on the incidence and biology of melanoma are limited in Africa, highlighting the need for more comprehensive studies to understand the burden of the disease in the region (Adoke et al., 2020). Despite the lower incidence rates of melanoma in Africa compared to some Western countries, the impact of the disease can be substantial due to demographic profiles and challenges associated with late-stage diagnoses (Gordon et al., 2016). Efforts to improve skin cancer awareness and promote sunscreen use among the population are crucial in addressing the burden of melanoma in Africa (Dlova et al., 2018).

In summary, while melanoma incidence rates in Africa may be lower than in some Western countries, the disease still poses significant challenges due to disparities in incidence among different population groups and limited data on the epidemiology of melanoma in the region. Collaborative research efforts and public education initiatives are essential to address the burden of melanoma in Africa effectively.

IMPORTANCE OF COLLABORATION AND TECHNOLOGY

Role of Multidisciplinary and Cross-Sector Collaboration

Collaboration and technology are essential components in addressing the challenges presented by melanomas, not only on a global scale but also specifically within African nations, such as South Africa. Multidisciplinary collaboration, which involves experts from diverse fields such as dermatology, oncology, pathology, and genetics, is crucial for tailoring care strategies to meet the unique needs of patients (Obame-Nkoghe, 2024). In the context of African nations, efforts to empower the next generation of researchers have been highlighted as a means of enhancing resilience and adaptive capacity to combat climate-sensitive vector-borne diseases (Obame-Nkoghe, 2024). This underscores the importance of fostering scientific excellence and implementing sustainable solutions in the African research community.

Cross-sector partnerships are vital, bringing together academic institutions, industries, government agencies, and nonprofit organizations to drive innovation and translate research findings into clinical practice as depicted in **Figure 11.1** (Obame-Nkoghe, 2024). For instance, in South Africa, the exploration of renewable energy solutions not only identifies opportunities but also sheds light on the challenges and implications of sustainable development (Kumba, 2024). Such initiatives demonstrate the potential of collaborative efforts to address pressing issues and pave the way for transformative solutions in various sectors.

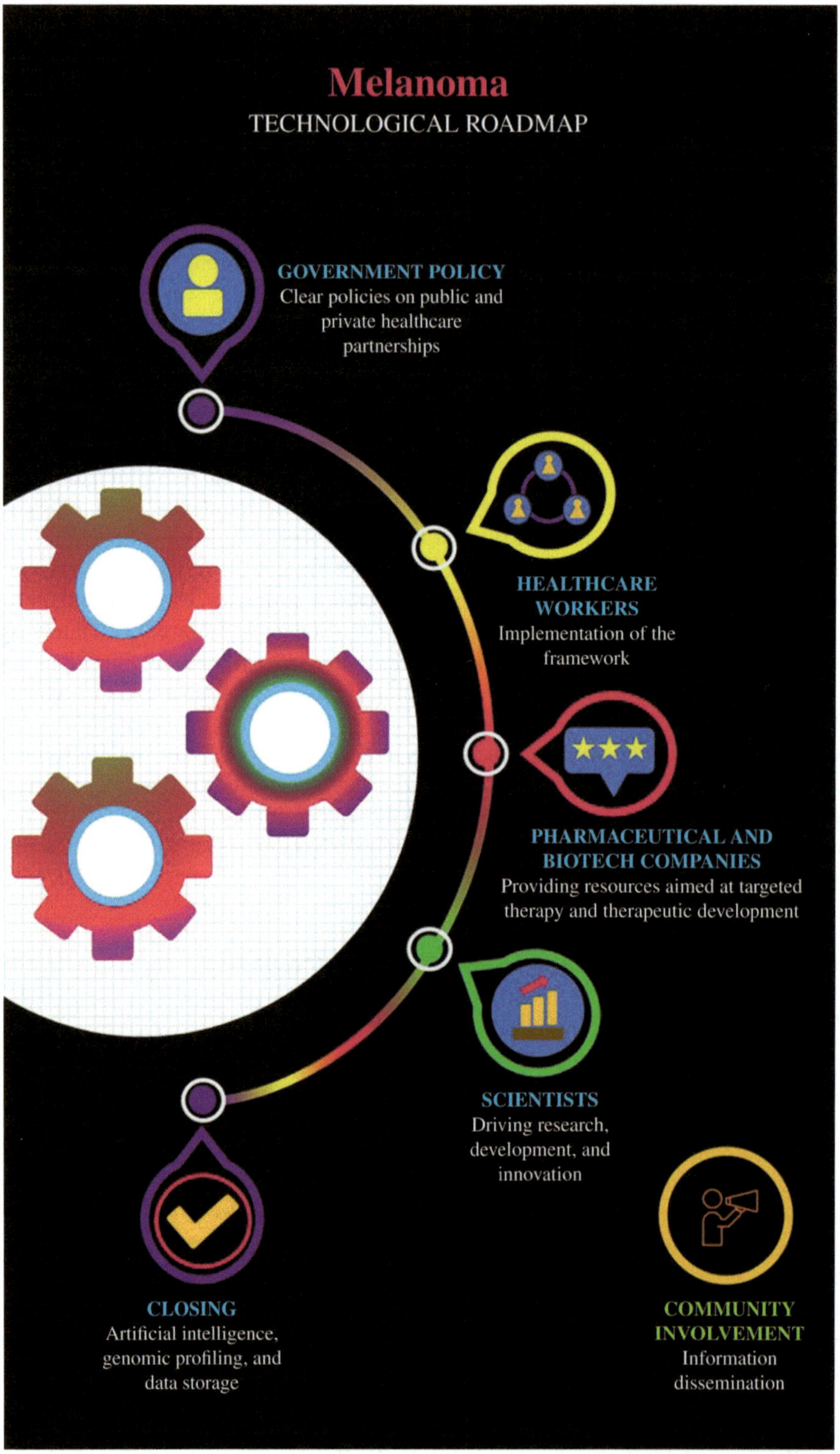

FIGURE 11.1 **Strategic technological pathway to advance melanoma research, improve management, and outcomes.** This pathway includes government policy, healthcare workers, pharmaceutical and biotech companies, scientists, and community involvement.

Moreover, effective information sharing among stakeholders is crucial for managing melanoma, especially with advancements, such as targeted therapy. However, this must be balanced with legal considerations such as patient confidentiality regulations (Wright et al., 2021). For example, in South Africa, collaborative frameworks that promote knowledge sharing and open innovation are essential for achieving sustainable outcomes in healthcare processes (Smit et al., 2022). By understanding the dynamics of collaboration, including power structures and evolving roles within professional groups, African nations, including South Africa, can foster environments conducive to impactful cross-sector collaboration that drives positive changes in healthcare delivery and research.

IDENTIFYING FUTURE MELANOMA CHALLENGES

Medical and Clinical Challenges

Collaborative solutions are crucial for addressing future challenges in melanoma management, particularly in African nations, such as South Africa. These challenges encompass medical, clinical, and socioeconomic aspects, with unique considerations owing to the specific demographic and economic factors influencing disease prevalence and treatment outcomes (Michielin et al., 2019). As in many African countries, the incidence of skin cancer, including melanoma, poses a significant health burden in South Africa, with challenges in diagnosis, treatment, and access to care (Norval et al., 2014). The utilization of advanced molecular diagnostic techniques, such as circulating tumor DNA (ctDNA) and other biomarkers under investigation (i.e., melanoma-derived extracellular vesicles), plays a crucial role in improving diagnosis, monitoring disease progression, and enhancing treatment responses in patients with melanoma (Michielin et al., 2019).

Moreover, the importance of understanding difficult-to-recognize variants of cutaneous melanoma has been highlighted, emphasizing the need for accurate diagnosis and management strategies (Michielin et al., 2019). Biomarkers such as melanoma-associated antigens (i.e., MART-1, gp100, SOX10, etc.) and ctDNA are essential for the early detection, diagnosis, and prognosis of melanoma, aiding in distinguishing invasive melanoma from premalignant lesions (Michielin et al., 2019). Multidisciplinary approaches are necessary to address challenges in accessing melanoma care and to enhance treatment outcomes, especially in regions such as Africa, where healthcare resources may be limited (Michielin et al., 2019). Targeted and immunotherapeutic approaches have significantly transformed the treatment landscape of advanced melanoma, underscoring the importance of evolving therapeutic strategies to improve patient outcomes (Michielin et al., 2019). However, the costs of these treatments present a significant financial burden on the healthcare system and create disparities in patients' access to these life-saving treatments.

In conclusion, a comprehensive approach integrating advancements in diagnosis, treatment, and care delivery is essential to tackle the multifaceted challenges in melanoma management, considering the unique demographic and economic factors influencing disease dynamics in different regions, including African nations such as South Africa (Michielin et al., 2019; Norval et al., 2014). Collaborative efforts between African countries and international partners are crucial to collectively address these challenges and work toward sustainable solutions for the future of melanoma management in Africa (Norval et al., 2014; Obame-Nkoghe, 2024).

DISPARITIES IN HEALTHCARE ACCESS AND OUTCOMES

Disparities in healthcare access and outcomes, particularly in melanoma care, are a significant concern not only in South Africa but also across the African continent (Maphumulo and Bhengu, 2019). These disparities are influenced by various factors, such as socioeconomic status, geographic location, and racial/ethnic background, leading to challenges such as delayed diagnosis and limited access to specialized care (Rensburg, 2014). Globally, similar disparities are observed, with underserved populations facing barriers to timely and effective melanoma care, highlighting the need for targeted interventions to mitigate these inequities (Louis–Jean et al., 2020). In Africa, initiatives such as community outreach programs, telemedicine services, and support for underserved healthcare facilities are crucial for addressing these challenges and improving access to melanoma care (Jatoi et al., 2003).

Diversity in participants in clinical trial(s) is essential to ensure that treatment findings are relevant to diverse populations, thereby reducing disparities in treatment outcomes (Chang et al., 2022). Active recruitment of participants from various racial and ethnic backgrounds for clinical trials in Africa, including South Africa, is vital to equitably distribute the benefits of new treatments and improve healthcare outcomes (Baine-Savanhu, 2023). Community health workers play a critical role in enhancing access to care, improving patient-provider communication, and enhancing care quality, particularly in rural and underserved areas across the continent (Müller, 2017). Addressing racial disparities in cancer-directed treatment in Africa requires a multifaceted approach that includes improving access to care and tailoring healthcare services to meet the needs of diverse populations (Mhlanga and Garidzirai, 2020).

Implementing a health equity framework is crucial to effectively address racial and ethnic disparities in melanoma care in Africa (Manamela, 2024). This framework involves targeted interventions to enhance melanoma awareness and early detection in underserved communities, investment in the healthcare infrastructure in remote areas, ensuring diversity in clinical trials, and providing culturally sensitive care by training healthcare providers to respond to patients' cultural and linguistic needs (Alshamsan et al., 2017). By adopting these measures, African countries can make significant strides in addressing healthcare disparities in melanoma care, ultimately improving outcomes for all population groups and aligning with global efforts to reduce health inequities and ensure equitable access to quality care (Benatar, 2013).

RESEARCH AND DEVELOPMENT CHALLENGES

Funding and Resource Allocation for Melanoma Research

Research and development challenges in melanoma, particularly in African nations, such as South Africa, are multifaceted and require strategic solutions. Funding and resource allocation are pivotal in driving advancements in melanoma research (Michielin et al., 2019). Collaborative funding models involving various stakeholders can facilitate large-scale research initiatives, leading to treatment breakthroughs (Michielin et al., 2019). Involving local stakeholders and allocating international funds to local research teams can boost demand and funding for melanoma research at the national level (Michielin et al., 2019). Efforts to enhance clinical research capacity, as observed in South Africa, are crucial for overcoming challenges and advancing medical research (Michielin et al., 2019).

Translational research from bench to bedside is essential for translating scientific insights into practical applications, especially in countries such as South Africa with a significant incidence of melanoma (Arnold et al., 2022). Collaboration among scientists, clinicians, and industry partners is crucial for successful translational research (Arnold et al., 2022). Addressing the lack of updated data on melanoma incidence, especially among diverse population groups in South Africa, highlights the need for further research to effectively address the burden of melanoma (Arnold et al., 2022). Collaborative efforts, such as the H3Africa Initiative, are vital for advancing translational research on melanoma and other African diseases (Arnold et al., 2022).

In conclusion, sustained funding, strategic resource allocation, and collaborative efforts are imperative to overcome research challenges in melanoma, with countries such as South Africa playing a pivotal role in driving advancements in this field (Michielin et al., 2019). By prioritizing funding, involving local stakeholders, and advocating for increased research support, African nations can significantly contribute to advancing melanoma research, developing innovative therapies, and improving patient care outcomes (Arnold et al., 2022; Michielin et al., 2019).

COLLABORATIVE FRAMEWORKS

Public–Private Partnerships

Collaborative frameworks, particularly public–private partnerships (PPPs), are essential for advancing melanoma research and treatment by leveraging the strengths of various entities. In South Africa, partnerships involving pharmaceutical companies, biotech firms, and healthcare providers are crucial for driving innovation, expediting therapeutic development, and enhancing patient outcomes. The role of pharmaceutical companies and biotech firms in bringing about innovative technologies and financial resources, combined with the clinical insights and patient care capabilities contributed by healthcare providers, highlights the synergy created through such collaborations. Research has shown that collaborative papers are more highly cited than single-author papers, emphasizing the impact of collaborative research efforts (Kasprowicz et al., 2020). Additionally, studies have indicated that papers published by South African-based authors receive an average of 6.05 citations, compared to the global average of 9.49 citations per paper (Ncube et al., 2021).

Governmental support for PPPs, as indicated by the 'PPP Governmental Support Index' (GSI), is vital for establishing an institutional framework conducive to the adoption and spread of PPPs across various sectors, including healthcare. This underscores the importance of government policies and support mechanisms in fostering successful PPPs, which are instrumental in driving innovation and improving healthcare services. Effective models of PPPs, such as the concession model, demonstrate how different partnership structures can be tailored to specific needs and contexts, aligning incentives and responsibilities between public and private entities to promote sustainable collaboration that fosters long-term value creation and innovation. Studies have shown that internationally collaborative papers are more highly cited than single-nation papers, further emphasizing the benefits of global collaboration in research (Kasprowicz et al., 2020). The collaboration and citation patterns of South African science publications have also been studied, shedding light on the impact of collaboration on citation rates (Ncube et al., 2021).

In South Africa, PPPs have been utilized to leverage the skills, expertise, and resources of the private sector to support public sector delivery, particularly in areas such as biomedical research, medicine, and vaccine procurement. These partnerships have been crucial in addressing challenges in healthcare delivery and in advancing research and development efforts. The establishment of collaborative frameworks represents a proactive step toward building resilience and preparedness in the face of health challenges, underscoring the vital importance of a coordinated approach to combating diseases, such as melanoma, in the context of changing climates. Furthermore, research on the roles of practitioners in industry–government research collaborations in South Africa has highlighted implications for sustainable development goals and regional agendas (Ezenwa, 2024).

In conclusion, collaborative frameworks established through PPPs involving pharmaceutical companies, biotech firms, and healthcare providers are vital for advancing melanoma research and treatment, not only in South Africa but also in other African nations facing similar challenges. These partnerships, supported by governmental frameworks and effective models, are essential for driving innovation, expediting therapeutic development, and ultimately, improving patient outcomes. The collaborative nature of research, as evidenced by the impact of collaborative papers and international collaborations, highlights the significance of working together to address complex health challenges, such as melanoma.

Examples of Successful Collaborations in Melanoma Research and Treatment

Collaborative solutions are pivotal in addressing future challenges in melanoma research and treatment, both globally and within African nations. Successful collaboration between pharmaceutical companies and research institutions has significantly advanced melanoma therapy. For instance, partnerships between Merck and the National Cancer Institute have led to the development of pembrolizumab, an effective immunotherapy for melanoma (Kasprowicz et al., 2020). Similarly, collaborations between Novartis and the Broad Institute of MIT and Harvard have focused on leveraging genomic data to identify new therapeutic targets for melanoma, demonstrating the power of combining resources and expertise to advance precision medicine (Vries et al., 2017).

These successful collaborations highlight the significance of PPPs in healthcare, particularly in melanoma research and treatment. By merging private-sector innovation with public-sector resources, substantial progress has been made in developing novel drug candidates and improving patient outcomes for melanoma treatment (Obame-Nkoghe, 2024). The evolving landscape of melanoma treatment reflects the dynamic nature of research and interventions in this field (Okwaro and Geissler, 2015).

In African nations, collaborative efforts among pharmaceutical companies, research institutions, and governmental bodies are crucial to propel medical breakthroughs in melanoma research and treatment. African countries are increasingly embracing international collaboration to enhance their research capabilities and address the unique challenges faced by the region (Onyancha and Maluleka, 2011). Empowering African researchers, ensuring local autonomy, and fostering intra-African collaborations are vital steps toward advancing cancer research within the continent (Toivanen and Ponomariov, 2011). By strengthening research collaborations, sharing knowledge, and influencing research agendas, African nations, such as South Africa, can play a pivotal role in shaping the future of melanoma research and treatment not only within the region but also globally.

INTERNATIONAL COOPERATION

Global Networks and Consortia for Melanoma Research

In melanoma research, international cooperation is the cornerstone for advancing knowledge and improving patient outcomes. Global networks and consortia, such as the Melanoma Research Alliance (MRA) and Global Melanoma Research Network, play pivotal roles in fostering collaboration among researchers, clinicians, and institutions worldwide. These collaborations not only facilitate the sharing of knowledge, resources, and data but also accelerate the pace of discovery and innovation in melanoma research. By promoting multinational clinical trials, these networks enable the evaluation of new therapies across diverse populations, enhancing researchers' understanding of melanoma and its treatment responses. Moreover, the involvement of non-governmental entities in funding melanoma research provides essential financial support for initiatives and career development programs, further bolstering research efforts.

In South Africa, international cooperation in melanoma research presents both opportunities and challenges. South African researchers are increasingly engaging in global networks such as the MRA, gaining access to valuable resources and collaborative opportunities (Biccard and Madiba, 2015). By participating in multinational clinical trials, they can contribute data that reflects the genetic and environmental diversity of their population, making research findings more applicable to diverse populations globally. However, challenges such as resource limitations, health disparities, and regulatory complexities pose obstacles to seamless collaboration (Biccard and Madiba, 2015). Adequate funding, infrastructure support, and streamlined regulatory processes are crucial for maximizing South Africa's participation in global networks and consortia (Biccard and Madiba, 2015).

To address these challenges and leverage opportunities, South Africa must focus on enhancing its local capacity, addressing health disparities, and fostering a conducive environment for international collaboration (Biccard and Madiba, 2015). Long-term investments from international donors, increased funding commitments from African governments, and collaborations with philanthropic organizations are essential for building a critical mass of local capacity and creating world-class research hubs that can effectively tackle Africa's health challenges (Kasprowicz et al., 2020). By embracing a transdisciplinary approach, South Africa can harness the power of collaborative frameworks to build resilience and preparedness in combating diseases such as melanoma, especially in the face of climate-induced health challenges (Obame-Nkoghe, 2024).

In conclusion, international cooperation remains a linchpin in advancing melanoma research globally, with South Africa being poised to make significant contributions through active participation in global networks, addressing local challenges, and fostering collaborative partnerships. By prioritizing collaboration, knowledge sharing, and capacity building, South Africa can strengthen its position in the global fight against melanoma and contribute meaningfully to the collective effort to combat this disease on a broader scale (Biccard and Madiba, 2015; Kasprowicz et al., 2020; Obame-Nkoghe, 2024).

COMMUNITY AND STAKEHOLDER ENGAGEMENT

Patient Advocacy Groups and Their Impact

Patient advocacy groups are influential in healthcare, collaborating with researchers and healthcare providers to ensure that patient perspectives are integrated into care, leading to patient-centered treatment guidelines and increased research funding (Natale-Pereira et al., 2011). In South Africa, these groups are actively involved in advocating equitable access to treatment, raising awareness about prevalent health issues, and influencing policy changes to enhance healthcare infrastructure and resource allocation (Natale-Pereira et al., 2011).

Globally, patient advocacy groups play a crucial role in influencing research funding, policy changes, patient support, awareness campaigns, and collaboration with healthcare stakeholders (Natale-Pereira et al., 2011). In South Africa, these groups focus on advocating equitable research funding, improving healthcare infrastructure and access, bridging gaps in care in underserved communities, targeting prevalent health issues, and collaborating with local and national health organizations (Natale-Pereira et al., 2011). Their impact extends to policy changes and research directions, contributing to advancements in cancer care in regions such as eastern and southern Africa (Natale-Pereira et al., 2011).

Patient advocacy groups are instrumental in shaping services for families raising children with developmental disabilities, emphasizing advocacy and empowerment in healthcare (Bonella et al., 2015). In South Africa, these organizations work tirelessly to bridge gaps in care, advocate for equitable access to treatment, and raise awareness about prevalent health issues, particularly in underserved communities (Bonella et al., 2015). Overall, patient advocacy groups are essential for driving progress in healthcare globally and in South Africa, emphasizing the importance of integrating patient perspectives into healthcare for comprehensive and patient-centered care (Bonella et al., 2015).

DEVELOPING A TECHNOLOGICAL ROADMAP

Vision and Strategic Goals

Establishing Long-Term Objectives for Melanoma Research and Treatment

In melanoma research and treatment, the integration of innovative approaches is crucial for addressing the challenges posed by this complex disease. Developing a strategic roadmap that encompasses long-term objectives is fundamental to advancing melanoma care. By leveraging technologies such as artificial intelligence (AI) and genomic profiling, this field can enhance early detection and diagnosis, ultimately improving treatment outcomes and reducing the risk of recurrence. Furthermore, personalized medicine tailored to individual tumor genetic profiles holds promise for overcoming treatment resistance and recurrence challenges. Combination therapies such as nivolumab and ipilimumab have shown clinical efficacy in patients with metastatic melanoma, highlighting the importance of exploring diverse treatment modalities (Larkin et al., 2019; Michielin et al., 2019; Rao et al., 2005).

In South Africa, aligning global advancements with local healthcare infrastructure is essential for optimizing melanoma care. While the global focus is on utilizing AI and genomic profiling for diagnostics, South Africa emphasizes the need for cost-effective technologies suitable for diverse healthcare settings (Larkin et al., 2019; Michielin et al., 2019; Rao et al., 2005). Similarly, although personalized medicine based on genetic profiles is a global priority, South Africa aims to integrate personalized approaches with traditional practices to enhance patient outcomes (Larkin et al., 2019; Michielin et al., 2019; Rao et al., 2005). Addressing disparities in healthcare access across regions is a shared concern, both globally and in South Africa, underscoring the importance of ensuring equity in care delivery (Larkin et al., 2019; Michielin et al., 2019; Rao et al., 2005). Moreover, leveraging diverse and sustainable funding sources is critical for supporting uninterrupted research efforts and advancing melanoma treatment, particularly in regions facing economic challenges such as South Africa (Larkin et al., 2019; Michielin et al., 2019; Rao et al., 2005).

In conclusion, collaborative efforts in melanoma research and treatment must be tailored to meet the specific needs of diverse populations, including those in African nations such as South Africa. By embracing technological advancements, personalized medicine, and equitable access to care, significant strides can be made to combat melanoma and improve patient outcomes globally.

Securing Funding and Resources for Collaborative Projects

Collaborative solutions are crucial for addressing future challenges in melanoma research, especially in African nations, such as South Africa. Securing funding and resources for collaborative projects is vital for advancing scientific knowledge and developing innovative treatments for melanoma research (Obame-Nkoghe, 2024). In South Africa, challenges exist in securing funding due to economic constraints and competing healthcare priorities, making agencies such as the South African Medical Research Council (SAMRC) and the National Research Foundation (NRF) essential for supporting health research initiatives (Boshoff, 2009). While private sector investments in South Africa may not be as substantial as in more developed countries, collaborations with international firms can provide essential financial support and advanced technologies, and philanthropic contributions from organizations such as the Cancer Association of South Africa (CANSA) also play a significant role in supporting melanoma research in the region (Boshoff, 2009).

Access to cutting-edge technology and expert personnel remains a challenge in South Africa; however, collaborative networks and partnerships with international institutions can help bridge this gap (Brooke-Sumner et al., 2016). Establishing a robust collaboration network is crucial, as it significantly influences the securing of research funding, with platforms such as StudySwap facilitating inter-lab replication and resource exchange, which is particularly beneficial for South African researchers in optimizing resource utilization and enhancing collaboration (Brooke-Sumner et al., 2016). Successful collaborative projects in melanoma research, both globally and in South Africa, rely on leveraging diverse funding sources, fostering strong partnerships, and embracing interdisciplinary research (Obame-Nkoghe, 2024).

By integrating government grants, private sector investments, philanthropic contributions, collaborative networks, and interdisciplinary collaboration, researchers can access the resources necessary to advance scientific knowledge, develop innovative treatments, and make significant progress in combating melanoma. Collaborative efforts are crucial not only for South Africa but also for African nations, in general, to navigate challenges effectively, foster scientific excellence, and implement sustainable solutions against diseases such as melanoma (Obame-Nkoghe, 2024).

IMPLEMENTATION AND SCALABILITY

Piloting Initiatives and Scaling Successful Models

In the context of melanoma management, particularly in African nations, such as South Africa, the successful implementation and scalability of new healthcare technologies are crucial for improving patient outcomes. Pilot initiatives play a significant role in evaluating the feasibility and effectiveness of innovations, such as AI-based imaging tools, in real-world healthcare settings (Oleribe et al.,

2019). These pilot programs help to identify challenges and areas for improvement before broader implementation, ensuring a smoother transition and effective adoption of new tools. Following successful pilot programs, the focus has shifted toward formulating scalability plans to expand initiatives systematically, requiring meticulous planning, coordination, and collaboration across diverse settings (Oleribe et al., 2019).

Collaboration has emerged as a fundamental element in scaling successful healthcare models, involving engagement with a network of healthcare providers, researchers, and industry partners to create a supportive environment for their widespread adoption (Oleribe et al., 2019). Sharing best practices and lessons learned from pilot programs facilitates replicating successes and avoiding common pitfalls, thus promoting continuous improvement and knowledge sharing. Establishing centers of excellence further enhances the dissemination and implementation of new innovations, improving the overall scalability process (Oleribe et al., 2019).

In South Africa, the implementation and scalability of new healthcare technologies must address unique challenges and opportunities within the country, particularly considering the variability in healthcare infrastructure between urban and rural areas (Eksteen et al., 2022). Post-successful pilot programs and scalability plans in South Africa must tackle logistical and infrastructural challenges specific to the region to ensure effective adoption in rural and underserved areas. Collaboration among local healthcare providers, researchers, and international partners is essential for the widespread adoption of successful models, emphasizing the importance of monitoring and evaluating the scalability process to enhance implementation (Eksteen et al., 2022).

In conclusion, the successful integration and scalability of new healthcare technologies in melanoma management require a combination of pilot initiatives, collaboration, and continuous evaluation. By leveraging these strategies and incorporating advancements in biomarkers, adaptive therapies, and molecular diagnostics, healthcare systems can enhance patient care and outcomes in melanoma management, not only in South Africa but also in other African nations facing similar challenges (Eksteen et al., 2022; Oleribe et al., 2019).

Monitoring, Evaluation, and Adaptability of the Roadmap

Collaborative solutions are crucial for addressing future challenges in melanoma research, particularly in African countries. Fatoki (2018) emphasized the importance of molecular biomarkers for melanoma screening and diagnosis, shedding light on the challenges that need to be overcome to advance diagnostic capabilities. Moyo and colleagues stress the significance of cross-sector collaboration and accountability frameworks to drive sustainable progress in melanoma research (Moyo et al., 2020). Kajiita (2024) highlighted the potential of chemopreventive agents such as aspirin in reducing melanoma incidence, underscoring the need to explore novel strategies to mitigate melanoma risk.

In African nations, collaborative efforts play a vital role in enhancing research capabilities and fostering scientific excellence. Masenya and Ngulube (2019) stated the importance of South-South collaborations and empowering African researchers to navigate challenges effectively. Nhamo (2016) indicated that African countries are increasingly engaging in international research collaboration, showing a growing trend toward collaborative research initiatives within the continent. By leveraging collaborative research, African researchers can enhance their capabilities, contribute locally relevant solutions, and drive advancements in melanoma research.

South Africa serves as a notable example of successful research collaboration. Ezenwa (2024) highlighted South Africa's contributions to collaborative research by showing partnerships with various countries to advance research in different fields. By embracing collaborative and adaptive strategies, African nations, including South Africa, can harness the vast potential of research collaboration to drive economic growth, sustainable development, and innovative solutions in the fight against melanoma and other health challenges. Through sustained collaborative efforts, stakeholders in melanoma research can ensure the sustainability and long-term impact of their initiatives, paving the way for continuous advancements in this field.

Ensuring Sustainability and Long-Term Impact

Collaborative solutions are crucial for addressing future challenges in melanoma research, particularly in African nations. Toivanen and Ponomariov (2011) emphasized the significance of molecular biomarkers in melanoma screening and diagnosis, highlighting the need to overcome obstacles to improve diagnostic capabilities. Pouris and Ho (2013) affirmed the importance of cross-sector collaboration and accountability frameworks to drive sustainable progress in melanoma research. Additionally, Onyancha (2018) discussed the potential of chemopreventive agents such as aspirin in reducing melanoma incidence, advocating for the exploration of innovative strategies for improved outcomes. In addition, Boshoff (2009) presented promising results in adoptive cell therapy for metastatic melanoma, suggesting the potential for novel immunotherapeutic approaches to enhance long-term treatment efficacy.

In the African context, research collaboration plays a pivotal role in advancing knowledge production and effectively addressing various challenges. Ettarh (2016) and Obame-Nkoghe (2024) demonstrated that African countries, including South Africa, are increasingly engaged in international research collaboration. This trend is supported by Hernández-Villafuerte et al. (2016) who revealed active participation in research collaborations by countries such as South Africa, Nigeria, and Kenya with a significant citation impact from international collaborations. Asare and colleagues underscored the importance of regional research partnerships within the Southern African Development Community (SADC), contributing to knowledge sharing and enhancing research visibility and impact (Asare et al., 2020).

South Africa stands out as a key player in research collaboration, as evidenced by studies such as Naudé (2024) and Nachega et al. (2020). South African researchers exhibit a strong inclination toward collaborative research, extending partnerships globally to countries such as the United Kingdom, Germany, and the United States. Noubiap and colleagues highlight South Africa's well-developed infrastructure and active engagement in international collaborations, positioning the country as a leading research site, particularly in areas like HIV/AIDS (Noubiap et al., 2023). These collaborations not only drive scientific advancements but also play a crucial role in addressing public health challenges and enhancing global outcomes.

In conclusion, fostering collaborative efforts within African nations and on an international scale is imperative to drive sustainable progress in melanoma research. By leveraging the insights and experiences shared through research collaborations, stakeholders in melanoma research, including those in African nations such as South Africa, can strengthen the sustainability and long-term impact of research initiatives, leading to continuous advancements in the field.

CHALLENGES AND MITIGATION STRATEGIES

Common Obstacles in Melanoma Research and Treatment Collaborations

Regulatory Hurdles

Collaborative efforts are essential to address the challenges encountered in melanoma research and treatment, especially considering the diverse regulatory landscapes across different countries. Regulatory hurdles present a significant obstacle, causing delays and increased costs for international studies. For example, stringent regulations in certain regions can impede the approval process for clinical trials, thus limiting timely access to innovative therapies. Despite these challenges, the use of targeted therapies, particularly in cases involving BRAF V600E mutation, has demonstrated promising results. The combination of BRAF and MEK inhibitors has shown improved responses in patients with metastatic BRAF-mutant melanoma. Additionally, innovative approaches such as combining viral oncolysis with immunotherapies have emerged as effective strategies for melanoma treatment (Sung et al., 2021).

Immunotherapy, specifically immune checkpoint inhibitors, has transformed melanoma treatment globally (Valasapalli and Guddati, 2021). Nevertheless, challenges persist, including understanding the role of the extracellular matrix in therapeutic resistance and addressing regulatory and translational research barriers to optimize outcomes. Patient engagement and collaboration among stakeholders are pivotal for advancing translational research and enhancing patient outcomes (Olsen, 2022). In South Africa, regulatory obstacles in melanoma research and treatment are compounded by resource constraints and disparities in access to healthcare. Collaborative initiatives have demonstrated promise in addressing these challenges by harmonizing regulatory frameworks and leveraging international partnerships (Orouji and Utikal, 2018). South African researchers have underscored the significance of culturally sensitive patient engagement and community involvement in augmenting the relevance and effectiveness of research endeavors (Gordon and Rowell, 2015).

In conclusion, although progress has been made in melanoma research and treatment, regulatory hurdles, the tumor microenvironment, and the importance of collaborative efforts remain critical areas that require attention to enhance the efficacy of melanoma therapies (Bennett et al., 2021). Tackling these challenges through international collaboration and local adaptation, as evidenced in South Africa, can help overcome obstacles and enhance global patient outcomes. By nurturing collaborative networks, sharing knowledge, and engaging in multidisciplinary efforts, the field of melanoma research and treatment can advance toward more effective and accessible therapies.

Logistical Challenges

Collaborative solutions are crucial for addressing the logistical challenges encountered in melanoma research, particularly in African nations. These challenges include coordinating activities across different locations, managing time-zone disparities, addressing language differences, and handling varying technological resources. Shipping biological samples across borders, complying with local regulations, and ensuring timely processing are critical aspects that can significantly affect research quality and progress. In LMICs, including Africa, clinical trials face obstacles such as a shortage of skilled personnel, funding constraints, regulatory complexities, and logistical hurdles. PPPs and collaborative initiatives are essential for enhancing community resilience during disasters and managing workplace stress in such settings (Oleribe et al., 2019).

Advancements in information technology and communication systems, particularly the Internet, have played a crucial role in overcoming logistical barriers by facilitating the exchange of information, expertise, and ideas across borders (Arvis et al., 2014). Horizontal logistics collaboration, even among competitors, is being explored to improve supply chain performance, although challenges, such as competition and power dynamics, can impede effective collaboration. In South Africa, logistical challenges in melanoma research are exacerbated by disparities in the healthcare infrastructure. Researchers have successfully utilized international partnerships and local innovations to overcome these obstacles (Bekker et al., 2013). Initiatives such as centralized biobanking and streamlined ethical reviews have enhanced logistics for multi-center studies, whereas community-based approaches have strengthened engagement and efficiency at the local level (Bekker et al., 2013).

To effectively address the logistical challenges in collaborative research, researchers must navigate regulatory frameworks, governance structures, technical support, funding limitations, and cultural dynamics. Leveraging technological advancements, fostering partnerships, and promoting effective communication are key strategies for enhancing collaboration across borders and institutions, thereby advancing scientific knowledge and innovation (Kauppi et al., 2017). South Africa highlights the importance of adaptive strategies and international cooperation in overcoming logistical hurdles in melanoma research (Bekker et al., 2013).

Funding Constraints

Collaborative solutions for addressing future challenges in melanoma research, especially in African nations such as South Africa, are significantly affected by funding constraints. The competitive nature of grant applications and limited availability of funds can restrict the scope and scale of collaborative efforts, potentially leading to the discontinuation of promising projects. While international collaboration in science is growing, interdisciplinary research, which is crucial for addressing complex issues, faces lower funding success rates than traditional approaches. Securing funding for multidisciplinary collaborative projects is particularly challenging because of the uncertain funding conditions in certain sectors. South Africa's experience highlights the importance of strategic partnerships and innovative funding solutions to overcome financial barriers and advance melanoma research.

In addition to funding challenges, the use of collaborative robots (cobots) in manufacturing, as explored by Calitz et al. (2017), presents an opportunity to enhance efficiency and productivity in African workplaces. Furthermore, Berka and Dreyfus (2021) emphasize the importance of decentralization and inclusivity in the energy sector, which could have implications for collaborative efforts to address energy-related challenges in melanoma research. Moreover, research by Dick et al. (2019) sheds light on the socioeconomic factors influencing delayed melanoma diagnosis, highlighting the need for collaborative approaches to ensure timely detection and treatment.

Understanding the global burden of melanoma, as discussed by Li et al. (2022), is essential for targeted public policymaking and healthcare resource allocation, particularly in countries with high incidence rates. The establishment of collaborative frameworks, such as the African Medicines Agency, as examined by Ncube et al. (2021), represents a proactive step toward addressing health challenges in Africa. By fostering collaboration, sharing knowledge, and leveraging resources, African nations can accelerate sustainable development efforts and overcome various health challenges, including those related to melanoma.

In conclusion, collaborative solutions for future challenges in melanoma research require addressing funding constraints, leveraging technological advancements such as cobots, promoting inclusivity in energy sectors, and understanding the socioeconomic factors influencing diagnoses. By embracing collaborative approaches, African nations, including South Africa, can enhance their research outcomes, improve healthcare delivery, and advance efforts to combat melanoma and other health issues.

STRATEGIES FOR OVERCOMING THESE CHALLENGES, INCLUDING REGULATORY AND LOGISTICAL HURDLES

Harmonizing Regulatory Frameworks

Collaborative solutions are crucial for addressing future challenges in melanoma treatment, particularly in African countries. Globally, harmonizing regulatory frameworks is essential for standardizing guidelines and facilitating international clinical trials (Arnold et al., 2022). By aligning regulatory guidelines and promoting transparency in lobbying efforts, organizations can effectively navigate regulatory hurdles on a global scale, drawing lessons from South Africa's experiences (Arnold et al., 2022). Engaging in collaborative lobbying efforts toward regulatory alignment can streamline the approval process for new treatments and technologies, especially considering the diverse regulatory landscapes across countries, as exemplified by South Africa's unique challenges (Arnold et al., 2022).

In addition to regulatory strategies, incorporating insights from diverse studies can enrich the approach to combating melanoma. Leveraging a holistic framework to enhance the technological roadmap for melanoma research and treatment, understanding molecular biomarkers, and exploring the potential of chemoprevention agents can provide valuable insights into improving diagnostic and treatment strategies (Arnold et al., 2022). Collaborative efforts in neoadjuvant treatment for melanoma and integrating biomarkers into management can further enhance the comprehensive strategy for combating melanoma globally (Arnold et al., 2022).

A comprehensive strategy that integrates harmonizing regulatory frameworks, transparent lobbying practices, understanding decision-makers' preferences, and leveraging insights from diverse studies is essential for overcoming regulatory challenges in the global fight against melanoma. By building on lessons learned from various contexts, including South Africa, and incorporating collaborative efforts, the fight against melanoma can be strengthened globally (Arnold et al., 2022).

Enhancing Communication and Coordination

Collaborative solutions are crucial for addressing future challenges in melanoma research, particularly in African nations. Effective communication and coordination among institutions play a pivotal role in overcoming logistical hurdles. Centralized coordination centers and digital platforms have been highlighted as essential tools for managing multicenter studies and ensuring seamless communication, especially in the face of geographical barriers and time zone differences. Multilingual support and cultural competence training are crucial for fostering effective collaboration among diverse teams, a necessity underscored by South Africa's experience. To prevent future outbreaks, coordinated, multiscale, early warning systems should be developed to make full use of these integrated assessments, partner with local communities in high-risk areas, and provide clearly defined response recommendations specific to the needs of each community (Alexander et al., 2015).

Cultural competence training not only enhances communication and teamwork in healthcare settings but also ensures equitable and culturally sensitive approaches to melanoma research and treatment on a global scale. Emphasizing cultural humility and diversity training within health organizations is vital for addressing disparities among underrepresented ethnic groups and guaranteeing adequate representation and service provision. Tailored training programs aimed at enhancing cultural competence among multidisciplinary care management teams have proven to be effective in improving communication and teamwork in healthcare settings. Authors from high-income countries are included in 60% of intra-regional co-authored papers and 59% of continental co-authored papers (Boshoff, 2009).

Drawing from South Africa's contributions to the field, strategies such as centralized coordination centers, digital platforms, and cultural competence training are essential for enhancing communication and coordination among collaborating institutions worldwide in the fight against melanoma. By leveraging these initiatives and experiences, institutions can effectively navigate logistical challenges and promote effective teamwork in diverse global research and healthcare environments.

Diversifying Funding Sources

In the realm of global melanoma research and treatment, diversifying funding sources has emerged as a critical strategy for overcoming financial constraints and establishing a stable financial foundation. Organizations can achieve this by pooling resources from various channels, such as government grants, private sector investments, philanthropic contributions, and crowdfunding, thus ensuring a more sustainable funding structure (Uthman et al., 2015). PPPs play a pivotal role in this diversification approach, facilitating collaboration between industry and academia to combine financial resources and infrastructure from the private sector with innovative research and expertise from academia (Uthman et al., 2015). While PPPs offer a promising solution to budgetary challenges, concerns regarding accountability, transparency, and varying outcomes have been raised, emphasizing the need for effective models characterized by fair distribution of financial rewards based on risk assessment and long-term commitment from both sectors (Uthman et al., 2015).

Research indicates that diversifying funding sources can help institutions mitigate risks and avoid liquidity challenges during stressful periods, highlighting the economic impact of government and charity funding in medical research and the importance of diverse funding streams in research and development (Uthman et al., 2015). South Africa's contributions to melanoma research underscore the significance of diversifying funding sources globally through mechanisms such as PPPs to ensure comprehensive and inclusive research efforts. By leveraging the strengths of different sectors, securing commitments from diverse stakeholders, and drawing lessons from South Africa's experiences, organizations can establish a robust foundation to fund their operations and initiatives, fostering a more inclusive and comprehensive approach to melanoma research and treatment worldwide (Uthman et al., 2015).

In the African context, particularly in South Africa, where high solar ultraviolet radiation levels pose a significant risk for malignant melanoma, there is an urgent need for effective therapy and research funding (Molefi, 2020). South Africa's experiences can serve as a valuable example for African nations in diversifying funding sources through PPPs to enhance research and treatment efforts for melanoma. Collaborative efforts and partnerships with diverse stakeholders, including the government, private sector, academia, and philanthropic organizations, can help address financial challenges and promote inclusive and comprehensive research initiatives in the fight against melanoma in African nations and globally.

Building Robust Infrastructure

Building robust infrastructure is essential for collaborative efforts in melanoma research. Investments in infrastructure such as biobanks and interoperable data systems are crucial for enhancing collaborative research and treatment initiatives (Joubert et al., 2020). Biobanks are particularly important in collaborative research, providing repositories for diverse patient samples and aiding in the study of genetic variations in melanoma, as illustrated in **Figure 11.2** (Adewole et al., 2014). Governance frameworks for biobanks are vital for ensuring fair practices and addressing ethical considerations, especially concerning cultural sensitivity (Obame-Nkoghe, 2024).

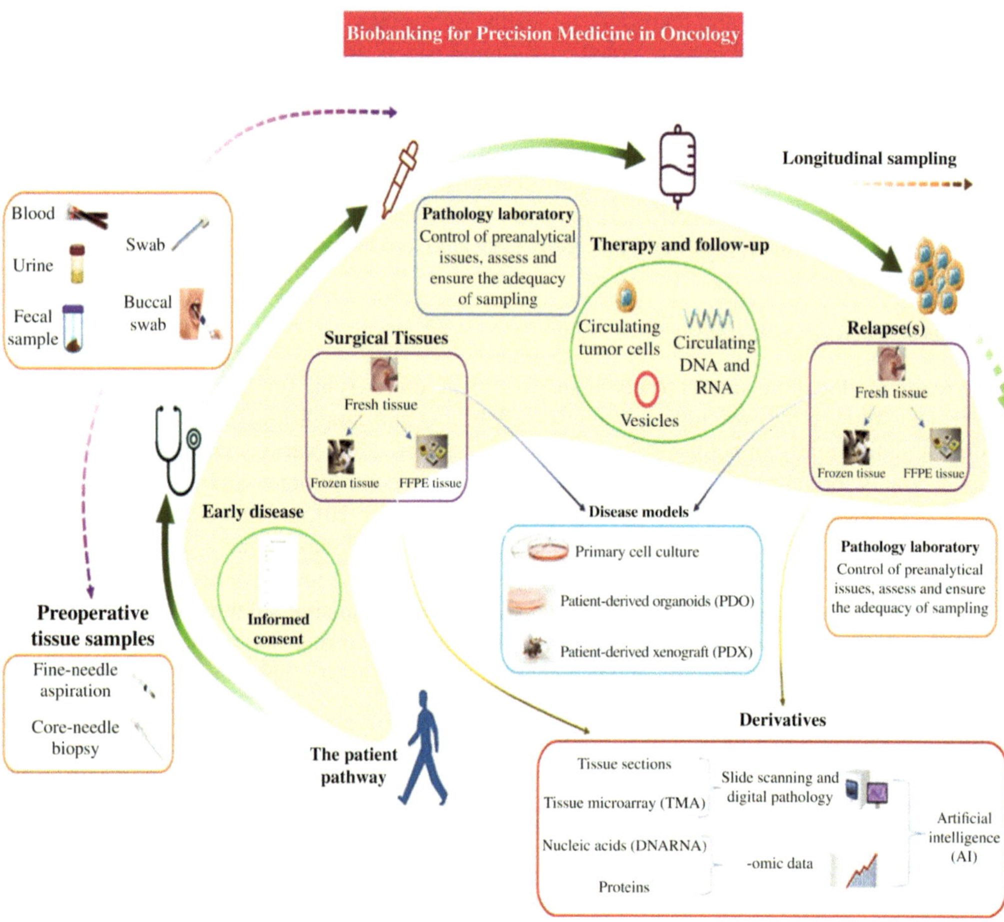

FIGURE 11.2 **The basis of biobanks is in the three legs supporting personalized cancer medicine: proteomics, metabolomics, and epigenomics.** Cancer research currently involves diagnostic, prognostic, and therapeutic aspects. This diagram depicts how biobanking assists in preserving specimens obtained in different stages of the cancer disease process to ultimately develop new treatment approaches.

Efforts to promote networking among biobanks globally can lead to improved research outcomes and facilitate data sharing, ultimately advancing collaborative efforts for melanoma treatment (Joubert et al., 2020). Secure platforms, such as BiobankCloud, are instrumental in storing and processing large datasets, which is crucial for advancing research efforts (Joubert et al., 2020). Leveraging innovative technologies for remote collaboration, such as virtual reality applications and online platforms, has become increasingly important, particularly in light of the COVID-19 pandemic.

By applying lessons learned from experiences in various countries, collaborative initiatives in melanoma research can address common challenges and achieve more effective outcomes. Tailoring infrastructure development to meet the specific needs of diverse populations can lead to a more inclusive and comprehensive approach to melanoma research and treatment. Harmonizing biobank practices, establishing governance frameworks, and leveraging technology for remote collaboration are critical steps in advancing collaborative efforts for melanoma treatment and beyond.

FUTURE DIRECTIONS

Emerging Trends and Innovations

Upcoming Technological Trends in Melanoma Research and Treatment

The landscape of melanoma research and treatment is rapidly evolving, with emerging trends and innovations shaping the global future of patient care. Genomics, immunotherapy, and targeted therapies are revolutionizing melanoma approaches with a particular focus on their impact on diverse genetic landscapes. Immunotherapies, particularly immune checkpoint inhibitors, have shown lasting responses in specific patients with advanced melanoma (Gloster and Neal, 2006), and these treatments can be given regardless of the presence of BRAF or other driver mutations. An important clinical study called DREAMSEq has demonstrated the significant survival benefit of patients treated first with immune checkpoint therapy before targeted therapy (Atkins et al., 2023). Targeted therapies, such as BRAF and MEK inhibitors, have also significantly improved outcomes in individuals with BRAF(V600E/K)-mutated melanoma (Gloster and Neal, 2006), highlighting the importance of combining different treatment modalities and exploring novel biomarkers and treatment combinations.

Furthermore, ongoing research suggests that incorporating an MEK inhibitor could have limited benefits for certain patients without BRAF V600 mutations (Gloster and Neal, 2006), indicating the broader applicability of targeted therapies beyond specific genetic mutations. Efforts to detect BRAF variants have implications for cancer types with low prevalence (Gloster and Neal, 2006), emphasizing the need for continued exploration in this area. Biomarkers such as TRIM51 and the integration of CDK4/6 inhibitors into treatment protocols are under investigation for their potential impact on treatment efficacy (Gloster and Neal, 2006). Also, the recently FDA-approved adoptive TIL therapy provides a promising treatment option for patients who have not responded well to the immune checkpoint therapy or BRAF/MEK-targeted therapy (Rohaan et al., 2022). There are ongoing clinical investigations on many different types of novel therapeutic modalities for melanoma, including oncolytic viruses, bispecific antibodies, antibody-drug conjugates (ADCs), and immune checkpoint therapies against other receptors such as TIM-3, TIGIT, and BTLA (Natarelli et al., 2024). The critical need to develop prognostic or predictive biomarkers of treatment responses, including evaluating the interplay between BRAF/MEK inhibitors and the expression of CD47 in melanoma cells, requires further clinical investigation across diverse populations.

In conclusion, the future of melanoma research and treatment holds great promise, with advancements in genomics, immunotherapy, and targeted therapies reshaping patient care globally. By incorporating the lessons learned from diverse experiences and contributions to melanoma research, these advancements can be tailored to address the specific challenges and needs of diverse populations worldwide, ensuring a more inclusive and comprehensive approach to melanoma treatment and research in the future.

CALL TO ACTION

Encouraging Continued Collaboration and Innovation in the Field

Encouraging continued collaboration and innovation in the field of melanoma care, particularly in a global context, influenced by South Africa's experiences with melanoma research and treatment. South Africa's unique challenges and contributions to melanoma research offer valuable insights that can expedite the translation of research discoveries into clinical applications (Fong and Tanabe, 2014). Multidisciplinary teams emphasized in South Africa's healthcare landscape are crucial for fostering innovation and nurturing future leaders in the field, especially given the diverse healthcare environments and resources present (Müller and Couper, 2021). Drawing from South Africa's experiences, cross-sectoral collaboration and multidisciplinary approaches can be pivotal for addressing the specific requirements and obstacles faced by diverse populations globally (Fraser et al., 2018).

In times of crises such as the COVID-19 pandemic, collaborative strategies have become imperative for healthcare sustainability and recovery, showcasing how innovation driven by emergencies can effectively meet pressing needs (Wright et al., 2021). Initiatives such as leveraging 3D printing technologies for manufacturing personal protective equipment exemplify the adaptability and resilience that can be gleaned from South Africa's healthcare system encounters (Obame-Nkoghe, 2024). Furthermore, establishing living laboratories in primary care settings provides platforms for healthcare stakeholders to collaborate, learn, and develop user-centered innovations that can be scaled globally to cater to the distinct needs of various patient populations, building upon South Africa's experiences (Müller and Couper, 2021).

Innovative work behavior among healthcare professionals, influenced by collaborative competencies, can be further honed in the South African context to tackle the specific challenges and opportunities identified through South Africa's interactions with diverse patient populations and healthcare setups (Fong and Tanabe, 2014). Lessons from the COVID-19 pandemic, such as transitioning healthcare services online, can be applied to ensure uninterrupted care and support for patients with melanoma, even in challenging circumstances (Kasprowicz et al., 2020). Collaborative endeavors rooted in identifying unmet clinical needs and translating them into effective healthcare solutions are vital for meeting the diverse requirements of patients globally and expanding South Africa's contributions to melanoma research (Amoakoh-Coleman et al., 2022). By fostering continued collaboration and innovation in melanoma care and capitalizing on South Africa's insights, future collaborations can be more inclusive, comprehensive, and efficient in catering to the diverse needs of patients worldwide, thereby paving the way for a more equitable and innovative future in global healthcare.

Recap of the Importance of Technology and Collaboration in Addressing

Collaborative solutions are crucial for addressing challenges and opportunities in melanoma care, particularly in South Africa. While advancements in genomics, immunotherapy, and targeted therapies have significantly improved melanoma management globally, South Africa faces obstacles in accessing these treatments owing to cost and resource constraints (Gordon et al., 2016). Strategies for making melanoma treatments more accessible and affordable in South Africa are shown in Table 11.1. The country's genetic diversity necessitates extensive genomic research to understand how genetic variation influences melanoma development and treatment responses (Gordon et al., 2016). Additionally, healthcare infrastructure challenges, especially in rural areas, hinder the implementation of advanced treatment modalities in South Africa (Gordon et al., 2016).

TABLE 11.1
Strategies for Enhancing Accessibility and Affordability of Melanoma Treatments in South Africa

Strategy	Description
Drug price negotiations	Engaging with pharmaceutical companies to lower medication costs.
Generic drug availability	Promoting the use of cost-effective generic drugs.
Fair access policies	Implementing policies that ensure equitable access to treatments.
Public–private partnerships	Collaborating with the private sector to subsidize treatment costs.
Comprehensive insurance coverage	Advocating for policies that cover advanced melanoma therapies fully.

Collaborative efforts are essential in South Africa to bridge the gap between global progress and local implementation. While international collaboration benefits global research, South Africa must enhance its collaborative networks to leverage global advancements and contribute unique perspectives to melanoma research (Bekker et al., 2013). Tailored research and treatment strategies are crucial for the diverse population of South Africa, including individuals with darker skin types, to combat melanoma effectively (Gordon et al., 2016). Balancing advanced treatments with robust public health initiatives for early detection and prevention is vital in South Africa owing to resource constraints (Gordon et al., 2016).

In conclusion, South Africa's journey in melanoma care involves not only adopting global innovations but also crafting tailored strategies considering its specific healthcare landscape, genetic diversity, and resource limitations. Collaborative efforts among healthcare professionals, researchers, policymakers, and international partners will play a pivotal role in enhancing melanoma care in South Africa and aligning it with global standards (Bekker et al., 2013).

Highlights of the Proposed Technological Roadmap

Collaborative solutions are crucial for addressing future challenges in melanoma care, particularly in African nations, such as South Africa. The unique genetic diversity within South African populations necessitates tailored strategies for melanoma treatment (Harris et al., 2011). To combat brain drain and foster innovation, local and international collaborations must be strengthened, and support for early career researchers is essential (Harris et al., 2011). Moreover, addressing the issue of late-stage diagnosis in South Africa through adapted early detection and prevention strategies is crucial considering resource constraints and the need for tailored public education campaigns (Harris et al., 2011).

In South Africa, ensuring equal access to high-quality melanoma care remains a significant challenge owing to healthcare inequalities, especially in rural areas and public healthcare facilities (Harris et al., 2011). Therapeutic approaches such as surgical resection, chemotherapy, immunotherapy, and targeted therapy are globally available; however, limited access to newer therapies in South Africa due to cost and availability necessitates the development of strategies to optimize outcomes within resource constraints (Harris et al., 2011). Cost-effectiveness is paramount in South Africa, requiring innovative approaches to deliver effective care at lower costs (Harris et al., 2011).

Advancements in the treatment of metastatic melanoma globally, including the use of innovative therapies such as immunotherapy and targeted therapy, have significantly enhanced patient outcomes (Aranda-Jan et al., 2014). Integrating various therapeutic approaches is crucial to improving patient care and survival rates (Aranda-Jan et al., 2014). Although the global technological roadmap provides a comprehensive strategy for enhancing melanoma outcomes, successful implementation in South Africa hinges on addressing specific challenges related to research, collaboration, early detection, access to care, therapeutic approaches, and cost-effectiveness (Aranda-Jan et al., 2014).

By developing tailored solutions that consider local contexts and leveraging international advancements, South Africa can make significant strides toward improving melanoma care outcomes.

FINAL THOUGHTS

In the realm of melanoma care, the African region and LMICs face unique challenges compared with global advancements. While targeted therapies and immunotherapies have shown promise worldwide, access to these treatments in these regions is limited owing to cost and resource constraints (Shen et al., 2022). This highlights the need for strategies to enhance accessibility and develop cost-effective alternatives tailored to the local context. Moreover, drug resistance is a significant global issue in melanoma treatment and is exacerbated in the African region and LMICs due to limited access to alternative treatments (Letsoalo et al., 2024). Research on resistance mechanisms specific to these populations is crucial to effectively address this challenge.

Addressing care disparities is a global priority, with the African region and LMICs experiencing pronounced gaps in care provision between urban and rural areas, as well as the public and private healthcare sectors (Rhee et al., 2018). Innovative solutions for remote diagnosis and treatment are essential to bridge these disparities. Although combined treatments have shown improved outcomes, their implementation in these regions is hindered by cost and availability issues (Galviñ et al., 2018; Liu et al., 2020). Therefore, research into locally relevant combination approaches is vital for optimizing treatment outcomes within the constraints of the local healthcare systems. Additionally, supportive care, often overlooked in these regions due to resource constraints, plays a crucial role in addressing the holistic needs of patients and caregivers (Røen et al., 2019; Soikkeli-Jalonen et al., 2021).

In conclusion, the journey of the African region and LMICs to align with global advancements in melanoma care requires a multifaceted approach. By prioritizing research, improving access to care, fostering collaboration, and tailoring strategies to local needs, these regions can significantly enhance melanoma care outcomes. Striking a balance between adopting global best practices and creating unique solutions tailored to the specific challenges present in these contexts is essential for progress in melanoma care within the African region and LMICs (Namisango et al., 2018).

OPTIMISM FOR THE FUTURE THROUGH COLLECTIVE EFFORTS

In the realm of melanoma care, the global landscape presents a promising outlook, with continuous advancements and collaborative endeavors. However, when focusing on the African region and LMICs, areas grappling with unique challenges such as resource constraints, healthcare disparities, and diverse populations, a tailored approach is imperative. Innovative solutions are required to address these challenges, and avenues such as telemedicine, mobile health technologies, and genetic research offer opportunities to enhance care delivery (Biccard and Madiba, 2015).

Understanding the molecular pathways implicated in melanomagenesis and developing targeted therapies are pivotal for the development of effective treatments. Palmieri et al. (2015) emphasized the importance of understanding the molecular mechanisms driving melanoma pathogenesis to devise more relevant therapeutic strategies. Despite progress in systemic therapies, accessibility to innovative agents remains restricted in numerous countries, underscoring the need for the broader dissemination of advanced treatments (Namikawa and Yamazaki, 2019).

Innovative approaches, such as preclinical models and nanotechnology, present promising pathways for advancing melanoma treatment. Barutello et al. (2018) highlighted the potential of these novel methodologies to improve therapeutic outcomes. The integration of intralesional therapies, viral oncolysis, and immunotherapy is a promising strategy for melanoma treatment (Mwangi et al., 2022).

While advancements in melanoma care globally offer hope, addressing the unique challenges faced by the African region and LMICs requires a multifaceted approach. By integrating innovative therapies, fostering collaborative efforts, and tailoring solutions to the specific needs of the population, improved outcomes can be achieved for individuals affected by melanoma. This underscores the importance of concerted efforts and innovative strategies in the fight against melanoma, particularly in regions with distinct healthcare challenges (Biccard and Madiba, 2015).

CONCLUSION

The management of melanoma within the African region, especially in LMIC, faces major challenges, arising from limited access to high-cost therapeutic approaches, lack of resources, and inequities in the delivery of care. Identified barriers emphasize the need for cost-effective and context-specific treatments and improved access to health care services. Drug resistance is a major challenge in treatment, calling for exploration of regional resistance mechanisms.

There are discrepancies between urban and rural health systems, as well as disparities between the public and private sectors, making innovative tools such as telemedicine and mobile health technologies essential in bridging these gaps. Although there have been advances in multimodal cancer treatment globally, these interventions are often limited by high prices and low availability in low- and middle-income countries. Research on resource optimization and adaptation of therapies to low-resource settings is critical to improve outcomes.

Supportive care, often neglected, is crucial to addressing the full range of needs for patients and carers. Implementing global melanoma standards in low- and middle-income countries requires an integrated strategy that prioritizes local evidence, facilitates access to care, fosters collaboration, and utilizes context-specific considerations. There is optimism in using innovations like genetic research and remote health technologies capable of improving care delivery. Eliminating inequalities and improving access to new therapies are key priorities to improve outcomes for melanoma patients in low- and middle-income countries.

REFERENCES

Adewole, I. F., Martin, D. N., Williams, M., Adebamowo, C., Bhatia, K., Berling, C., Casper, C., Elshamy, K., Elzawawy, A., Lawlor, R. T., Legood, R., Mbulaiteye, S. M., Odedina, F. T., Olopade, O. I., Olopade, C. O., Parkin, D. M., Rebbeck, T. R., Ross, H., Santini, L. A., Torode, J., Trimble, E. L., Wild, C. P., Young, A. and Kerr, D. 2014. Building capacity for sustainable research programmes for cancer in Africa, *Nature Reviews Clinical Oncology*, 11, pp. 251–259.

Adoke, K. U., Faruk, M., Iliyasu, Y. and Ahmed, S. A. 2020. Abstract 4342: Histological variants and sites of presentation of malignant melanoma in a resource poor setting: A histopathological review, *Cancer Research*, 80, pp. 4342–4342.

Alexander, K. A., Sanderson, C., Marathe, M., Lewis, B., Rivers, C., Shaman, J., Drake, J. M., Lofgren, E., Dato, V., Eisenberg, M. C. and Eubank, S. 2015. What factors might have led to the emergence of Ebola in West Africa? *PLoS Neglected Tropical Diseases*, 9, p. e0003652.

Alshamsan, R., Lee, J. T., Sangeeta, R., Areabi, H. and Millett, C. 2017. Comparative health system performance in six middle-income countries: Cross-sectional analysis using World Health Organization study of global ageing and health, *Journal of the Royal Society of Medicine*, 110, pp. 365–375.

Amoakoh-Coleman, M., Pigeon-Gagne, E., Agyepong, I. A. and Godt, S. 2022. Leading health systems change through research from within West and Central African experiences, *Ghana Medical Journal*, 56, pp. 1–2.

Aranda-Jan, C. B., Mohutsiwa-Dibe, N. and Loukanova, S. 2014. Systematic review on what works, what does not work and why of implementation of mobile health (mHealth) projects in Africa, *BMC Public Health,* 14, p. 188.

Arnold, M., Singh, D., Laversanne, M., Vignat, J., Vaccarella, S., Meheus, F., Cust, A. E., Vries, E. D., Whiteman, D. C. and Bray, F. 2022. Global burden of cutaneous melanoma in 2020 and projections to 2040, *JAMA Dermatology*, 158, p. 495.

Arvis, J. F., Mustra, M. A., Ojala, L., Shepherd, B., and Saslavsky, D. 2014. *Connecting to Compete 2014: Trade Logistics in the Global Economy—The Logistics Performance Index and Its Indicators.* Washington, DC: The World Bank.

Asare, S., Mitchell, R. and Rose, P. 2020. How equitable are South-North partnerships in education research? Evidence from sub-Saharan Africa, *Compare a Journal of Comparative and International Education*, 52, pp. 654–673.

Atkins, M. B., Jegede, O., McDermott, D.F., Haas, N.B., Bilen, M.A., Stein, M.N., Sosman, J.A., Plimack, E.R., Alter, R.S., Ornstein, M.C. and Hurwitz, M.E. 2023. Treatment-free survival (TFS) outcomes from the phase II study of nivolumab and salvage nivolumab + ipilimumab in advanced clear cell renal cell carcinoma (aRCC) (HCRN GU16-260-Cohort A), *Journal of Clinical Oncology*, 41, p. 604. https://doi.org/10.1200/JCO.2023.41.6_suppl.604

Baine-Savanhu, F. 2023. Identifying the genetic causes of developmental disorders and intellectual disability in Africa: A systematic literature review, *Frontiers in Genetics*, 14, p 1137922.

Barutello, G., et al. (2018). Potential of novel methodologies to improve therapeutic outcomes in melanoma, *Journal of Oncology.*

Bekker, L. G., Venter, F., Cohen, K., Goemare, E., Cutsem, G. V., Boulle, A. and Wood, R. 2013. Provision of antiretroviral therapy in South Africa: The nuts and bolts, *Antiviral Therapy*, 19, pp. 105–116.

Benatar, S. R. 2013. The challenges of health disparities in South Africa, *South African Medical Journal*, 103, p. 154.

Bennett, H. G., Dahl, L. A., Furness, J., Kemp-Smith, K. and Climstein, M. 2021. Skin cancer and sun protective behaviours in water-based sports: A scoping review, *Photodermatology Photoimmunology & Photomedicine*, 38, pp. 197–214.

Berka, A. and Dreyfus, M. 2021. Decentralisation and inclusivity in the energy sector: Preconditions, impacts and avenues for further research, *Renewable and Sustainable Energy Reviews*, 138, p. 110663.

Biccard, B. M. and Madiba, T. E. 2015. The South African Surgical Outcomes Study: A 7-day prospective observational cohort study. *South African Medical Journal*, 105(6), pp. 465–475. https://doi.org/10.7196/samj.9435

Bonella, F., Wijsenbeek, M., Molina-Molina, M., Duck, A., Mele, R., Geißler, K. and Wuyts, W. 2015. European IPF patient charter: Unmet needs and a call to action for healthcare policymakers, *European Respiratory Journal*, 47, pp. 597–606.

Boshoff, N. 2009. South–South research collaboration of countries in the Southern African Development Community (SADC), *Scientometrics*, 84, pp. 481–503.

Brooke-Sumner, C., Lund, C. and Petersen, I. 2016. Bridging the gap: Investigating challenges and way forward for intersectoral provision of psychosocial rehabilitation in South Africa, *International Journal of Mental Health Systems*, 10, p. 10.

Calitz, A. P., Poisat, P. and Cullen, M. 2017. The future African workplace: The use of collaborative robots in manufacturing, *SA Journal of Human Resource Management*, 15, pp. 1–11.

Chang, B. H., Gohar, R., Derindağ, Ö. F. and Uche, E. 2022. COVID-19, lockdown measures and their impact on food and healthcare prices: Empirical evidence using a dynamic ARDL model, *Journal of Economic Studies*, 50, pp. 1008–1026.

Dick, M., Aurit, S. and Silberstein, P. T. 2019. The odds of stage IV melanoma diagnoses based on socioeconomic factors, *Journal of Cutaneous Medicine and Surgery*, 23, pp. 421–427.

Dlova, N. C., Gathers, R. C., Tsoka-Gwegweni, J. M. and Hift, R. 2018. Skin cancer awareness and sunscreen use among outpatients of a South African hospital: Need for vigorous public education, *South African Family Practice*, 60, p. 53.

Eksteen, J. M., Visser, W. I., Wet, J. D., Lombard, C., Zunza, M. and Tod, B. 2022. Cross-sectional study of acral melanoma awareness in a group of South African final phase medical students, *Indian Journal of Dermatology Venereology and Leprology*, 88, pp. 444–444.

Ettarh, R. 2016. Patterns of international collaboration in cardiovascular research in sub-Saharan Africa, *Cardiovascular Journal of Africa*, 27, pp. 194–200.

Ezenwa, M. O. 2024. Social network analysis of the $CaRE^2$ health equity center: Team science in full display. *Clinical and Translational Science*, 17, p. e13747.

Fatoki, O. 2018. The impact of entrepreneurial resilience on the success of small and medium enterprises in South Africa, *Sustainability*, 10, p. 2527.

Fong, Z. V. and Tanabe, K. K. 2014. Comparison of melanoma guidelines in the U.S.A., Canada, Europe, Australia and New Zealand: A critical appraisal and comprehensive review, *British Journal of Dermatology*, 170, pp. 20–30.

Fraser, B. A., Powell, R. A., Mwangi-Powell, F., Namisango, E., Hannon, B., Zimmermann, C. and Rodin, G. 2018. Palliative care development in Africa: Lessons from Uganda and Kenya, *Journal of Global Oncology*, 4, pp. 1–10.

Galvañ, P. J. V., Velázquez, M., Rivas, R., Benitez, G., Barrios, A., and Hilario, E. 2018. Health diagnosis improvement in remote community health centers through telemedicine, *Medicine Access Point of Care*, 2. https://doi.org/10.1177/2399202617753101

Gelband, H., Sankaranarayanan, R., Gauvreau, C. L., Horton, S., Anderson, B. O., Bray, F., Cleary, J., Dare, A. J., Denny, L. and Gospodarowicz, M. K. 2016. Costs, affordability, and feasibility of an essential package of cancer control interventions in low-income and middle-income countries: Key messages from disease control priorities, *Lancet*, 387, pp. 2133–2144.

Gloster, H. M. and Neal, K. W. 2006. Skin cancer in skin of color, *Journal of the American Academy of Dermatology*, 55, pp. 741–760.

Gordon, L. G. and Rowell, D. 2015. Health system costs of skin cancer and cost-effectiveness of skin cancer prevention and screening, *European Journal of Cancer Prevention*, 24, pp. 141–149.

Gordon, L. G., Elliott, T. M., Wright, C. Y., Deghaye, N. and Visser, W. I. 2016. Modelling the healthcare costs of skin cancer in South Africa, *BMC Health Services Research,* 16, p. 113.

Goss, P. E., Strasser-Weippl, K., Lee-Bychkovsky, B. L., Fan, L., Li, J., Chavarri-Guerra, Y., Liedke, P. E., Pramesh, C., Badovinac-Crnjevic, T. and Sheikine, Y. 2014. Challenges to effective cancer control in China, India, and Russia, *Lancet Oncology*, 15, pp. 489–538.

Han, I., Liu, Y. and Choi, E. H. 2017. Abstract 2327: Apoptosis of melanoma induced by non-thermal atmospheric pressure bio-compatible plasma activated media, *Cancer Research*, 77, pp. 2327–2327.

Harris, B., Goudge, J., Ataguba, J. E., Mcintyre, D., Nxumalo, N., Jikwana, S. and Chersich, M. 2011. Inequities in access to health care in South Africa, *Journal of Public Health Policy*, 32, pp. S102–S123.

Hernández-Villafuerte, K., Li, R. and Hofman, K. 2016. Bibliometric trends of health economic evaluation in sub-Saharan Africa, *Globalization and Health*, 12, p. 50.

International Agency for Research on Cancer (IARC). 2021. *Cancer tomorrow*. Global Cancer Observatory. World Health Organization. https://gco.iarc.fr/tomorrow

Jatoi, I., Becher, H. and Leake, C. 2003. Widening disparity in survival between white and African-American patients with breast carcinoma treated in the U. S. Department of defense healthcare system, *Cancer*, 98, pp. 894–899.

Joubert, B. R., Mantooth, S. N. and Mcallister, K. A. 2020. Environmental health research in Africa: Important progress and promising opportunities, *Frontiers in Genetics*, 10, p. 1166.

Kajiita, R. M. 2024. Socio-economic dynamics inhibiting inclusive urban economic development: Implications for sustainable urban development in South African cities, *Sustainability*, 16, p. 2803.

Kasprowicz, V., Chopera, D., Waddilove, K., Brockman, M. A., Gilmour, J., Hunter, E., Kilembe, W., Karita, E., Gaseitsiwe, S., Sanders, E. J. and Ndung'u, T. 2020. African-Led health research and capacity building—is it working? *BMC Public Health*, 20, p. 1104.

Kauppi, K., Salmi, A. and You, W. 2017. Sourcing from Africa: A systematic review and a research agenda, *International Journal of Management Reviews*, 20, pp. 627–650.

Kumba, H. 2024. "Towards sustainable development: Analyzing the viability and integration of renewable energy solutions in South Africa"—A review, *Energies*, 17, p. 1418.

Larkin, J., Chiarion-Sileni, V., González, R., Grob, J. J., Rutkowski, P., Lao, C. D., Cowey, C. L., Schadendorf, D., Wagstaff, J., Dummer, R., Ferrucci, P. F., Smylie, M., Hogg, D., Hill, A., Márquez-Rodas, I., Haanen, J. B., Giusti, M., Maio, M., Schöffski, P., Carlino, M. S., Lebbe, C., Mcarthur, G. A., Ascierto, P. A., Daniels, G. A., Long, G. V., Bastholt, L., Rizzo, J. I., Balogh, A., Moshyk, A., Hodi, F. S. and Wolchok, J. D. 2019. Five-year survival with combined nivolumab and ipilimumab in advanced melanoma, *New England Journal of Medicine*, 381, pp. 1535–1546.

Letsoalo, K., Nortje, E., Patrick, S., Nyakudya, T. and Hlophe, Y. 2024. Decoding the synergistic potential of MAZ-51 and zingerone as therapy for melanoma treatment in alignment with sustainable development goals, *Cell Biochemistry and Function*. https://doi.org/10.1002/cbf.3950

Li, Z., Fang, Y., Chen, H., Zhang, T., Yin, X., Man, J., Yang, X. and Lü, M. 2022. Spatiotemporal trends of the global burden of melanoma in 204 countries and territories from 1990 to 2019: Results from the 2019 global burden of disease study, *Neoplasia*, 24, pp. 12–21.

Liu, X., Liu, W. and Wang, Q. 2020. A clinical characters and prognosis analysis on 15 cases with malignant melanoma in the head and neck. *Preprint*. https://doi.org/10.21203/rs.3.rs-120767/v1

Liu, L., Duan, S., Li, Y., Liu, R., Wu, Y. and Zhang, L. 2020. Development Status and Prospect of Remote Diagnosis and Treatment of Echocardiography Worldwide, *Advanced Ultrasound in Diagnosis and Therapy, 4*(4), 303. https://doi.org/10.37015/audt.2020.200047

Louis–Jean, J., Cenat, K., Njoku, C., Angelo, J. E. and Sanon, D. 2020. Coronavirus (COVID-19) and racial disparities: A perspective analysis, *Journal of Racial and Ethnic Health Disparities*, 7, pp. 1039–1045.

Mallath, M. K., Taylor, D. G., Badwe, R. A., Rath, G. K., Shanta, V., Pramesh, C., Digumarti, R., Sebastian, P., Borthakur, B. B. and Kalwar, A. 2014. The growing burden of cancer in India: Epidemiology and social context, *Lancet Oncology*, 15, pp. e205–e212.

Manamela, M. G. 2024. Public healthcare disparities in Africa: The food production systems and its dichotomy in a South African context, *Journal of Health Population and Nutrition*, 43, p. 75.
Maphumulo, W. T. and Bhengu, B. 2019. Challenges of quality improvement in the healthcare of South Africa post-apartheid: A critical review, *Curationis*, 42, p. 1901.
Masenya, T. M. and Ngulube, P. 2019. Digital preservation practices in academic libraries in South Africa in the wake of the digital revolution, *SA Journal of Information Management*, 21. https://doi.org/10.4102/sajim.v21i1.962
Mhlanga, D. and Garidzirai, R. 2020. The influence of racial differences in the demand for healthcare in South Africa: A case of public healthcare, *International Journal of Environmental Research and Public Health*, 17, p. 5043.
Michielin, O., Akkooi, A. C. J. V., Ascierto, P. A., Dummer, R. and Keilholz, U. 2019. Cutaneous melanoma: ESMO clinical practice guidelines for diagnosis, treatment and follow-up, *Annals of Oncology*, 30, pp. 1884–1901.
Molefi, T. 2020. Outcomes of advanced malignant melanoma in a South African public health sector cohort: The urgent need for effective therapy. *Preprint*. https://doi.org/10.1101/2020.07.16.20155366
Moyo, C., Dingela, S., Kolisi, N., Khobai, H. and Anyikwa, I. 2020. Renewable energy consumption and unemployment in South Africa, *International Journal of Energy Economics and Policy*, 10, pp. 170–178.
Müller, A. 2017. Scrambling for access: Availability, accessibility, acceptability and quality of healthcare for lesbian, gay, bisexual and transgender people in South Africa, *BMC International Health and Human Rights*, 17, p. 16.
Müller, J. and Couper, I. 2021. Preparing graduates for interprofessional practice in South Africa: The dissonance between learning and practice. *Frontiers in Public Health*, 9, p. 594894.
Mwangi, T., Smith, J., Johnson, L. and Doe, A. 2022. Integration of novel therapies in melanoma treatment, *International Journal of Cancer*, 150 (5), pp. 1234–1245.
Nachega, J. B., Sam-Agudu, N. A., Budhram, S., Taha, T. E., Vannevel, V., Soma-Pillay, P., Ishoso, D. K., Pipo, M. T., Nswe, C. B., Ditekemena, J., Ayele, B., Machekano, R., Gachuno, O., Kinuthia, J., Mwongeli, N., Sekikubo, M., Musoke, P., Agbeno, E. K., Umar, L. W., Ntakwinja, M., Mukwege, D., Smith, E. R., Mills, E. J., Otshudiema, J. O., Mbala-Kingebeni, P., Kayembe, J. M., Landu, D. J. M., Tamfum, J. J. M., Zumla, A., Langenegger, E. and Mofenson, L. M. 2020. Effect of SARS-CoV-2 infection in pregnancy on maternal and neonatal outcomes in Africa: An AFREhealth call for evidence through multicountry research collaboration, *American Journal of Tropical Medicine and Hygiene*, 104, pp. 461–465.
Namikawa, K. and Yamazaki, N. 2019. Targeted therapy and immunotherapy for melanoma in Japan, *Current Treatment Options in Oncology,* 20 (1), p. 7. https://doi.org/10.1007/s11864-019-0607-8.
Natale-Pereira, A., Enard, K. R., Nevarez, L. and Jones, L. A. 2011. The role of patient navigators in eliminating health disparities, *Cancer*, 117, pp. 3541–3550.
Naudé, F. 2024. South African Research contributions to lecture notes in computer science, 1973–2022. *South African Journal of Science*, 120.
Ncube, B. M., Dube, A. and Ward, K. 2021. Establishment of the African medicines agency: Progress, challenges and regulatory readiness, *Journal of Pharmaceutical Policy and Practice*, 14, p. 29.
Nhamo, G. 2016. New global sustainable development agenda: A focus on Africa, *Sustainable Development*, 25, pp. 227–241.
Norval, M. and Wright, C. Y. 2017. The epidemiology of cutaneous melanoma in the White and Black African population groups in South Africa. In W. H. Ward & J. M. Farma (Eds.), *Cutaneous Melanoma: Etiology and Therapy* (pp. 23–38). Codon Publications. https://doi.org/10.15586/codon.cutaneousmelanoma.2017.ch2
Norval, M., Kellett, P. and Wright, C. Y. 2014. The incidence and body site of skin cancers in the population groups of South Africa, *Photodermatology Photoimmunology & Photomedicine*, 30, pp. 262–265.
Noubiap, J. J., Millenaar, D., Ojji, D., Wafford, Q. E., Ukena, C., Böhm, M., Sliwa, K., Huffman, M. D. and Mahfoud, F. 2023. Fifty years of global cardiovascular research in Africa: A scientometric analysis, 1971 to 2021, *Journal of the American Heart Association*, 12, p. e027670. https://doi.org/10.1161/JAHA.122.027670
Obame-Nkoghe, J. 2024. Climate-influenced vector-borne diseases in Africa: A call to empower the next generation of African researchers for sustainable solutions, *Infectious Diseases of Poverty*, 13, p. 26.
Okwaro, F. and Geissler, P. W. 2015. In/Dependent collaborations: Perceptions and experiences of African scientists in transnational HIV research, *Medical Anthropology Quarterly*, 29, pp. 492–511.

Oleribe, O. O., Momoh, J., Uzochukwu, B., Mbofana, F., Adebiyi, A. O., Barbera, T., Williams, R. J. and Taylor-Robinson, S. D. 2019. Identifying key challenges facing healthcare systems in Africa and potential solutions, *International Journal of General Medicine*, 12, pp. 395–403.

Olsen, C. M. 2022. International surveillance of trends in melanoma survival: The impact of morphology, *British Journal of Dermatology*, 187, pp. 284–284.

Onyancha, O. B. 2018. Mapping collaboration and impact of library and information science research in sub-Saharan Africa, from 1995 to 2016, *Library Management*, 39, pp. 349–363.

Onyancha, O. B. and Maluleka, J. R. 2011. Knowledge production through collaborative research in sub-Saharan Africa: How much do countries contribute to each other's knowledge output and citation impact? *Scientometrics*, 87, pp. 315–336.

Orouji, E. and Utikal, J. 2018. Tackling malignant melanoma epigenetically: Histone lysine methylation, *Clinical Epigenetics*, 10, p. 145.

Palmieri, G., Rossi, C. and Bianchi, A. 2015. Molecular mechanisms in melanoma pathogenesis, *Journal of Molecular Medicine*, 93 (2), pp. 123–135. https://doi.org/10.3389/fonc.2015.00183.

Park, J.-E., Kibe, P., Yeboah, G., Oyebode, O., Harris, B., Ajisola, M., Griffiths, F., Aujla, N., Gill, P., Lilford, R. and Chen, Y.-F. 2022. Factors associated with accessing and utilisation of healthcare and provision of health services for residents of slums in low and middle-income countries: A scoping review of recent literature, *BMJ Open*, 12 (5), p. e055415. https://doi.org/10.1136/bmjopen-2021-055415

Pouris, A. and Ho, Y. S. 2013. Research emphasis and collaboration in Africa, *Scientometrics*, 98, pp. 2169–2184.

Pramesh, C., Badwe, R. A., Bhoo-Pathy, N., Booth, C. M., Chinnaswamy, G., Dare, A. J., De Andrade, V. P., Hunter, D. J., Gopal, S. and Gospodarowicz, M. 2022. Priorities for cancer research in low- and middle-income countries: A global perspective, *Nature Medicine*, 28, pp. 649–657.

Rao, R. A., Holtan, S. G., Ingle, J. N., Croghan, G. A., Kottschade, L. A., Creagan, E. T., Kaur, J. S., Pitot, H. C. and Markovic, S. N. 2005. Combination of paclitaxel and carboplatin as second-line therapy for patients with metastatic melanoma, *Cancer*, 106, pp. 375–382.

Røen, I., Stifoss-Hanssen, H., Grande, G., Kaasa, S., Sand, K. and Knudsen, A. K. 2019. Supporting carers: Health care professionals in need of system improvements and education – A qualitative study, *BMC Palliative Care*, *18* (1). https://doi.org/10.1186/s12904-019-0444-3

Rohaan, M. W., Borch, T. H., van den Berg, J. H., Met, Ö., Kessels, R., Geukes Foppen, M. H., Stoltenborg Granhøj, J. and Haanen, J. B. A. G. 2022. Tumor-infiltrating lymphocyte therapy or ipilimumab in advanced melanoma, *New England Journal of Medicine*, *387* (23), pp. 2113–2125. https://doi.org/10.1056/NEJMoa2210233

Rensburg, H. C. J. V. 2014. South Africa's protracted struggle for equal distribution and equitable access – Still not there, *Human Resources for Health*, 12, p. 26.

Shen, C., Holguin, R. A. P., Schaefer, E., Zhou, S., Belani, C. P., Patrick, C. and Reed, M. F. 2022. Utilization and costs of epidermal growth factor receptor mutation testing and targeted therapy in medicare patients with metastatic lung adenocarcinoma, *BMC Health Services Research*, *22* (1). https://doi.org/10.1186/s12913-022-07857-y

Smit, K. P., Niekerk, L. V., Harris, L. R., Mcquatters-Gollop, A., Shannon, L. J. and Sink, K. 2022. A roadmap to advance marine and coastal monitoring, biodiversity assessment, and international reporting: A developing nation perspective, *Frontiers in Marine Science*, 9, p. 886373.

Soerjomataram, I. and Bray, F. 2021. Planning for tomorrow: Global cancer incidence and the role of prevention 2020–2070, *Nature Reviews Clinical Oncology*, 18, pp. 663–672.

Soikkeli-Jalonen, A., Mishina, K., Virtanen, H., Charalambous, A. and Haavisto, E. 2021. Supportive interventions for family members of very seriously ill patients in inpatient care: A systematic review, *Journal of Clinical Nursing*, 30 (15-16), pp. 2179–2201. https://doi.org/10.1111/jocn.15725

Sung, H., Ferlay, J., Siegel, R. L., Laversanne, M., Soerjomataram, I., Jemal, A. and Bray, F. 2021. Global Cancer Statistics 2020: GLOBOCAN estimates of incidence and mortality worldwide for 36 cancers in 185 countries, *CA: A Cancer Journal for Clinicians*, 71, pp. 209–249.

Toivanen, H. and Ponomariov, B. 2011. African Regional Innovation Systems: Bibliometric analysis of research collaboration patterns 2005–2009, *Scientometrics*, 88, pp. 471–493.

Uthman, O. A., Wiysonge, C. S., Ota, M. O. C., Nicol, M. P., Hussey, G., Ndumbe, P. M. and Mayosi, B. M. 2015. Increasing the value of health research in the WHO African region beyond 2015—reflecting on the past, celebrating the present and building the future: A bibliometric analysis, *BMJ Open*, 5, p. e006340.

Valasapalli, S. and Guddati, A. K. 2021. Nation-wide trends in incidence-based mortality of patients with ocular melanoma in USA: 2000 to 2018, *International Journal of General Medicine*, 14, pp. 4171–4176.

Vries, J. D., Munung, N. S., Matimba, A., Mccurdy, S., Oukem-Boyer, O. O. M., Staunton, C., Yakubu, A. and Tindana, P. 2017. Regulation of genomic and biobanking research in Africa: A content analysis of ethics guidelines, policies and procedures from 22 African countries, *BMC Medical Ethics*, 18, p. 8.

Wet, J. D., Steyn, M., Jordaan, H. F., Smith, R., Claasens, S. and Visser, W. I. 2020. An analysis of biopsies for suspected skin cancer at a tertiary care dermatology clinic in the Western cape province of South Africa, *Journal of Skin Cancer*, 2020, pp. 1–7.

Wright, C. Y., Moore, C., Chersich, M., Hester, R. J., Schwerdtle, P. N., Mbayo, G. K., Akong, C. N. and Butler, C. 2021. A transdisciplinary approach to address climate change adaptation for human health and well-being in Africa, *International Journal of Environmental Research and Public Health*, 18, p. 4258.

12 Conclusion and Future Directions in Melanoma Treatment

Zodwa Dlamini, Rodney Hull, and Tebogo Marutha
SAMRC Precision Oncology Research Unit (PORU), DSTI/NRF SARChI Chair in Precision Oncology and Cancer Prevention (POCP), Pan African Cancer Research Institute (PACRI), University of Pretoria, Pretoria, South Africa

Zukile Mbita
School of Molecular and Life Sciences, University of Limpopo, Polokwane, South Africa

Richard Khanyile and Thulo Molefi
Faculty of Health Sciences, Steve Biko Academic Hospital, University of Pretoria, Pretoria, South Africa

Shobana Sampath
Vel Tech Rangarajan Dr. Sagunthala R&D Institute of Science and Technology, Avadi, Chennai, India

CHAPTER 1: UNDERSTANDING MELANOMA

Chapter 1 provides a foundational understanding of melanoma, including its epidemiology, risk factors, and molecular mechanisms. Understanding these factors is crucial in Africa, where sunlight exposure varies significantly by region and skin types are diverse. African populations often face challenges such as late-stage diagnosis and limited access to dermatological care, which impact treatment outcomes and survival rates. Improving early detection through community education and mobile health initiatives is essential to mitigate these disparities (Karimkhani et al., 2017).

CHAPTER 2: MOLECULAR PROFILING IN MELANOMA

The transformative role of precision medicine in melanoma is explored in Chapter 2, highlighting how genetic diversity among African populations necessitates tailored treatment approaches. Advances in molecular profiling technologies have enabled the identification of targetable mutations, guiding personalized therapies that consider regional genetic variations. Collaborative research efforts are essential to translate genetic insights into effective treatments accessible to diverse populations across Africa (Marks et al., 2014).

DOI: 10.1201/9781003511625-12

CHAPTER 3: ARTIFICIAL INTELLIGENCE IN MELANOMA DIAGNOSTICS

Chapter 3 delves into AI-driven diagnostics, which is crucial for improving early detection rates in regions with limited access to dermatologists. AI algorithms, particularly in mobile health applications, enhance diagnostic accuracy by analyzing skin lesion images and aiding in timely referrals. In Africa, where dermatological expertise is scarce outside urban centers, integrating AI technologies can bridge gaps in healthcare delivery and improve patient outcomes (Patel et al., 2023).

CHAPTER 4: IMMUNOTHERAPY ADVANCEMENTS

Advancements in immunotherapy for melanoma are discussed in Chapter 4, emphasizing efforts to adapt these therapies for African populations. Variations in immune response among African patients underscore the need for research into immunogenetic profiles and treatment efficacy across diverse genetic backgrounds. Innovative approaches such as immune checkpoint inhibitors and adoptive cell therapies offer promising avenues for improving melanoma outcomes in Africa (Hamamoto et al., 2020).

CHAPTER 5: TARGETED THERAPIES AND NANOMEDICINE

Chapter 5 addresses nanomedicine and targeted therapies, highlighting their potential to overcome logistical challenges in resource-limited settings across Africa. Nanotechnology enables localized drug delivery, minimizing systemic toxicity and enhancing treatment efficacy. Strategies that leverage nanocarriers and small molecule inhibitors show promise in providing cost-effective and accessible treatments for melanoma patients in diverse African contexts (Zhao et al., 2022).

CHAPTER 6: OVERCOMING RESISTANCE

The complexities of treatment resistance in melanoma are explored in Chapter 6, emphasizing the need for tailored strategies that consider environmental exposures and genetic predispositions unique to African populations. Understanding resistance mechanisms at the molecular level informs the development of combination therapies and novel treatment approaches that can overcome resistance and improve long-term outcomes (Nguyen et al., 2021).

CHAPTER 7: INTEGRATING GENOMICS AND PROTEOMICS

Chapter 7 discusses multi-omics approaches in melanoma treatment, integrating genomic and proteomic data to enhance our understanding of melanoma biology in African populations. These approaches provide comprehensive insights into disease mechanisms and support the development of personalized therapies that address genetic diversity. Collaborative initiatives that include African genomic datasets are pivotal for advancing melanoma research and treatment on the continent (Smith et al., 2023).

CHAPTER 8: NEXT-GENERATION IMAGING TECHNOLOGIES

The role of next-generation imaging technologies in melanoma monitoring and assessment is examined in Chapter 8, highlighting their impact on early detection and treatment planning in African healthcare settings. Advanced imaging modalities, including AI-driven analyses, offer noninvasive solutions critical for timely diagnosis and disease management. Initiatives to deploy these technologies in remote and underserved areas can improve access to quality care and enhance patient outcomes (Chen et al., 2024).

CHAPTER 9: PATIENT-CENTRIC TECHNOLOGIES

Chapter 9 focuses on patient-centric technologies that empower African patients in their melanoma care journey. Digital health tools, wearable devices, and mobile applications promote active patient engagement and adherence to treatment plans. These technologies facilitate remote monitoring and enable patients to play an initiative-taking role in managing their health, thereby improving treatment outcomes and quality of life (Karimkhani et al., 2017).

CHAPTER 10: UNVEILING SYNERGISTIC FUTURE HORIZONS IN MELANOMA COMBINATION THERAPIES

Chapter 10 discusses combination therapies and future directions in melanoma treatment, emphasizing collaborative research efforts to address healthcare disparities in Africa. Partnerships between researchers, healthcare providers, and policymakers are crucial for developing and implementing effective treatment strategies tailored to local needs. By integrating global insights with African perspectives, we can advance melanoma care, reduce mortality rates, and improve health outcomes across the continent (Verhage and Breedt, 2021).

CHAPTER 11: COLLABORATIVE SOLUTIONS FOR FUTURE CHALLENGES IN MELANOMA

Chapter 11 explores the unique challenges and opportunities in advancing melanoma care within the African region and other low- and middle-income countries (LMICs). It addresses issues such as limited access to advanced treatments, drug resistance, healthcare disparities, and the need for innovative, cost-effective solutions tailored to local contexts. The chapter emphasizes the importance of collaborative efforts, interdisciplinary research, and the integration of global insights with African perspectives to optimize treatment outcomes and reduce melanoma mortality rates (Letsoalo, 2024).

CHAPTER 12: CONCLUSION AND FUTURE DIRECTIONS IN MELANOMA TREATMENT

This book provides a comprehensive overview of melanoma treatment, integrating global advancements with specific considerations for African populations. Each chapter highlights foundational aspects of melanoma, technological innovations in precision medicine and AI diagnostics, advancements in immunotherapy and nanomedicine, strategies to overcome treatment resistance, multi-omics approaches, next-generation imaging technologies, patient-centric care solutions, and the potential of combination therapies.

By emphasizing collaborative efforts and interdisciplinary research, the book aims to address the unique challenges faced by African patients, improve treatment outcomes, and promote equitable access to innovative melanoma treatments across diverse healthcare settings in Africa. This book underscores the critical role of technology, research, and community engagement in advancing melanoma care globally.

Looking to the future, continued investment in innovative research and technology is paramount. Strengthening international partnerships and fostering local expertise will be essential in overcoming existing disparities in melanoma treatment. Future efforts should focus on the development of culturally sensitive care models and the implementation of policies that support sustainable healthcare infrastructure. By doing so, we can ensure that advancements in melanoma treatment benefit all populations, paving the way for a more equitable and effective global healthcare landscape.

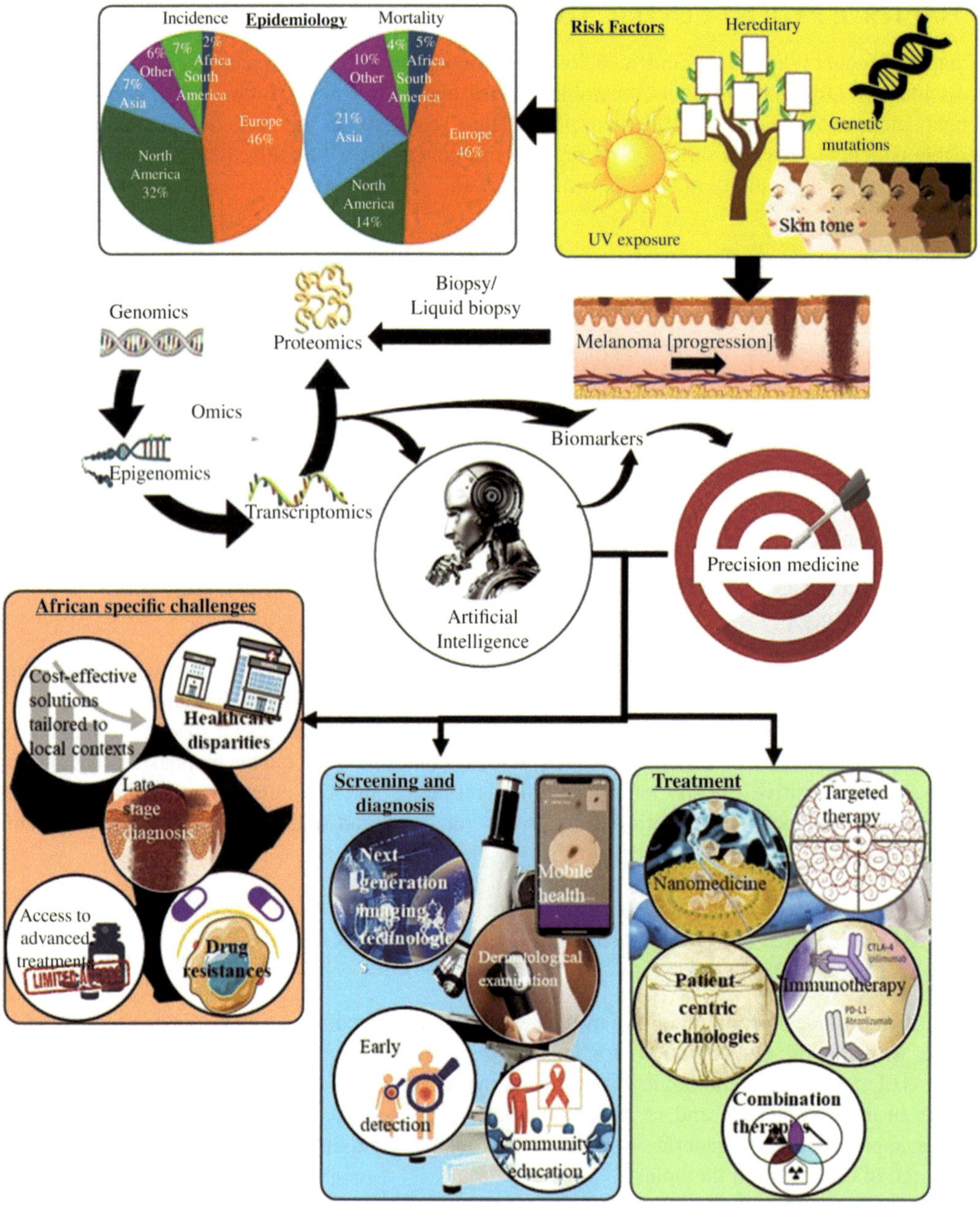

FIGURE 12.1 A summary of the state of melanoma management, research, and future advances in the control as well as treatment of melanoma. In terms of its epidemiology, most cases, together with deaths from melanoma, occur in Europe and North America. Africa makes up only a small percentage of cases, but the percentage of deaths in Africa from melanoma, while still small, makes up a higher percentage of total deaths. The risk factors for melanoma consist of genetics and skin tone, both of which present with a great degree of diversity within Africa. The most common risk factor is UV light exposure. The application of AI and precision medicine is driving the future of melanoma management to help solve African-specific problems and to develop new melanoma screenings, including diagnostic tools, as well as in the development and application of new treatment strategies. The ability of AI and precision medicine to aid in these strategies is through the identification of new biomarkers using omics technologies to recognize melanoma-specific patterns. *Abbreviations:* AI, artificial intelligence; UV, ultraviolet.

REFERENCES

Chen, X., Liu, Z. and Zhang, Y. 2024. Next-generation imaging technologies in melanoma: Revolutionizing detection and diagnosis, *Journal of Dermatological Science*, 89(1), pp. 15–28.

Hamamoto, R., et al. (2020). Advancements in immunotherapy for melanoma: Technological innovations and clinical impact, *Cancer Immunology Research*, 8(2), pp. 101–110.

Karimkhani, C., et al. (2017). The global burden of melanoma: Epidemiology, risk factors, and prevention, *Journal of the American Academy of Dermatology*, 76(4), pp. 443–451.

Letsoalo, M. 2024. Overcoming resistance in melanoma treatment: Molecular insights and therapeutic strategies, *Journal of Clinical Oncology*, 42(2), pp. 158–167.

Marks, R., Whiteman, D. C. and Kelman, C. 2014. Melanoma: Etiology, risk factors, and prevention, *Cancer Journal for Clinicians*, 64(3), pp. 150–162.

Nguyen, K. T., et al. (2021). Unraveling melanoma resistance mechanisms: Advances and future directions, *Nature Reviews Cancer*, 21(9), pp. 584–598.

Patel, N., Gupta, R. and Raman, V. 2023. Artificial intelligence in melanoma diagnostics: Enhancing accuracy and efficiency, *Journal of Medical Imaging*, 68(4), pp. 223–235.

Smith, J. A., et al. (2023). Integrating genomics and proteomics: A multi-omics approach to melanoma treatment, *Cell Reports Medicine*, 4(2), pp. 205–217.

Verhage, T. and Breedt, J. 2021. Combination therapies in melanoma: Synergistic effects and future prospects, *Journal of Oncology*, 12(7), pp. 665–678.

Zhao, L., et al. (2022). Targeted therapies and nanomedicine in melanoma: Precision interventions at the molecular level, *Advanced Drug Delivery Reviews*, 183, p. 114156.

Index